'This new book is an immaculately researched guide to living with dementia in England in the 21st century, covering the subject from policy to lived experience, but always with consideration and compassion. There is no better introduction to the challenges and complexities that dementia brings to individuals, families and society.'

– *Geoff Huggins, Director of Health and Social Care Integration, Scottish Government*

'This book is informative and challenging in equal measure. It not only provides a thorough analysis of the issues currently facing dementia care, but it also offers a refreshing and thoughtful critique of the many challenges. Each chapter carefully combines research evidence, practice issues and policy influences, and contextualises these within the experience of those living with dementia, including their carers.

Whilst this book is complex and thought-provoking, I believe it is a highly welcome counterbalance to current thinking on how to improve the lives of all those who are affected by dementia. It will force the reader to challenge their own thinking about dementia, not just as an illness but as a social construct, and as such I would highly recommend it.'

– *Rachel Thompson, Professional and Practice Development Lead for Admiral Nursing, Dementia UK*

'Shibley Rahman follows his first brilliant book on dementia with this fascinating publication, containing insight and empathy in equal measure. This book will help readers – health professionals and the public alike – to understand people in their lives with dementia, guiding you through everything you ever wanted to know about dementia and could possibly want to ask. Shibley guides you through the challenges of caring for people and living with dementia. He doesn't shy away from the topics that are uncomfortable, but he also gives space to examples of good living and practice that leave the reader with hope and positivity.'

– *Jenni Middleton, editor, Nursing Times*

'I commend Shibley for this valuable addition to the current thinking and discussion on what it is to live with dementia. This text builds quite significantly on his original work and continues to challenge professionals on issues of importance for families affected by dementia. I find his frank and open style refreshing, unreserved in his willingness to question both the semantics used in practice and assumptions that are too easily made on what it might be like to live with dementia. I doubt this will be the last contribution we see from him.'

– *Karen Harrison Dening, Director of Admiral Nursing, Dementia UK*

Living Better with Dementia

of related interest

Dementia, Culture and Ethnicity Issues for All
Edited by Julia Botsford and Karen Harrison Dening
Foreword by Alistair Burns
ISBN 978 1 84905 486 7
eISBN 978 0 85700 881 7

Intellectual Disability and Dementia: Research into Practice
Edited by Karen Watchman
ISBN 978 1 84905 422 5
eISBN 978 0 85700 796 4

How We Think About Dementia Personhood, Rights, Ethics, the Arts and What They Mean for Care
Julian C. Hughes
ISBN 978 1 84905 477 5
eISBN 978 0 85700 855 8

Key Issues in Evolving Dementia Care
International Theory-based Policy and Practice
Edited by Anthea Innes, Fiona Kelly and Louise McCabe
ISBN 978 1 84905 242 9
eISBN 978 0 85700 503 8

Living Better with Dementia

— Good Practice and Innovation for the Future —

Dr Shibley Rahman

Queen's Scholar; BA (1st Class Honours) MB BChir PhD (all Cambridge); MRCP(UK); LLB (Hons) (BPP Law School); LLM (with commendation) (University of Law of England and Wales); MBA (BPP Business School); Postgraduate Diploma in Law (BPP Law School)

Forewords by Kate Swaffer, Chris Roberts and Beth Britton

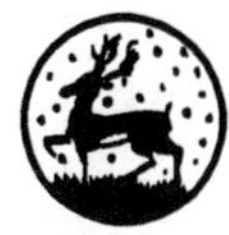

Jessica Kingsley *Publishers*
London and Philadelphia

Copyright permissions are listed on page 24.

First published in 2015
by Jessica Kingsley Publishers
73 Collier Street
London N1 9BE, UK
and
400 Market Street, Suite 400
Philadelphia, PA 19106, USA

www.jkp.com

Library of Congress Cataloging in Publication Data
Rahman, Shibley, author.
Living better with dementia : looking to the future / Shibley Rahman ; forewords by Kate Swaffer, Chris Roberts, and Peter Gordon.
p. ; cm.
Includes bibliographical references and index.
ISBN 978-1-84905-600-7 (alk. paper)
I. Title.
[DNLM: 1. Dementia--rehabilitation. 2. Quality of Life. WM 220]
RC521
616.8'3--dc23
2015003541

British Library Cataloguing in Publication Data
A CIP catalogue record for this book is available from the British Library

ISBN 978 1 84905 600 7
eISBN 978 1 78450 062 7

Printed and bound in Great Britain

This book is dedicated to my late father

CONTENTS

	Foreword by Kate Swaffer	11
	Foreword by Chris Roberts	13
	Foreword by Beth Britton	15
	Preface	17
	Copyright Acknowledgements	24
Chapter 1	Introduction	25
Chapter 2	Stigma, Citizenship and Living Better with Dementia	51
Chapter 3	Culture and Diversity in Living Better with Dementia	63
Chapter 4	Global Strategies for Living Better with Dementia	81
Chapter 5	What Might Living Better with Young-Onset Dementia Mean?	98
Chapter 6	Delirium and Living Better with Dementia	113
Chapter 7	Care and Support Networks for Living Better with Dementia	128
Chapter 8	Eating and Living Better with Dementia	164
Chapter 9	Incontinence and Living Better with Dementia	179
Chapter 10	How is 'Whole-Person Care' Relevant to a Person Living Better with Dementia?	193

Chapter 11 Inequalities and Living Better with Dementia: A Focus on Housing 225

Chapter 12 Does GPS Tracking Have a Role to Play in Living Better with Dementia? 242

Chapter 13 Rights-Based Approaches, Personal Budgets and Living Better with Dementia 258

Chapter 14 Art, Music and Creativity for Living Better with Dementia 289

Chapter 15 Explaining the Triggering of Sporting Memories in People Living Better with Dementia 304

Chapter 16 Innovation, Antipsychotics and Living Better with Dementia 321

Chapter 17 Promoting Leadership for Living Better with Dementia 341

Chapter 18 Conclusion 356

Subject Index 382

Author Index 389

FOREWORD

Kate Swaffer, Chair, Dementia Alliance International

It is my great honour and a real privilege to have been asked to write a foreword for this very important book. When reading Shibley's previous book, the title *Living Well with Dementia* initially irked me very slightly, as I knew he personally was not living with dementia. However, as I have come to know this gentle man, who is now a close friend as well as a colleague and an academic in the field of dementia, I fully believe he was right to use that title.

That book and this latest one are all about teaching others, including doctors and healthcare professionals, to empower and teach people like me, people who are diagnosed and living with dementia, to live well. It is also a book for people living with dementia and family carers, being highly accessible, in spite of the narrative coming from a very impressive evidence-based perspective.

This book, like the last one, is highly relevant and highly readable. We have, I believe, taught each other a great deal about dementia.

One might wonder: Why do we need to teach others it is possible to live well with dementia? From my personal experience and perspective, the current post-diagnostic support begins with Prescribed Disengagement™, which supports aged care and dying, rather than living.

Shibley is one of the few healthcare professionals and academics who believes passionately that it is not only possible but also necessary for us to be treated with autonomy and without stigma. This is urgently required if the escalating number of new diagnoses of dementia is to be believed. He is often willing to speak up for things outside of the boundaries of what perhaps his colleagues or others might think are current practice; his deep concerns for the value of individuals and his desire to support us (people with dementia) to live well resonate throughout this book.

The overriding messages about living well, of our most basic of human rights, and of the legal perspectives relating to the treatment and care of people with disabilities, which includes people with dementia, recognises that we are as full and equal human beings as every other group of people. It instructs and teaches from a rights-based perspective, with humanity and a deep and sincere interest in the wellbeing of the person.

Whilst some might see it as a medical book, it does not medicalise the support of people with dementia. The discussions on autonomy, discrimination, prejudice, citizenship and stigma must be absorbed, not just read, and in the context of equality and not just living well, but living better with dementia.

He quotes me in Chapter 5: 'It is time all people with dementia and their families stood up for better advice and services that enhance well being.' It is my firm belief that this book does a great job towards achieving that. Alzheimer's Disease International has a charter: *I can live well with dementia*. Dr Rahman is one of the very few who not only believes this is possible, but has chosen, quite often, to go against the tide and speak up for it. Thank you, Shibley.

Kate Swaffer
Co-chair and co-founder, Dementia Alliance International
Chair, Alzheimer's Australia Dementia Advisory Committee
Co-chair, Alzheimer's Australia Consumer Dementia Research Network
December 2014

FOREWORD

Chris Roberts, Dementia Alliance International, Dementia Friends Champion

There are a lot of books out there on dementia but none as informative as this one.

It is an excellent follow-on from Dr Rahman's first book, *Living Well with Dementia*. I read his first, which we found a considerable help, especially as I have mixed dementia.

After reading it I had a thirst for more knowledge about the dementias and how I could live better.

This book has just satisfied that!

It goes into great detail, using his academic knowledge and using the experiences of other carers.

More importantly, he has used the experience of people who are living with dementia to explore different therapies and self-help to achieve this.

It explores disability rights, dementia-friendly communities, and even advocacy. It talks about some subjects hardly ever touched before. It's a great guide for anyone exploring dementia for whatever reason, bringing about discussions as well as factual information.

It is possible to 'live better with dementia' using this book as a reference to answer questions as to what is to come and how you can be involved in your own destiny.

I highly recommend this book as a great starting point on your journey after your diagnosis, aimed at those with a dementia, carers, families and professionals – and care homes.

It reminds us that there is a beginning and a middle before the end, and, using every resource to hand, once you have read this book and explored therapies out there, you can live well and better with dementia.

I would like to thank Dr Rahman for bringing about such a useful book and for being a very good friend to my wife and me.

Chris Roberts, aged 53
Living well and better with dementia
Rhuddlan, Wales
December 2014

FOREWORD

Beth Britton, Freelance Campaigner, Consultant, Writer and Blogger

It is an exceptionally difficult task to write a foreword that could add anything more to a book that is already packed full of the very best in ideas, examples and articulation of the essence of living better with dementia. The title is particularly apt, and I applaud Shibley for reasoning that the concept of 'living better' has an inclusivity about it that reflects some of the immense difficulties many people who are living with dementia, and their families, are going through.

I feel passionately that this book has huge potential to provide hope to people who are living with dementia and their families – hope, that alongside love, helped to sustain me and my family during my father's nineteen years with vascular dementia, a period of time that included my teens and twenties. Having gone ten years without a diagnosis, the last nine years of my father's life were spent in three different care homes before he passed away in April 2012, aged 85. My hope now is that his memory lives on through my work as a campaigner, consultant, writer and blogger.

During those nineteen years we faced some extremely traumatic times as a family. The stroke that left my father collapsed at home, the aftermath of his diagnosis and the search for care homes, alongside variable standards of health and social care, and my father battling with critical chest and urinary tract infections all had aspects of heartbreak and challenge about them.

Yet in the midst of great sadness and difficulty we unexpectedly found even more joy – indeed, sharing some of the positives from our experiences was my inspiration for beginning my D4Dementia blog which has subsequently led onto all the work I do now. Within this book, Shibley has devoted key chapters to some of the most important elements that enabled my father to live better, namely:

» Food and eating. For many years, with no teeth and eventually having to cope with dysphagia, my father had the best appetite in his care home.

» Art and creativity, which enhanced my father's life immeasurably and proved to be far more effective than medications.

» Reminiscence and sport, both of which played a significant part in helping us remain connected with my father as a family through to the end of his life.

Vitally, I feel, Shibley also tackles some of the more taboo topics around dementia, most notably incontinence. My father became doubly incontinent in the aftermath of his largest stroke (the stroke that led to his diagnosis of vascular dementia), and lived with that incontinence throughout his nine years in care homes. For the person themselves, their carer(s) and family, shining a light on this difficult topic can only help to improve care and support.

I am also heartened to see Shibley including a chapter on 'wandering' and widening this out to look at the debates around GPS systems. My father was labelled a 'wanderer' just because he wanted and needed to walk, this despite the fact that in his earlier years he had led an active outdoor life as a farmer. Only when he was diagnosed with dementia did his life-long love of walking suddenly become labelled as 'wandering', something I felt was hugely disrespectful.

The need for dignity and respect runs throughout my work, and never more so than when highlighting the need for diagnosis to go hand-in-hand with appropriate, personalised post-diagnostic support that gives the person with dementia and their family the very best chance of living better with dementia. With this in mind, I am delighted that the largest chapter in this book is devoted to care and support networks, a topic that I know Shibley is very passionate about.

I congratulate Shibley on writing a book that brings together so many of the challenges facing people who are living with dementia, their families, and professionals from many different disciplines, and takes them forward in a critically thoughtful way. This is a book that truly points the way to a future where living better is a reality for everyone affected by dementia.

Beth Britton
Freelance Campaigner,
Consultant, Writer and Blogger
www.bethbritton.com
February 2015

PREFACE

> 'Include us in the activities of community organisations, particularly those addressing dementia. Are we on your committees, boards, seminar organising groups and suchlike? Unlike people with other diseases, we seem to be written off from active participation in addressing our own needs.'
>
> Christine Bryden, *Dancing with Dementia: My Story of Living Positively with Dementia* (2005)

Unfortunately, this issue has not gone away in the ten years since Christine published her famous book in 2005.

When I first published *Living Well with Dementia* at the beginning of January 2014, there were few accounts looking at the whole policy arena of living well with dementia (Rahman, 2014). There are still few accounts; books tend to be slightly out of date, or occupy particular focal areas of interest. The policy of dementia-friendly communities is finding its first feet in England, and Chapter 17 of my book *Living Well with Dementia*, I feel, reflects its young nature. Now that it is gathering momentum, alongside a concerted global effort on dementia, it is an opportune time to think about what people with dementia want out of dementia-friendly communities.

The wish for people who have been given a diagnosis of dementia to live as full a life as possible is not an unreasonable one. Anything can happen to anyone at any time. While talk seemingly has centred around 'opportunities' from dementia, it is very easy to see dementia as a business case. But being a person gives you your identity, your legal and ethical rights. I have spent a lot of the last year meeting people living with dementia in conversations about what 'living well' might be. I have, nonetheless, kept myself interested in latest advances in molecular biology and pharmacology too, as it has become clear, from attending international conferences recently for Alzheimer Europe and the Alzheimer's Association in Glasgow and Copenhagen, that living well and basic science-based approaches are not in fact mutually exclusive.

I have marvelled at the evolution of language regarding people at all sorts of stages of life after diagnosis. I looked at the global backdrop to the current dementia strategies in Chapter 5 of my first book *Living Well with Dementia* (Rahman, 2014). How the World Dementia Council, only recently founded, existed for so long without a person living well with dementia representing that community is a testament to the stigma and discrimination against people with dementia, which major charities and the caring professions can unwittingly perpetuate. Certain parts of the human brain are known to be redundant in function (Glassman, 1987). But it would be utterly unacceptable for people living well with dementia simply to become 'window dressing' in the global dementia agenda. Already pimping out expensive drugs, some of which are clearly not efficacious in some living with dementia, is not without its remarkable opportunity cost compared with people striving to live well with dementia, assisted to some extent by 'regulatory capture' (Heller and Heller, 2013). 'Reserve' is a phenomenon where the brain has a bit of leeway before functioning abnormally in an observable way (Stern, 2012). One wonders how many people living with dementia you could lose from implementation of the approach of appearing to prioritise cure for the future ahead of care for the people who are currently living with dementia without certain beneficiaries of the approach being significantly affected.

It is unreasonable to object on principle to the main aspects of the policy plank that is dementia-friendly communities, in a world which otherwise does not include or accommodate the person living with dementia. But the policy runs the risk of homogenising people. And this is not on. It's exactly the same criticism that 'black-friendly communities' faced four decades ago (Cohen, 1970). Instead of promoting seamless integration, it might inadvertently promote division. As a broad-brush tool, the promotion of equality is totally in line with dementia being considered as a disability. The root of this is found legally in the United Nations Convention on the Rights of Persons with Disabilities.

It is easy to sell the idea of dementia-friendly communities to employers who can seek advantage against competitors in a revamped 'nudge' for dementia (for a neat account of the nudge doctrine in policy, the reader is directed to an excellent review by Johnson and colleagues, 2012). But this would be to use dementia-friendly communities as a 'community brand', a tamer form of the corporate brand (Füller, 2014). It is textbook 'diversity marketing', one could argue (Murray, O'Driscoll and Torres, 2002). But I feel it is more of a challenge to think about how an employee living with dementia may be given an altogether different task he or she might be happier with; celebrating diversity has to be balanced against the wish of the employer to lose the employee altogether. But this represents a general societal issue of whether employment favours the employer or the employee. The promotion of equality has always rested uneasily with the lack of promotion of diversity. The tension between the business case and social justice approaches forms a crucial point of debate in the diversity and equality field (Tomlinson and Schwabenland, 2010).

It is clear that too many assumptions in policy strands are much more problematic than they would first appear. For example, there seems to be legally some mythical cut-off at 65 whereby people with young-onset dementia are literally excluded from dementia services. This, of course, is potentially subject to 'judicial review', but it should not have to be. And the relentless drive to 'successful ageing', where all citizens have to be productive, potentially belittles the value of a person with dementia simply in terms of how much money he or she can contribute to failing economies.

The equality of wellbeing

> 'Equality of wellbeing would ensure the exercise of fundamental citizenship rights by all citizens independent of their economic and social contribution.'
>
> Marcia H. Rioux, 'Towards a concept of equality of wellbeing: overcoming the social and legal construction of inequality' (1994)

The value of people living with dementia, some of whom have quite remarkable visual and artistic talents unleashed, can get somewhat strangulated by discussion and by tomes of bulky cost estimates of how much 'dementia' is a crisis and will cost the earth in future. But these estimates are not without their considerable methodological problems, such as the extent to which risk factors for dementia of the Alzheimer type, the most common type of dementia globally, are truly independent. Such a 'shock doctrine approach', while well suited to fundraising, can be built on flaky arguments.

This book

In this book, I should like to initiate a reboot of v.2.0 of Dementia-Friendly Communities, putting the person living with dementia in the driving seat. And the carer, whether paid or unpaid, needs to be in that seat too. It is difficult to reconcile campaigning for increased dividends of Pharma in the future against a social care system on its knees currently; otherwise re-articulated as the meme 'care for today, cure for tomorrow'.

I feel the book takes me much further into issues I barely touched upon in my first book, *Living Well with Dementia: The Importance of the Person and the Environment for Wellbeing* (2014).

Contents

Chapter 1 provides an introduction to policy in England as it currently stands, including a review of the need for a 'timely diagnosis' as well as a right to timely post-diagnostic care. This has been a vocal concern of Baroness Sally Greengross, the current Chair of the All-Party Parliamentary Group on Dementia. This chapter also provides an overview of the current evidence base of the hugely popular Dementia Friends campaign run very successfully by the Alzheimer's Society and Public Health England, to raise awareness about five key 'facts' about dementia.

Chapter 2 comprises a preliminary analysis of stigma, citizenship and the notion of 'living better with dementia'. This chapter explains the urgency of the need to 'frame the narrative' properly. This chapter also introduces the Dementia Alliance International group, which has fast become a highly influential campaigning force *by* people living with dementia *for* people living with dementia.

Chapter 3 looks at the various issues facing the timely diagnosis and post-diagnostic support of people living with dementia from diverse cultural backgrounds, including people from black, Asian and ethnic minority backgrounds, people who are lesbian, bisexual, gay or transsexual, and people with intellectual difficulties. Attention is paid to the various intricate ways in which culture can impact not only on the timely diagnosis of dementia but also on post-diagnostic care.

Chapter 4 looks at the issue of how different jurisdictions around the world have formulated their national dementia strategies. There is remarkable convergence in the efforts of various jurisdictions, and it is here I first introduce the critical importance of collaboration.

Chapter 5 looks at the intense care versus cure debate which has now surfaced in young-onset dementia. There is a potentially problematic schism between resources being allocated to drugs for today and resources being used to fund adequately contemporary care to allow people to live better with dementia.

Chapter 6 focuses on delirium, or the acute confusional state, and dementia. It attempts to explain why delirium and dementia might converge in policy, after all.

Chapter 7 is the longest chapter in this book, and takes as its theme care and support networks. I make no apologies for the length of this chapter, as I have been hugely influenced by the Dementia Action Alliance Carers' Call to Action in the last year. I have used the word 'carers' in this chapter, but I am mindful that alternative terms are commonly used especially in other jurisdictions, such as 'caregivers', 'family carers', 'paid or unpaid carers' or even 'care partners'.

Chapter 8 considers eating for living well with dementia. The main focus of the chapter is how people with dementia might present with alterations in their eating behaviour, and how the mealtime environment must be a vital consideration for living better with dementia.

Chapter 9 looks at a particular co-morbidity: incontinence. Focusing on the various co-morbidities will be an opportunity for a whole-person approach for a person living with dementia, during health as well as illness.

Chapter 10 argues how the needs for people living better with dementia would be best served by a fully integrated health and social care service in the form of 'whole-person care'.

Chapter 11 considers the importance of the social determinants of health. The framework, I argue, is eminently sensible for organising one's thoughts about dementia-friendly communities. Housing for living well with dementia is not just about buildings, and is pivotally enmeshed with the person-centred care philosophy of projected English policy.

With such a broad-brush tool as equality and dementia-friendly communities, the scope for squashing diversity is enormous. Few topics enter the realms of 'one glove does not fit all' to the same degree as the potential use of global positioning systems (GPS) for dementia. Chapter 12 considers whether 'wandering' is the most appropriate term. The main emphasis of this chapter is the legal and ethical considerations in the use of GPS in enhancing the quality of life of persons with dementia and their closest ones.

Chapter 13 considers head-on a number of important contemporary issues, with the main emphasis on human rights and 'rights-based approaches'. While there is no universal right to a budget, the implementation of personal budgets is discussed.

Too often the debate about dementia can be engulfed in a diatribe about 'cost', not 'value'. Persons living better with dementia wish to contribute effectively with the outside world, and the feeling is mutual. Chapter 14 is primarily concerned with art and creativity, which can be incredibly empowering for some people trying to live better with dementia.

The focus in international policies is too often on medications. Chapter 15 looks at the triggering of football sporting memories in people living well with dementia. This chapter considers the cognitive neuroscience behind this.

Chapter 16 looks at the impact of various innovations in English dementia policy, including service provision (such as the policy on reducing inappropriate use of antipsychotics or the policy in timely diagnosis) and research.

Chapter 17 looks at how leadership could be promoted by people living with dementia themselves. I first introduce the need for this in Chapter 2. Chapter 17 considers who might lead the change, where and when, and why this change might be necessary to 'recalibrate' the current global debate about dementia.

Finally, I attempt a conclusion in Chapter 18.

And finally...

I should like to give a special mention to Kate Swaffer. I have just heard that Kate has been recommended for the degree of Master of Science in dementia care from the University of Wollongong, Australia. It is a real honour to know Kate. She has informed my book like no other.

I hope you find the issues I discuss thought-provoking.

The issue is not about what conferences you can turn up to, how many commissions you can get, how many courses you can flog, or how many papers you can publish on dementia.

It's all about whether you feel you have made a real difference.

In England, the Conservative Party Manifesto 2015 included as one of its manifesto pledges the integration of health and social care through the Better Care Fund (p.37) and 'to scrap the Human Rights Act' (p.58). As the Conservative Party won a majority in the 2015 general election, these pledges have to be taken into account when looking to the future of English dementia policy. Some of the debates will arouse fierce emotions. I think to understand living better with dementia you do need to draw on the strengths of contributions from more than one discipline. This may seem to the uninitiated a rather 'Swiss army knife' approach, but the only way to promote living better with dementia, for people who have received this diagnosis, is to break out of the restricted mentality of the biomedical model. I must emphasise that no part of this book is to be taken as medical or legal advice in any jurisdiction, and that you should be able to use this text in conjunction with other texts to make up your mind about the emerging narrative.

I should like personally to thank the following over permission to reproduce material relevant to my book: All-Party Parliamentary Group for Dementia, Alzheimer's Disease International, Alzheimer Scotland, British Psychological Society, Carers Trust, Dementia Action Alliance, Gráinne McGettrick, Housing Learning and Improvement Network, Institute for Futures Studies (Stockholm), John Snow Inc., Kate Swaffer, National Housing Federation, the Scottish Government and Simone Willig. Where material is reproduced under the Open

Government Licence, every effort has been taken to comply with the terms and conditions of the relevant licences.

You are strongly advised to read the original references cited if you should wish to pursue any points of discussion. I have tried to represent all narratives as accurately as possible, to the best of my knowledge.

Thank you, and good luck!

Dr Shibley Rahman
London
December 2014

References

Bryden, C. (2005) Dancing with Dementia: My Story of Living Positively with Dementia. London: Jessica Kingsley Publishers.

Cohen, D. (1970) Advertising and the black community. Journal of Marketing, 34, 8–11.

Conservative Party (2015) The Conservative Party Manifesto 2015. Available at https://s3-eu-west-1.amazonaws.com/manifesto2015/ConservativeManifesto2015.pdf (accessed 18 May 2015).

Füller, J. (2014) For us: the charm of community brands. GfK Marketing Intelligence Review, 6, 2, 40–5.

Glassman, R.N. (1987) An hypothesis about redundancy and reliability in the brains of higher species: analogies with genes, internal organs, and engineering systems. Neuroscience and Behavioural Reviews, 11, 275–85.

Heller, T. and Heller, L. (2003) First among equals? Does drug treatment for dementia claim more than its fair share of resources? Dementia, 2, 7–19.

Johnson, E.J., Shu, S.B., Delleart, B.G.C., Fox, C. *et al.* (2012) Beyond nudges: tools of a choice architecture. Marketing Letters, 23, 487–504.

Murray, J.A., O'Driscoll, A. and Torres, A. (2002) Discovering diversity in marketing practice. European Journal of Marketing, 36, 3, 373–90.

Rahman, S. (2014) Living Well with Dementia: The Importance of the Person and the Environment for Wellbeing. Oxford: Radcliffe Health.

Rioux, M.H. (1994) Towards a concept of equality of wellbeing: overcoming the social and legal construction of inequality. Canadian Journal of Law and Jurisprudence, 7, 1, 127–47.

Stern, Y. (2012) Cognitive reserve in ageing and Alzheimer's disease. Lancet Neurology, 11, 11, 1006–12.

Tomlinson, F. and Schwabenland, C. (2010) Reconciling competing discourses of diversity? The UK non-profit sector between social justice and the business case. Organisation, 17, 101.

COPYRIGHT ACKNOWLEDGEMENTS

Boxes 1.1 and 3.1 are reproduced by kind permission of the Secretariat of the All-Party Group on Dementia for the UK parliament.
Figures 1.1 and 8.1 and Box 11.1 are reproduced under the Open Government Licence v3.0.
Figure 2.1 and Box 4.1 are reproduced by kind permission of Alzheimer's Disease International.
Boxes 4.2 and 13.2 are reproduced by kind permission of Alzheimer Scotland.
Figure 7.1 is reproduced by kind permission of the Carers Trust.
Boxes 7.1 and 7.2 are reproduced by kind permission of the Dementia Action Alliance.
Figure 11.2 is reproduced by kind permission of the Institute for Futures Studies, Stockholm, Sweden.
Figure 11.3 is reproduced by kind permission of the Housing Learning and Improvement Network.
Figure 13.1 is reproduced by kind permission of Kate Swaffer.
Figure 13.2 is reproduced by kind permission of the Scottish Government.
Figure 16.1 is reproduced by kind permission of the British Psychological Society.
Box 11.2 is reproduced by kind permission of Dementia Services Centre, Stirling.
Extract on page 275 is reproduced by kind permission of Griánne McGettrick.
Extract on page 299 is reproduced by kind permission of Simone Willig.

Chapter 1

INTRODUCTION

> 'It was the best of times, it was the worst of times, it was the age of wisdom, it was the age of foolishness, it was the epoch of belief, it was the epoch of incredulity, it was the season of Light, it was the season of Darkness, it was the spring of hope, it was the winter of despair, we had everything before us, we had nothing before us, we were all going direct to Heaven, we were all going direct the other way – in short, the period was so far like the present period, that some of its noisiest authorities insisted on its being received, for good or for evil, in the superlative degree of comparison only.'
>
> Charles Dickens, *A Tale of Two Cities* (1859)

Professor Sube Banerjee, instrumental in the first English dementia strategy direction, recently referred to Sun Tzu's *The Art of War*, citing the apocryphal quote, 'Strategy without tactics is the slowest route to victory. Tactics without strategy is the noise before defeat.' The sentiment is deeply felt by most reasonable persons. It would be difficult to imagine there being no dementia strategy to follow on from the current one for England, 'Living well with dementia' (2009–14).

Introduction to current policy in England

England is one country of many that has a programme allowing persons with dementia to live as well as possible; an overview of other global policies is provided in Chapter 4. The last few years have indeed seen some considerable shifts in policy, concurrent with operational changes in service provision and research in the dementias in England in the last few years. It is wonderful to observe a real sense of innovation (Chapter 16) and leadership (Chapter 17) in the current

English policy. The last few years have indeed been traumatic, given the nature of operational changes in the service provision of the National Health Service in England, Scotland and Wales (see, for example, Holland, 2012). The clinical syndrome of dementia has several aetiologies of which dementia of the Alzheimer type is the most common globally. There have undoubtedly been major successes, ranging from the large (e.g. increases in research funding) to the 'small gains' (e.g. individual nurses feeling more confident on individual wards in working with people with dementia).

The relatively recent starting point for all is 'Living well with dementia', the strategy document published in 2009 for English dementia policy. The National Dementia Strategy for England aims to help ensure that uniform care is delivered to patients with dementia and that standards are maintained at a nationally agreed level (Koch and Iliffe, 2011). And indeed it was one of the first strategies of its kind in the world. It established a standard for improving the lives of people with dementia, for their families and their carers, through raising awareness, encouraging earlier diagnosis and providing high-quality treatment and care.

In a *British Medical Journal* editorial entitled 'The National Dementia Strategy in England', the current clinical lead for dementia in England, Professor Alistair Burns, summarised the background to this document as a '"smorgasbord" of evidence, economics, and obligation' and convincingly explained how the policy recommendations had emerged from the existent literature (Burns and Robert, 2009).

Pervasive strands of the English dementia policy

The Prime Minister's Dementia Challenge was developed as a successor to the National Dementia Strategy, with the challenge of delivering major improvements in dementia care, support and research.

It ran until March 2015. There are four core strands of improving health and social care policy in Europe following the Prime Minister's Dementia Challenge to create dementia-friendly communities and research.

1. Timely diagnosis

The initial timely diagnosis of dementia can itself bring considerable stigma (stigma is a focus of Chapter 3).

Primary care teams and general practitioners (GPs) play an important role in the diagnosis and care of dementia patients and their families (Brodaty *et al.*, 1994;

Downs *et al.*, 2003). Kmietowicz (2014) reported in the *British Medical Journal* that, according to the official figures, the number of people with a diagnosis of dementia in England has risen by 62% in the past seven years, from 213,000 in 2006–07 to 344,000 in 2013–14. In March 2012, the Prime Minister David Cameron issued a 'dementia challenge', which called for the United Kingdom to become a world leader in dementia care (Kmietowicz, 2012).

Various arguments for a timely diagnosis of dementia were proposed by De Lepeleire and colleagues (2008). These have stood the 'test of time', despite landmark global events, including potential benefits for the person with dementia, family, health professionals, friends, family and society as a whole.

Historically, there has been an increasing medical and public consensus that diagnosis of dementia should be made as early as possible in the illness trajectory; the consensus has included the feeling that early identification of symptoms is beneficial to both users and their relatives (National Audit Office, 2007). Notwithstanding this, Milne (2010) warns that early diagnosis also carries risks: loss of status, acquisition of a stigmatising label, loss of employment and, for a minority, depression. Interestingly, however, Milne points to a finding that, whether one is for or against early intervention in dementia, a defining feature of most of the key arguments to date is that they are located within the medical sphere and in the context of a healthcare provision driven by evidence-based practice (Lupton, 1999).

The All-Party Parliamentary Group (APPG) on Dementia outlined a series of recommendations in their report of July 2012, 'Unlocking diagnosis: the key to improving the lives of people with dementia' (see Box 1.1).

At the time of a letter on progress on the Prime Minister's Dementia Challenge, dated May 2014, there were approaching 60 services accredited with the Royal College of Psychiatrists' Memory Services National Accreditation programme out of 94 members who are currently part of the programme. The Department of Health had commissioned the Royal College of Psychiatrists to undertake a survey of memory clinics and this reported in November 2013. The audit reported that the number of people being assessed by memory clinics had risen four-fold since 2010–11, with just under half of the people diagnosed with dementia over the previous 12 months being in the early stages of the condition.

David Cameron had said that only 42% of people with dementia had a formal diagnosis and that this varied significantly by region, from 29% in some areas to 67% in those with the most diagnoses. In March 2014, NHS England announced a £90 million (€113 million; $152 million) package in an effort to meet the Prime Minister's challenge to give a diagnosis to two-thirds of people with dementia by March 2015 (Wise, 2014). However, critics expressed concerns about this policy, saying that no convincing evidence had shown earlier diagnosis to be helpful for patients and that setting diagnosis targets was an unproven strategy that could lead to over-diagnosis (Brunet, 2014). Currently, as articulated well by Ionicioiu and colleagues (2014), a meta-analysis shows overall that psychosocial interventions are effective in dementia care in general, but more evidence is needed for specific psychosocial interventions.

Box 1.1 Recommendations from the APPG report of July 2012: 'Unlocking diagnosis: the key to improving the lives of people with dementia'

Recommendation 1. Invest in a sustained public dementia awareness campaign.

Recommendation 2. A quantified ambition that increases the percentage of people with dementia who have a formal diagnosis should be embedded in the NHS and used to lever change.

Recommendation 3. Public health directors across the UK should make early dementia diagnosis a priority.

Recommendation 4. Primary care workers and other health and social care professionals in contact with people in groups with an established risk of dementia should routinely ask questions to identify symptoms of dementia.

Recommendation 5. UK-wide, all health and social care professionals working in a general capacity with people at risk of dementia should have pre- and post-registration training in identifying and understanding dementia.

Recommendation 6. Issues with the assessment tools used by UK GPs and other primary care professionals should be explored and addressed.

Recommendation 7. Across the UK, commissioners should invest in appropriate memory service resources to cater to the needs of their population.

Recommendation 8. Strengthen the role of the Memory Services Accreditation Programme.

Recommendation 9. Adequate information and one-to-one support should be provided to patients and their families immediately following diagnosis.

Source: APPG on Dementia, 2012 (pp.10–13) (reproduced by kind permission of the Secretariat of the All-Party Group on Dementia for the UK parliament)

2. Post-diagnostic care and support, including inappropriate use of antipsychotic medication

The landscape of post-diagnostic care and support is extremely important, and is the focus of Chapter 7 of this book. Recently, there has been a growing realisation that the service needs to be designed around people, not around traditional interest groups (NHS Confederation, 2014). This necessarily puts a large emphasis on the ethical issues of caring.

As described by Gauthier and colleagues (2013), the ethical debates up to 2005 included:

» disclosure of the diagnosis of dementia and related consequences (e.g. stigma, discrimination)

» the cost/benefit of symptomatic drugs in mild to moderate stages of dementia

» the efficacy of these drugs in the severe stages of dementia, and the clinical criteria to stop them.

Since 2005, however, the ethical issues have indeed become elaborate: the disclosure of a diagnosis of dementia of Alzheimer type (DAT) in asymptomatic or minimally symptomatic persons with full insight, an uncertainty of a diagnosis based on biomarkers without full validation, and the social stigma of very mild DAT (Gauthier *et al.*, 2013). Converging evidence now from both genetically at-risk cohorts and clinically normal older individuals suggests that the pathophysiological process of DAT begins years, if not decades, before the diagnosis of clinical dementia (Morris, 2005). Working groups in the past established by the National Institute on Aging/Alzheimer's Association have focused on developing diagnostic criteria for the clinical stages of mild cognitive impairment as well as dementia due to an underlying 'AD-pathophysiological process' (Albert *et al.*, 2011; McKhann *et al.*, 2011).

The current nursing strategy for dementia, 'Making a Difference in Dementia: Nursing Vision and Strategy', emphasises the '6Cs' of nursing: care, compassion, competence, communication, courage and commitment. This resource was introduced by the Department of Health (2013) to raise the profile of the wider nursing contribution to dementia care, and to describe what is expected of all nurses to meet the level and quality of care expected in all care settings. There are diverse opportunities and challenges for good-quality care for persons with dementia, including eating (Chapter 8) and incontinence (Chapter 9). Activities involving art and creativity can be incorporated in good-quality care (Chapter 14), or activities might involve reminiscence of football memories (Chapter 15).

It is anticipated that, under the current Department of Health nursing strategy, nurses will contribute to implementing nursing care by working in partnership and in all environments of care to ensure they work collaboratively with GPs and primary care practitioners (including practice nurses) to manage the interface with wider community services: in a person's home, hospitals, housing (Chapter 11) including care homes, care homes with nursing, hospice services, community (social care) and the voluntary sector organisations, and 'out of hours' organisations. Pro-active case management, from the initial timely diagnosis right up to end-of-life care, is likely to grow in prominence in the person-centred approach of whole-person care. This strategy provides a useful backdrop for the large transformational change anticipated for England (Chapter 10). In Chapter 2 of my previous book, *Living Well with Dementia*, I considered what 'living well' is; I then went on to consider how you could measure it in Chapter 3 of the same book. This will be increasingly significant as commissioners get involved with services promoting wellbeing in accordance with current English law.

Nurses of all grades are therefore anticipated to contribute to the implementation of the English dementia strategy:

1. Dementia awareness – all nurses.
2. Dementia skilled workforce – all providing nursing to people living with dementia directly.
3. Dementia specialists – experts in the field of dementia care.

This is shown schematically in Figure 1.1.

In 2012 the Dementia Action Alliance (DAA) and the NHS Institute for Innovation and Improvement launched a campaign entitled 'The Right Prescription: a call to action on the use of antipsychotic drugs for people with dementia' (DAA and the NHS Institute for Innovation and Improvement, 2012).

The rationale for this campaign is that the inappropriate prescribing of antipsychotic medication can have significant consequences for the person, and that antipsychotic medications can increase people's symptoms of dementia and cause dizziness and unsteadiness, leading to falls and injuries and robbing people of their quality of life. In November 2009, the Banerjee report highlighted these risks, and concluded that antipsychotics are too often used as a first-line response to behavioural difficulty in dementia rather than as a considered second-line treatment when other non-pharmacological approaches have failed (Banerjee, 2009). I have given an overview of these complex issues in Chapter 16, with a central focus on a need for systemic innovation.

Usual care with support (e.g. district nurse, practice nurse, PHN)
Dementia awareness – all nurses

Assisted care or care management (e.g. mental health nurses, liaison nurse, community matron, care home nurse, hospital nurse)
Dementia skilled workforce – all providing nursing to people living with dementia directly

Intensive or case management (e.g. Admiral Nurses, dementia specialist nurse)
Dementia specialists – experts in the field of dementia care

Figure 1.1 Model of dementia nursing

Source: Adapted from Department of Health, 2013
(reproduced under the Open Government Licence v3.0)

Pharmacotherapeutic interventions in dementia have found a rocky road in recent years, and it is hoped that a drive for new treatments will not be to the detriment of looking after people currently living with dementia. Since amyloid clearly has a major role, the focus on disease-modifying treatments has centred on those pathways. The number of careful analyses of resource allocation and opportunity costs of pharmacologically oriented approaches is currently very poor for England.

Disease-modifying approaches, including the targeting of amyloid processing, aggregation of tau, insulin signalling, neuroinflammation and neurotransmitter dysfunction, have, most people agree, been disappointing (Cunningham and Passmore, 2013). Harmonisation of legislation across different jurisdictions may be necessary to advance this. For a summary of possible current lines of therapy, please refer to Box 1.2.

Of course, interventions in post-diagnostic care and support are not confined to pharmacology. There are a number of non-pharmacological approaches to promote living well with dementia, and successful implementation of these will require a sophisticated analysis of risk. Chapter 12 provides a discussion of some of the issues involved in GPS tracking of people living well with dementia, which, whilst advancing independence, has risks of its own. Meanwhile, Chapter 13 considers what the future of personal budgets might be for people living with dementia.

Box 1.2 Potential future therapeutic approaches for dementia

* Targets of tam or amyloid, including immunotherapies
* Modifying insulin signalling
* Neurotrophic agents
* Neurotransmitter approaches
* Dietary modification

SOURCE: ADAPTED FROM CUNNINGHAM AND PASSMORE, 2013

3. Research

At the G8 Dementia Summit (as it was then) on 8 December 2013, the Prime Minister pledged to double the funding for research for dementia by 2025. There are important drivers to research stemming from the Prime Minister's Dementia Challenge, as follows:

» an increase in actual funding

» an increase in capacity (this might include nursing research, Big Data, or Brain Bank research)

» a broadening of the research agenda (this might include primary prevention, treatments, research into living well with dementia, efficacy of gerotechnology interventions)

» improvement in access to research.

Three broad theoretical models underpin dementia care policy (as well as practice and research): biomedical, psychosocial and social-gerontological (Innes and Manthorpe, 2013). The discipline of social gerontology, in particular 'critical social gerontology', has raised critiques of biomedical approaches to dementia (Bond, 1992; Lyman, 1989). Its proponents argue that the wider social context of dementia experiences (Bowling, 2007) may best be seen and responded to within a social model of disability rather than a disease model. But dementia is not solely about old people; indeed, Chapter 5 discusses what the notion of living well with dementia means for young-onset dementia. This approach to disability, with its concomitant sequelae for the legal protection of rights for people with dementia, will be a core theme of this book, particularly in Chapter 13.

Effective 'service user involvement' requires that flexibility is incorporated into research design. It has been suggested that quantitative research methodologies do not capture patient-centred elements of health care such as the subjective views of service users (Jenkins *et al.*, 2005; Redman and Lynn, 2004; Vileland, 2002). Tischler and colleagues (2010) observe that the terms 'patient involvement' and 'patient-centred' are increasingly being incorporated into research and clinical governance strategies.

A 'research champion group' has latterly been formed in England to oversee the implementation of the commitments on dementia research in the Dementia Challenge. The group includes some of the country's leading dementia scientists and its work builds on the previous work of the Ministerial Advisory Group on Dementia Research.

The key achievements in research in the Prime Minister's Dementia Challenge, as stated in the letter to the Prime Minister dated 7 May 2014, are stated in Box 1.3.

Box 1.3 The key achievements in research in the Prime Minister's Dementia Challenge, as stated by key stakeholders in the letter to the Prime Minister dated 7 May 2014

* Continuing progress towards achieving the doubling of public sector research funding £20m for research on living well with dementia
* Further progress towards recruiting 10% of patients into clinical studies
* Further progress on international initiatives in neurodegenerative disease research
* NIHR has appointed Professor Martin Rossor (Clinical Neurology, University College London) as the NIHR National Director for Dementia Research
* Developing 'readiness' cohorts of patients
* Identifying and validating therapeutic targets
* Maintaining a broad focus on cognitive health and impairments
* Development of innovative trials and innovative funding models
* Creating 'self-sustaining' capacity development

* Contributing to the development of an international action plan for research
* Living well with dementia

SOURCE: CARRUTHERS ET AL., 2014 (PP.5–7)

4. Dementia-friendly communities

In summary, dementia-friendly communities were supposed to encourage independent living well by people who had received a diagnosis of dementia, and to raise public awareness so as to combat the stigma and discrimination often faced by people living with dementia (Department of Health, 2012). Profound loneliness can accompany a diagnosis of dementia. For such individuals, loneliness becomes inescapable, and it is for these individuals that interventions are perhaps most necessary (Masi *et al.*, 2011). However, the focus on communities, in my opinion, tends to ignore 'networks' (Rahman, 2014).

Prevention of the dementias

As described by Khachaturian and colleagues (2011), the fourth Leon Thal Symposium was convened in Toulouse, France, on 3 November 2010. This symposium reviewed design parameters that are necessary to develop comprehensive national databases on healthy ageing.

Such relevant datasets are aimed to offer the potential to serve as the foundation for a systems-approach to solve the dual public health problems of:

» early detection of people who are at elevated risk for Alzheimer's disease

» the development of interventions to delay onset of, or prevent, late-life dementia.

There is no doubt that tackling prevention or risk factors for dementia has gained momentum in recent years.

Following a meeting of various stakeholders, including public health practitioners, policy makers, voluntary and community representatives, and researchers hosted by the UK Health Prevention Forum and Public Health England in London on 30 January 2014, consensus was reached on the potential for incorporation of dementia risk reduction into current approaches for non-communicable diseases (Public Health England and the UK Health Prevention Forum, 2014): this is known as the 'Blackfriars Consensus Statement'. The authors of this joint statement argued that dementia risk reduction should begin to be incorporated into both national and global policies to tackle non-communicable diseases, ideally beginning with the interventions where the evidence is most robust. The point from Lincoln and colleagues (2014) that a substantial proportion of dementia might be delayed or averted if modifiable risk factors are effectively addressed is a particularly meritorious one potentially.

Timely interventions targeted at these non-genetic risk factors may offer opportunities for prevention and treatment of DAT. There has been major interest in the role of cardiovascular risk factors in the development of this type of dementia. Diabetes, hypertension, hypercholesterolaemia, smoking and obesity in mid-life are all associated with late-onset DAT. Lower education, less social interaction and a more sedentary lifestyle also confer risk (Daviglus *et al.*, 2010; Ligthart *et al.*, 2010). The 'memory clinic', for example, might become a cost-effective opportunity to develop preventive multi-domain approaches for patients with higher risk of cognitive impairment (particularly patients with subjective memory complaint, family history of DAT or vascular and metabolic risk factors) (Vellas, Gillette-Guyonnet and Andrieu, 2008).

Norton and colleagues (2014), writing in *Lancet Neurology*, argued that around one-third of Alzheimer's disease cases worldwide might be attributable to potentially modifiable risk factors. They argued that the incidence of DAT might be reduced through improved access to education and use of effective methods targeted at reducing the prevalence of vascular risk factors and depression. Interestingly, Geert Jan Biessels from the Brain Center Rudolf Magnus at Utrecht emphasises that:

> Norton and colleagues show that Alzheimer's disease, just like many other disorders in late life, is at least partially preventable and that several known risk factors for poor health also substantially contribute to dementia risk. In fact, the potential for prevention might be even larger if other modifiable risk factors for dementia (e.g. diet and leisure activities) are considered. (Biessels, 2014, p.752)

Clinical trials: PREVENT and AT

Two epidemiological studies, described below, indicate that significant decreases in the incidence of DAT may be obtained by targeting multiple middle-age risk factors.

The 'PREVENT trial' is a prospective cohort study examining biomarker status at mid-life in at least 150 individuals genetically at high, medium or low risk of late-onset DAT. Participants are children of individuals with or without a diagnosed DAT allocated to high, medium and low-risk groups according to parental clinical status and APOE genotype (Ritchie and Ritchie, 2012). The 'AT trial', on the other hand, a secondary prevention trial in older people with amyloid accumulation at high risk for DAT, should provide insights into whether anti-amyloid therapy can delay cognitive decline (Sperling *et al.*, 2014).

An overview of some hypothesised risk factors, important in the prevention of the dementias, including dementia of the Alzheimer type, is shown in Box 1.4.

Box 1.4 An overview of the risk factors for the dementias/possible targets for prevention of the dementias

1. Age
2. Family history
3. Social networks and education
4. Exercise
5. Stroke and vascular risk factors
6. Psychological stress
7. Being overweight and obese
8. Smoking and alcohol
9. Diet
10. Zinc
11. Psychological symptoms

---

1. Age

Dementia does not just occur in old people, although age is possibly the strongest risk factor for dementia. The incidence of dementia has been found to rise exponentially from 65 to 90 years of age (Jorm and Jolley, 1998). It is possible that older individuals have longer exposure to putative environmental and genetic influence (McCullagh *et al.*, 2001). Recent work suggests that the acceleration of incidence rates for DAT slows down in very old age (although there is no evidence of a rate decline), the corollary thus being that DAT is age-related rather than age-dependent (Gao *et al.*, 1998).

2. Family history

Dementia risk can increase two- to four-fold among individuals who have at least one first-degree relative with dementia (Devi *et al.*, 1999; van Duijn *et al.*, 1991). This effect is thought to be stronger for those where a relative had early onset and with increased longevity. Risk increases from 5% up to the age of 70 and to 33% up to the age of 90 years (Lautenschlager *et al.*, 1996). However, while the familial occurrence of dementia may reflect shared environmental factors, there is also strong evidence to support a genetic link (Black, Patterson and Feightner, 2001).

3. Social networks and education

Social characteristics refer to a wide range of attributes. For example, high social networking, purpose in life, supporting social interactions, lifelong learning and stimulation in later life, high education and socioeconomic position, involvement in cognitively challenging tasks and being in a relationship have all been claimed to be protective against DAT.

A useful recent review is provided by Imtiaz and colleagues (2014). Education, in spite of some methodological complications, has been associated with a reduction in the risk of incident dementia (Ngandu *et al.*, 2007b; Stern *et al.*, 1994). Better education apparently confers protection against the clinical manifestation of dementia/DAT even in individuals with an unfavourable genetic background (i.e. APOE ε4 carriers) (Wang *et al.*, 2012). The potential protective role of education for dementia is an area of major interest and has been looked at in detail by EClipSE (Epidemiological Clinicopathological Studies in Europe). More education did not protect individuals from developing neurodegenerative and vascular neuropathology by the time they died, but it did appear to mitigate the impact of pathology on the clinical expression of dementia before death (EClipSE *et al.*, 2010).

I will discuss social networks extensively in the chapter on care and support networks (Chapter 7).

4. Exercise

Physical activity in midlife decreased the risk of dementia studied 26 years later, which can be explained by the decline in the cardiovascular risk profile and a reduction in brain tissue loss (Chang *et al.*, 2010). High- and moderate-intensity physical activity decreased the risk of cognitive decline in healthy individuals by up to 38% and 35% respectively (Sofi *et al.*, 2011). Aerobic exercise has been found to reduce the risk of cognitive impairment and dementia, which can be explained by either a direct neurotrophic effect of exercise or by an improvement in the cerebrovascular and cardiovascular risk profiles (Ahlskog *et al.*, 2011).

5. Stroke and vascular risk factors

There may be a vascular component to many dementias. Therefore, interventions to address vascular risk factors (such as tobacco, poor diet, physical inactivity and alcohol; and intermediate disease precursors such as raised blood pressure, raised blood cholesterol, obesity and diabetes which arise from behavioural and other factors) should theoretically also help reduce the risk, progression and severity of dementia (Public Health England and the UK Health Prevention Forum, 2014). Stroke is a common cause of cognitive impairment and dementia. However, effective strategies for reducing the risk of post-stroke dementia remain somewhat undefined at present. Potential strategies include intensive lowering of blood pressure and/or lipids. The PODCAST trial is ongoing, with 78 patients recruited to date from 22 sites (Blackburn *et al.*, 2013).

As reviewed by Ruth Peters, several intervention trials have been carried out with antihypertensives and have shown mixed results with regard to cognitive and dementia outcomes (both dementia overall and that of the vascular and Alzheimer type) (Peters, 2012). Hypertension is the most important remediable risk factor for stroke (especially lacunar infarction) and vascular dementia (Lindsay, Hébert and Rockwood, 1997). Along with hyperlipidaemia, diabetes is associated with a reduction in cerebral perfusion due to microangiopathy, often resulting in lacunar infarctions (Desmond *et al.*, 1993). However, no relationship has been found between lipid levels and the risk of probable Alzheimer's disease, suggesting that dyslipidaemia may be most relevant to the occurrence of dementia with a vascular component (Moroney *et al.*, 1999).

6. Psychological stress

Lena Johansson and colleagues (2010) found an association between psychological stress in middle-aged women and development of dementia, especially DAT.

Previous research had revealed that psychological stress could plausibly lead to neural degeneration and development of cognitive impairment via changes in hormonal and immune system functions (Leonard, 2006). Stress may be related to cognitive decline and dementia by its activation of the hypothalamic–pituitary–adrenal axis, and increasing levels of glucocorticoid hormones (Sapolsky, 1996). Promising preliminary evidence has indeed been presented that corticotropin-releasing factor receptor (CRFR) signalling mechanisms can also influence mechanisms of DAT pathogenesis by affecting tau-P and solubility in the hippocampus. This identifies CRFR1 as a potential target for intervention in DAT (Kehne, 2007).

7. Being overweight and obese

Based on a number of observations, DAT has been proposed to be a generalised metabolic disorder. For example, some studies have suggested that being overweight or obese in middle age is a risk for the later development of cognitive decline (e.g. Beydoun, Beydoun and Wang, 2008). It is well known that obesity increases the risk for vascular disorders such as atherosclerosis, chronic heart disease, hypertension and diabetes (Kopelman, 2000). It has been suggested that these vascular disorders increase the probability that dementia will develop, particularly DAT and vascular dementias (VaD) (Hofman *et al.*, 1997; Skoog, Kalaria and Breteler, 1999). A high BMI late in life is associated with a low risk of dementia (Buchman *et al.*, 2005; Gustafson *et al.*, 2009), while a high BMI in midlife is associated with a higher risk of dementia (Kivipelto *et al.*, 2005).

8. Smoking and alcohol

Studies on the association of smoking and alcohol intake with cognition have yielded inconsistent results. There may be a complicated gene–environment interplay between smoking and dementia risk (Rusanen *et al.*, 2010). According to Ngandu and colleagues, alcohol drinking both at midlife and later is favourably related to the function in several cognitive domains, including episodic memory, psychomotor speed and executive function, in late life (Ngandu *et al.*, 2007a). It overall appears that mild-to-moderate alcohol intake is protective against dementia while excessive consumption increases the risk of cognitive decline and dementia. Kim and colleagues (2012) provide that, from studies published from 1971 to 2011 related to alcohol and cognition in the elderly reviewed using a desktop search, alcohol may have both a neurotoxic and neuroprotective effect. Difficulties in making conclusive conclusions may relate to methodological issues (Panza *et al.*, 2012).

9. Diet

Saturated fats have been found to increase the risk of DAT, while healthy dietary patterns such as diets rich in fruits and vegetables, adherence to a Mediterranean diet, intake of antioxidants and omega-3 fatty acids have been found to decrease the dementia risk. Dietary fatty acids and antioxidants may contribute to decrease dementia risk, but epidemiological data remain controversial.

A huge total of 8085 participants without dementia aged 65 and over were included in the 'Three-City cohort study' in Bordeaux, Dijon and Montpellier (France) in 1999–2000 and had at least one re-examination over four years. An independent committee of neurologists validated 281 incident cases of dementia (including 183 DAT) (Barberger-Gateau *et al.*, 2007). It was found that frequent consumption of fruits and vegetables, fish and oils rich in omega-3 may decrease the risk of dementia and Alzheimer's disease, especially among APOE ε4 non-carriers.

Previously, the Rotterdam Study found that higher dietary intakes of vitamins E and C related to lower risk of dementia including DAT over six years of follow-up, but a further study showed, with a mean follow-up period of 9.6 years, that dietary intake levels of vitamin C, beta carotene and flavonoids were not associated with dementia risk after multivariate adjustment, but a higher intake of foods rich in vitamin E may modestly reduce long-term risk of dementia including DAT (Devore *et al.*, 2010). Furthermore, Scarmeas and colleagues (2006) concluded that higher adherence to a Mediterranean diet is associated with a reduction in risk for DAT. There had been a paucity of data regarding the effect of composite dietary patterns (rather than individual foods or nutrients) on the risk for DAT. Leptin (from the Greek word λεπτός, *leptos*, 'thin'), the 'satiety hormone', is a hormone made by fat cells which regulates the amount of fat stored in the body. It does this by adjusting both the sensation of hunger and energy expenditure. Low leptin levels in older adults have been associated with the development of DAT and other dementias (Lieb *et al.*, 2009). However, other studies were unable to show a difference in leptin between persons with DAT and controls, unless an APOE ε4 allele was present (Warren, Hynan and Weiner, 2012).

I return to the potential significance of a Mediterranean diet and dementia in my chapter on eating and living better with dementia (Chapter 8).

10. Zinc

The brain acquires metals and exploits their unique biochemistry as part of its normal functioning (Zecca *et al.*, 2004). Metals such as iron, copper and zinc act as essential cofactors in metalloproteins required for the normal functioning of the nervous tissue, with unique importance in myelin synthesis and neurotransmission, while heavy metals such as mercury and lead are known 'neurotoxins' (poisonous to nerve cells). Zinc is one of the most prevalent trace elements in the human body: it is an essential nutrient, and is also central to many key molecular and cellular reactions critical for innate and adaptive immune system function (Haase and Rink, 2009; Szewczyk, 2013). Zinc deficiency is common in older people and contributes to many clinical disorders such as growth retardation, immune dysfunction and cognitive impairment, affecting up to two billion people worldwide (Prasad, 2009). Zinc supplementation is reported to be beneficial at ameliorating the effects of these disorders and in many infectious and non-infectious diseases (Prasad, 2009). Crucially, accumulation of zinc has been implicated in the accumulation of beta amyloid in DAT (for a good review, please refer to Szewczyk, 2013).

11. Psychological symptoms

Behavioural and psychological symptoms are common in the older population and may be an indication of early dementia. Van der Linde and colleagues (2013) concluded that some psychiatric symptoms are associated with increased short-term progression to dementia in those with low cognition. Previous clinical studies of such cohorts had reported mixed findings (Monastero *et al.*, 2009).

Head trauma with loss of consciousness is also a risk factor for dementia in some, but not all, studies.

Inequalities

Inequalities or 'the social determinants of health' concern the conditions in which people are born, grow, live, work and age. These circumstances are shaped by the distribution of money, power and resources at global, national and local levels. They include water and sanitation, agriculture and food, access to health and social care services, unemployment and welfare, working conditions, housing and living environment, education and transport.

The 'social determinants of health' are mostly responsible for health inequities – the unfair and avoidable differences in health status seen within and between countries (for a statement, see World Health Organization, 2013). Therefore, certainly, intervention studies that address inequalities in health are a priority area for future public health research (Bambra *et al.*, 2010).

The importance of housing in living better with dementia cannot be understated, I believe. An analysis of some of the key issues are provided in Chapter 11. Working in policy silos, it can be rather too easy to overlook the social determinants of health in the dementia-friendly communities policy, both domestically and internationally. Conversely, a mature account will be to enmesh the social narratives of health and the inequalities narrative properly with dementia-friendly communities one day in the future.

Dementia Friends

It was noted in the APPG report 'Unlocking diagnosis' that 'poor public understanding of dementia was an overwhelming theme' (2012, p.22). The APPG concluded that a key barrier to early diagnosis identified by professionals, people with dementia and carers was the length of time between symptoms such as memory problems first arising and the seeking of professional advice – from a GP, for example.

A large-scale public awareness campaign about dementia was settled upon, with the APPG report citing the evidence of Professor Sube Banerjee, now Chair of Dementia at Brighton and Sussex Medical School. It was decided in the Prime Minister's Dementia Challenge that the Department of Health and Social Care Fund would invest in a nationwide campaign to raise awareness of dementia, to be sustained to 2015. This would build on lessons learned from previous campaigns and inform future investment.

According to the progress letter to the Prime Minister (dated 7 May 2014), the launch of the Dementia Friends campaign, a major new campaign led by the Alzheimer's Society and Public Health England, would mobilise the whole country to tackle one of the biggest health issues of our time. The campaign was intended to raise awareness of dementia, improve attitudes towards the condition and create a more dementia-friendly society by encouraging one million people to become Dementia Friends. The number of Dementia Friends is indeed progressing impressively, including, with support from Public Health England, Dementia Friends from private businesses.

The five statements surrounding Dementia Friends (Alzheimer's Society, 2012) are extremely useful.

1. Dementia is not a natural part of ageing

This is an extremely important message. However, it is known that the greatest risk factor for dementias overall is increasing age. The majority of people with

Alzheimer's disease, typically manifesting as problems in new learning and short-term memory, are indeed 65 and older. But dementia is not just a disease of old age. A rare type of dementia called the variant Creutzfeldt-Jakob disease (vCJD) was first reported in 1996; the youngest patient developed symptoms at 16 years of age (reviewed in Verity *et al.*, 2000). As described in a World Health Organization factsheet (2012), vCJD is a rare and fatal human neurodegenerative condition which is classified as a transmissible spongiform encephalopathy (TSE) because of its ability to be transmitted and the characteristic spongy degeneration of the brain that it causes. Its diagnosis does need to be in very specialist hands.

I will be focusing on the policy for dementias which occur at a younger age in Chapter 5.

2. Dementia is caused by diseases of the brain

That 'dementia is caused by diseases of the brain' may seem like a pretty innocuous statement. There have been numerous attempts to look at the prevalence of the different causes of dementia, varying in overall success over the years.

One study – 'Prevalence of dementia subtypes: a 30-year retrospective survey of neuropathological reports' – came from Hans Brunnström and colleagues in 2008. The authors investigated the distribution of neuropathologically defined dementia subtypes among individuals with a dementia. The neuropathological diagnosis was dementia of the Alzheimer type in 42% of the cases, vascular dementia in 23.7%, dementia of combined Alzheimer and vascular pathology in 21.6%, and frontotemporal dementia in 4% of the patients.

3. Dementia is not just about losing your memory

Dementia is a general term for a number of progressive diseases affecting, it is estimated, more than 800,000 people living in the UK. The heart pumps blood around the circulation. The liver is involved in making things and breaking down things in metabolism. The brain combines these separate attributes into one giant perception, known as 'gestalt'. What an individual with dementia notices differently compared with before, on account of his or her dementia, will depend on the part of the brain that is affected. Indeed, cognitive neurologists are able to identify which part of the brain is likely to be affected from this constellation of symptoms, in much the same way that cardiologists can identify the precise defect in the heart from hearing a murmur with a stethoscope. In a dementia known as 'posterior cortical atrophy', the part of the brain involved with higher-order visual processing can be affected, leading to real problems in perception.

4. It's possible to live well with dementia

When asked to think of words associated with dementia, members of the public often suggest:

> 'Suffering.'
>
> 'Horrible.'
>
> 'Terrible.'
>
> 'Tsunami.'
>
> 'Epidemic.'
>
> 'Tidal wave.'

And indeed it would be wrong to ignore how distressing a diagnosis of dementia can be for certain individuals with dementia. Take, for example, people with diffuse Lewy body disease, typically individuals in the younger age bracket, in their 50s, who have complete insight into the condition, realise that their memory might be going and are exasperated at the 'night terrors'.

'Living well with dementia', conversely, is supposed to counteract the negative word associations many people have about dementia. It is felt that such negative connotations contribute to the stigma individuals with dementia can experience after their diagnosis.

5. There is more to the person than the dementia

This is an extremely important message. Equally, people who are physically disabled might not wish to be defined by their diagnoses. I sometimes feel that medics get totally lost in their own clinical diagnoses, backed up by a history, examination and relevant investigations, and they become focused on treating the diagnosis rather than the person. But once you've met one person living with dementia, you've done exactly that: you've met only one person living with dementia.

Big data

There is growing acknowledgement of the sheer enormity of knowledge which exists for research into dementia, including genetics, image and epidemiology, and there is now a genuine drive for international cooperation in other areas of biomedical research, mostly in infectious and other acute diseases.

An important way to progress will be to build upon ongoing projects and integrate existing resources to establish an International Database for Longitudinal Studies on Aging and Dementia (Alzheimer's Association Expert Advisory Workgroup on NAPA, 2012). Specifically, whole-genome techniques can now potentially be applied in dementia in different settings (diagnosis in patients with symptoms, research, pharmacogenomics, presymptomatic testing and population screening programmes), each of which raises different questions (van El *et al.*, 2013).

Conclusion

There are currently many reasons to be cheerful in England regarding our dementia policy. There has been a spotlight thrown on the dementias arguably like never before, and, credit where credit is due, whatever your own particular inclination, the UK has been instrumental on the world stage in promoting the dementias. It is easy to see, in evaluating critically the last five years in the English dementia policy, the progress that has been made.

The Dementia Friends campaign in England was supposed to target stigma and to encourage a sense of solidarity and citizenship. It is clear that this has been a huge success. It seems sensible to me, therefore, to start with stigma and citizenship in Chapter 2, before I advance my thesis that dementia-friendly communities should promote diversity and reflect legal obligations of equality and human rights.

References

Ahlskog, J.E., Geda, Y.E., Graff-Radford, N.R. and Petersen, R.C. (2011) Physical exercise as a preventive or disease-modifying treatment of dementia and brain aging. Mayo Clinic Proceedings, 86, 9, 876–84.

Albert, M.S., DeKosky, S.T., Dickson, D., Dubois, B. *et al.* (2011) The diagnosis of mild cognitive impairment due to Alzheimer's disease: recommendations from the National Institute on Aging–Alzheimer's Association workgroups on diagnostic guidelines for Alzheimer's disease. Alzheimer's and Dementia, 7, 270–9.

All-Party Parliamentary Group (APPG) on Dementia (2012) Unlocking diagnosis: the key to improving the lives of people with dementia. Available at www.alzheimers.org.uk/site/scripts/download_info.php?fileID=1457 (accessed 6 December 2014).

Alzheimer's Association Expert Advisory Workgroup on NAPA (2012) Workgroup on NAPA's scientific agenda for a national initiative on Alzheimer's disease. Alzheimer's and Dementia, 8, 357–61.

Alzheimer's Society (2012) Five things you should know about dementia. Available at www.alzheimers.org.uk/site/scripts/documents_info.php?documentID=1816 (accessed 30 April 2015).

Bambra, C., Gibson, M., Sowden, A., Wright, K., Whitehead, M. and Petticrew, M. (2010) Tackling the wider social determinants of health and health inequalities: evidence from systematic reviews. Journal of Epidemiology and Community Health, 64, 4, 284–91.

Banerjee, S. (2009) The use of antipsychotic medication for people with dementia: time for action. Available at http://webarchive.nationalarchives.gov.uk/20130107105354/http:/www.dh.gov.uk/en/Publicationsandstatistics/Publications/PublicationsPolicyAndGuidance/DH_108303 (accessed 6 December 2014).

Barberger-Gateau, P., Raffaitin, C., Letenneur, L., Berr, C. *et al.* (2007) Dietary patterns and risk of dementia: the Three-City cohort study. Neurology, 69, 20, 1921–30.

Beydoun, M.A., Beydoun, H.A. and Wang, Y. (2008) Obesity and central obesity as risk factors for incident dementia and its subtypes: a systematic review and meta-analysis. Obesity Reviews, 9, 204–18.

Biessels, G.J. (2014) Capitalising on modifiable risk factors for Alzheimer's disease. Lancet Neurology, 13, 8, 752–3.

Black, S.E., Patterson, C. and Feightner, J. (2001) Preventing dementia. Canadian Journal of Neurology Science, 28, Suppl. 1, S56–66.

Blackburn, D.J., Krishnan, K., Fox, L., Ballard, C. *et al.* (2013) Prevention of Decline in Cognition after Stroke Trial (PODCAST): a study protocol for a factorial randomised controlled trial of intensive versus guideline lowering of blood pressure and lipids. Trials, 14, 401.

Bond, J. (1992) The medicalization of dementia. Journal of Aging Studies, 6, 397–403.

Bowling, A. (2007) Aspirations for old age in the 21st century: what is successful aging? International Journal of Aging and Human Development, 64, 263–97.

Brodaty, H., Howarth, G., Mant, A. and Kurle, S. (1994) General practice and dementia: a national survey of Australian GPs. Medical Journal of Australia, 160, 10–14.

Brunet, M. (2014) Targets for dementia diagnoses will lead to over-diagnosis. British Medical Journal, 348, g2224.

Brunnström, H., Gustafson, L., Passant, U. and Englund, E. (2008) Prevalence of dementia subtypes: a 30-year retrospective survey of neuropathological reports. Archives of Gerontology and Geriatrics, 49, 1, 146–9.

Buchman, A.S., Wilson, R.S., Bienias, J.L., Shah, R.C., Evans, D.A. and Bennett, D.A. (2005) Change in body mass index and risk of incident Alzheimer disease. Neurology, 65, 892–7.

Burns, A. and Robert, P. (2009) The National Dementia Strategy in England. British Medical Journal, 338, b931.

Carruthers, I., Pickup, S., Rippon, A., Hughes, J., Maxwell, P. and Davies, S. (2014) Progress on the Prime Minister's Challenge on Dementia: Year Two. Available at https://s3-eu-west-1.amazonaws.com/media.dh.gov.uk/network/353/files/2014/05/10092-2902335-TSO-Dementia-Letter-to-PM-ACCESSIBLE.pdf (accessed 14 May 2015).

Chang, M., Jonsson, P.V., Snaedal, J., Bjornsson, S. *et al.* (2010) The effect of midlife physical activity on cognitive function among older adults: AGES – Reykjavik study. Journals of Gerontology, Series A, Biological Sciences and Medical Sciences, 65, 12, 1369–74.

Cunningham, E.L. and Passmore, A.P. (2013) Drug development in dementia. Maturitas, 76, 3, 260–6.

Daviglus, M.L., Bell, C.C., Berrettini, W., Bowen, P.E. *et al.* (2010) National Institutes of Health state-of-the-science conference statement: preventing Alzheimer disease and cognitive decline. Annals of Internal Medicine, 153, 3, 176–81.

De Lepeleire, J., Wind, A., Iliffe, S., Moniz-Cook, E. *et al.* (2008) The primary care diagnosis of dementia in Europe: an analysis using multi-disciplinary, multi-national expert groups. Aging and Mental Health, 12, 5, 568–76.

Dementia Action Alliance (DAA) and the NHS Institute for Innovation and Improvement (2012) The Right Prescription: a call to action on the use of antipsychotic drugs for people with dementia. Available at www.institute.nhs.uk/qipp/calls_to_action/Dementia_and_antipsychotic_drugs.html (accessed on 6 December 2014).

Department of Health (2012) Prime Minister's challenge on dementia: delivering major improvements in dementia care and research by 2015. Available at www.gov.uk/government/uploads/system/uploads/attachment_data/file/215101/dh_133176.pdf (accessed 6 December 2014).

Department of Health (2013) Making a Difference in Dementia: Nursing Vision and Strategy. Available at www.gov.uk/government/uploads/system/uploads/attachment_data/file/147956/Making_a_Difference_in_Dementia_Nursing_Vision_and_Strategy.pdf (accessed 6 December 2014).

Desmond, D.W., Tatemichi, T.K., Paik, M. and Stern, Y. (1993) Risk factors for cerebrovascular disease as correlates of cognitive function in a stroke free cohort. Archives of Neurology, 50, 162–6.

Devi, G., Ottman, R., Tang, M., Marder, K. *et al.* (1999) Influence of APOE genotype on familial aggregation of AD in an urban population. Neurology, 53, 789.

Devore, E.E., Grodstein, F., van Rooij, F.J., Hofman, A. *et al.* (2010) Dietary antioxidants and long-term risk of dementia. Archives of Neurology, 67, 7, 819–25.

Downs, M., Turner, S., Iliffe, S., Bryans, M., Wilcock, J. and Keady, J. (2003) Improving the response of primary care practitioners to people with dementia and their families: a randomised controlled trial of educational interventions, Final Report to the UK Alzheimer's Society. Bradford: UK Alzheimer's Society.

EClipSE Collaborative Members, Brayne, C., Ince, P.G., Keage, H.A. *et al.* (2010) Education, the brain and dementia: neuroprotection or compensation? Brain, 133, 8, 2210–16.

Gao, S., Hendrie, H.C., Hall, K.S. and Hui, S. (1998) The relationships between age, sex, and the incidence of dementia and Alzheimer disease: a meta-analysis. Archives of General Psychiatry, 55, 809–15.

Gauthier, S., Leuzy, A., Racine, E. and Rosa-Neto, P. (2013) Diagnosis and management of Alzheimer's disease: past, present and future ethical issues. Progress in Neurobiology, 110, 102–13.

Gustafson, D.R., Backman, K., Waern, M., Ostling, S. *et al.* (2009) Adiposity indicators and dementia over 32 years in Sweden. Neurology, 73, 1559–66.

Haase, H. and Rink, L. (2009) Functional significance of zinc-related signaling pathways in immune cells. Annual Review of Nutrition, 29, 133–52.

Hofman, A., Ott, A., Breteler, M.M., Bots, M.L. *et al.* (1997) Atherosclerosis, apolipoprotein E, and prevalence of dementia and Alzheimer's disease in the Rotterdam Study. Lancet, 349, 151–4.

Holland, W. (2012) Competition or collaboration? A comparison of health services in the UK. Clinical Medicine, 10, 5, 431–3.

Imtiaz, B., Tolppanen, A.M., Kivipelto, M. and Soininen, H. (2014) Future directions in Alzheimer's disease from risk factors to prevention. Biochemical Pharmacology, 88, 4, 661–70.

Innes, A. and Manthorpe, J. (2013) Developing theoretical understandings of dementia and their application to dementia care policy in the UK. Dementia (London), 12, 6, 682–96.

Ionicioiu, I., David, D. and Szamosközi, S. (2014) A quantitative meta-analysis of the effectiveness of psychosocial interventions in dementia. Procedia – Social and Behavioural Sciences, 27, 591–4.

Jenkins, C.R., Thien, F.C.K., Wheatley, J.R. and Reddel, H.K. (2005) Traditional and patient-centred outcomes with three classes of asthma medication. European Respiratory Journal, 26, 1, 36–44.

Johansson, L., Guo, X., Waern, M., Ostling, S. *et al.* (2010) Midlife psychological stress and risk of dementia: a 35-year longitudinal population study. Brain, 133, 8, 2217–24.

Jorm, A.F. and Jolley, D. (1998) The incidence of dementia: a meta-analysis. Neurology, 51, 728–33.

Kehne, J.H. (2007) The CRF1 receptor: a novel target for the treatment of depression, anxiety, and stress-related disorders. CNS and Neurological Disorders – Drug Targets, 6, 163–82.

Khachaturian, Z.S., Petersen, R.C., Snyder, P.J., Khachaturian, A.S. *et al.* (2011) Developing a global strategy to prevent Alzheimer's disease: Leon Thal Symposium 2010. Alzheimer's and Dementia, 7, 2, 127–32.

Kim, J.W., Lee, D.Y., Lee, B.C., Jung, M.H. *et al.* (2012) Alcohol and cognition in the elderly: a review. Psychiatry Investigation, 9, 1, 8–16.

Kivipelto, M., Ngandu, T., Fratiglioni, L., Viitanen, M. *et al.* (2005) Obesity and vascular risk factors at midlife and the risk of dementia and Alzheimer disease. Archives of Neurology, 62, 1556–60.

Kmietowicz, Z. (2012) Cameron launches challenge to end 'national crisis' of poor dementia care. British Medical Journal, 344, e2347.

Kmietowicz, Z. (2014) Recorded diagnosis of dementia in England increases by 62% since 2006. British Medical Journal, 349, g4911.

Koch, T. and Iliffe, S. (2011) Implementing the National Dementia Strategy in England: evaluating innovative practices using a case study methodology. Dementia, 10, 4, 487–98.

Kopelman, P.G. (2000) Obesity as a medical problem. Nature, 404, 635–43.

Lautenschlager, N.T., Cupples, L.A., Rao, V.S., Auerbach, S.A. *et al.* (1996) Risk of dementia among relatives of Alzheimer's disease patients in the MIRAGE study: what is in store for the oldest old? Neurology, 46, 641–50.

Leonard, B.E. (2006) HPA and immune axes in stress: involvement of the serotonergic system. Neuroimmunomodulation, 13, 268–76.

Letter to the Prime Minister charting progress on the Prime Minister's Dementia Challenge (dated 7 May 2014). Available at https://s3-eu-west-1.amazonaws.com/media.dh.gov.uk/network/353/files/2014/05/10092-2902335-TSO-Dementia-Letter-to-PM-ACCESSIBLE.pdf (accessed 6 December 2014).

Lieb, W., Beiser, A.S., Vasan, R.S., Tan, Z.S. *et al.* (2009) Association of plasma leptin levels with incident Alzheimer disease and MRI measures of brain aging. Journal of the American Medical Association, 302, 2565–72.

Ligthart, S.A., Moll van Charante, E.P., van Gool, W.A. and Richard, E. (2010) Treatment of cardio-vascular risk factors to prevent cognitive decline and dementia: a systematic review. Vascular Health and Risk Management, 6, 775–85.

Lincoln, P., Fenton, K., Alessi, C., Prince, M. *et al.* (2014) The Blackfriars Consensus on brain health and dementia. Lancet, 383, 9931, 1805–6.

Lindsay, J., Hébert, R. and Rockwood, K. (1997) The Canadian Study of Health and Aging: risk factors for vascular dementia. Stroke, 28, 526–30.

Lupton, D. (1999) Risk. London: Routledge.

Lyman, K.A. (1989) Bringing the social back in: a critique of the bio-medicalisation of dementia. Gerontologist, 29, 597–604.

Masi, C.M., Chen, H.Y., Hawkley, L.C. and Cacioppo, J.T. (2011) A meta-analysis of interventions to reduce loneliness. Personality and Social Psychology Review, 15, 3, 219–66.

McCullagh, C.D., Craig, D., Mollroy, S.P. and Passmore, A.P. (2001) Risk factors for dementia. Advances in Psychiatric Treatment, 7, 24–31.

McKhann, G.M., Knopman, D.S., Chertkow, H., Hyman, B.T. *et al.* (2011) The diagnosis of dementia due to Alzheimer's disease: recommendations from the National Institute on Aging–Alzheimer's Association workgroups on diagnostic guidelines for Alzheimer's disease. Alzheimer's and Dementia, 7, 263–9.

Milne, A. (2010) Dementia screening and early diagnosis: the case for and against. Health, Risk and Society, 12, 1, 65–76.
Monastero, R., Mangialasche, F., Camarda, C., Ercolani, S. and Camarda, R. (2009) A systematic review of neuropsychiatric symptoms in mild cognitive impairment. Journal of Alzheimer's Disease, 18, 1, 11–30.
Moroney, J.T., Tang, M.X., Berglund, L., Small, S. *et al.* (1999) Low-density lipoprotein cholesterol and the risk of dementia with stroke. Journal of the American Medical Association, 282, 254–60.
Morris, J.C. (2005) Early-stage and preclinical Alzheimer disease. Alzheimer Disease and Associated Disorders, 19, 3, 163–5.
National Audit Office (2007) Improving Services and Support for People with Dementia. London: The Statioeary Office.
Ngandu, T., Helkala, E.L., Soininen, H., Winblad, B. *et al.* (2007a) Alcohol drinking and cognitive functions: findings from the Cardiovascular Risk Factors Aging and Dementia (CAIDE) Study. Dementia and Geriatric Cognitive Disorders, 23, 3, 140–9.
Ngandu, T., von Strauss, E., Helkala, E.L., Winblad, B. *et al.* (2007b) Education and dementia: what lies behind the association? Neurology, 69, 14, 1442–50.
NHS Confederation (2014) A people-centred response to the 2015 Challenge is vital for the future of health and care, says Jeremy Taylor. Available at www.nhsconfed.org/blog/2014/06/a-people-centred-response-to-the-2015-challenge-is-vital-for-the-future-of-health-and-care (accessed 6 December 2014).
Norton, S., Matthews, F.E., Barnes, D.E., Yaffe, K. and Brayne, C. (2014) Potential for primary prevention of Alzheimer's disease: an analysis of population-based data. Lancet Neurology, 13, 8, 788–94.
Panza, F., Frisardi, V., Seripa, D., Logroscino, G. *et al.* (2012) Alcohol consumption in mild cognitive impairment and dementia: harmful or neuroprotective? International Journal of Geriatric Psychiatry, 27, 12, 1218–38.
Peters, R. (2012) Blood pressure, smoking and alcohol use, association with vascular dementia. Experimental Gerontology, 47, 11, 865–72.
Prasad, A.S. (2009) Impact of the discovery of human zinc deficiency on health. Journal of the American College of Nutrition, 28, 257–65.
Public Health England and the UK Health Prevention Forum (2014) The Blackfriars Consensus on promoting brain health: reducing risks for dementia in the population ('Blackfriars Consensus Statement'). Available at http://nhfshare.heartforum.org.uk/RMAssets/Reports/Blackfriars%20consensus%20%20_V18.pdf (accessed 6 December 2014).
Rahman, S. (2014) It's time we talked about 'dementia friendly communities'. Living well with dementia blog, 25 March 2014. Available at http://livingwelldementia.org/2014/03/25/its-time-we-talked-about-dementia-friendly-communities (accessed 6 December 2014).
Redman, R.W. and Lynn, M.R. (2004) Advancing patient-centred care through knowledge development. Canadian Journal of Nursing Research, 36, 3, 116–29.
Ritchie, C.W. and Ritchie, K. (2012) The PREVENT study: a prospective cohort study to identify mid-life biomarkers of late-onset Alzheimer's disease. BMJ Open, 2, 6, e001893.
Rusanen, M., Rovio, S., Ngandu, T., Nissinen, A. *et al.* (2010) Midlife smoking, apolipoprotein E and risk of dementia and Alzheimer's disease: a population-based cardiovascular risk factors, aging and dementia study. Dementia and Geriatric Cognitive Disorders, 30, 3, 277–84.
Sapolsky, R.M. (1996) Why stress is bad for your brain. Science, 273, 749–50.
Scarmeas, N., Stern, Y., Tang, M.X., Mayeux, R. and Luchsinger, J.A. (2006) Mediterranean diet and risk for Alzheimer's disease. Annals of Neurology, 59, 6, 912–21.
Skoog, I., Kalaria, R.N. and Breteler, M.M. (1999) Vascular factors and Alzheimer disease. Alzheimer Disease and Associated Disorders, 13, 3 Suppl., S106–11.

Sofi, F., Valecchi, D., Bacci, D., Abbate, R. *et al.* (2011) Physical activity and risk of cognitive decline: a meta-analysis of prospective studies. Journal of Internal Medicine, 269, 1, 107–17.
Sperling, R.A., Rentz, D.M., Johnson, K.A., Karlawish, J. *et al.* (2014) The A4 study: topping AD before symptoms begin? Science Translational Medicine, 6, 228, 228fs13.
Stern, Y., Gurland, B., Tatemichi, T.K., Tang, M.X., Wilder, D. and Mayeux, R. (1994) Influence of education and occupation on the incidence of Alzheimer's disease. Journal of the American Medical Association, 271, 13, 1004–10.
Szewczyk, B. (2013) Zinc homeostasis and neurodegenerative disorders. Frontiers in Aging Neuroscience, 5, 33.
Tischler, V., D'Silva, K., Cheetham, A., Goring, M. and Calton, T. (2010) Involving patients in research: the challenge of patient-centredness. International Journal of Social Psychiatry, 56, 6, 623–33.
van der Linde, R.M., Stephan, B.C., Matthews, F.E., Brayne, C. and Savva, G.M. (2013) Medical Research Council Cognitive Function and Study. The presence of behavioural and psychological symptoms and progression to dementia in the cognitively impaired older population. International Journal of Geriatric Psychiatry, 28, 7, 700–9.
van Duijn, C.M., Hendriks, L., Cruts, M., Hardy, J.A. and Hofman, A. (1991) Amyloid precursor protein gene mutation in early-onset Alzheimer's disease. Lancet, 337, 8747, 978
van El, C.G., Cornel, M.C., Borry, P., Hastings, R.J. *et al.* (2013) Whole-genome sequencing in health care: recommendations of the European Society of Human Genetics. European Journal of Human Genetics, 21, 6, 580–4.
Vellas, B., Gillette-Guyonnet, S. and Andrieu, S. (2008) Memory health clinics: a first step to prevention. Alzheimer's and Dementia, 4, Suppl. 1, S144–9.
Verity, C.M., Nicoll, A., Will, R.G., Devereux, G. and Stellitano, L. (2000) Variant Creutzfeldt Jakob disease in UK children: a national surveillance study. Lancet, 356, 9237, 1224–7.
Vileland, T. (2002) Managing chronic disease: evidence-based medicine or patient-centred medicine? Health Care Analysis, 10, 3, 289–98.
Wang, H.X., Gustafson, D.R., Kivipelto, M., Pedersen, N.L. *et al.* (2012) Education halves the risk of dementia due to apolipoprotein ε4 allele: a collaborative study from the Swedish brain power initiative. Neurobiology of Aging, 33, 5, 1007.e1–7.
Warren, M.W., Hynan, L.S. and Weiner, M.F. (2012) Lipids and adipokines as risk factors for Alzheimer's disease. Journal of Alzheimer's Disease, 29, 151–7.
Wise, J. (2014) £90m package to improve dementia care is announced in England. British Medical Journal, 348, g1879.
World Health Organization (2012) Variant Creutzfeldt-Jakob disease: factsheet no. 180. Available at www.who.int/mediacentre/factsheets/fs180/en (accessed 6 December 2014).
World Health Organization (2013) Social Determinants of Health: The Solid Facts (R. Wilkinson and M. Marmot, eds). Available at www.euro.who.int/__data/assets/pdf_file/0005/98438/e81384.pdf (accessed 6 December 2014).
Zecca, L., Youdim, M.B., Riederer, P., Connor, J.R. and Crichton, R.R. (2004) Iron, brain ageing and neurodegenerative disorders. Nature Reviews Neuroscience, 5, 863–73.

Chapter 2

STIGMA, CITIZENSHIP AND LIVING BETTER WITH DEMENTIA

> Last scene of all,
> That ends this strange eventful history,
> Is second childishness and mere oblivion,
> Sans teeth, sans eyes, sans taste, sans everything.
>
> William Shakespeare, *As You Like It*, Act 2, Scene 7

Introduction

Persons living well with dementia have sometimes described themselves as 'objects' of their illness, rather than active 'participants' in it (Cottrell and Schulz, 1993). The current global drive towards a 'cure' has left many people currently trying to live well with dementia in a rather disenfranchised way. The reaction of civil servants and the media has been to construct the slogan 'Care for today, but cure for tomorrow', but the racking up of the 'horrors' of dementia in the media rests very uneasily with people living with dementia, and all carers, in the current media drive. The variance between the scare tactics and the living well narrative has been disarming at the very least.

The word 'stigma' is defined as 'a mark of disgrace associated with a particular circumstance, quality or person' (*Oxford English Dictionary*). People living with dementia do not wish to feel 'stigmatised' or 'disgraced', and yet this can be exactly the consequence of many mainstream reports. This might be intended or unintended. The mainstream media are clearly critical in 'framing the narrative', and their raising awareness of dementia, including headlines referring to 'dementia sufferers', is a source of unpleasant cognitive dissonance.

Stigma, discrimination and prejudice

Some time ago, Professor Simon Wessely, current President of the Royal College of Psychiatrists, in discussion of Norman Sartorius who had championed a global campaign by the World Psychiatric Association to reduce the stigma associated with schizophrenia, observed that dementia, whilst having been 'a once neglected subject', is 'now at the cutting edge of research and investment' (Wessely, 2005, p.196).

We all tend to use 'shortcuts' in our thinking (or, as they tend to be called in the decision-making literature, 'heuristics'). Healthcare professionals use diagnostic labels to classify individuals for both treatment and research purposes. Despite their clear benefits in summarising a lot of information quickly, it is now increasingly being acknowledged that diagnostic labels also serve as cues that can activate stigma and stereotypes (Garand *et al.*, 2009).

In the *World Alzheimer Report: Overcoming the Stigma of Dementia*, Batsch and Mittelman (2012) argued that identifying stigma is crucial because stigma often prevents affected individuals from acknowledging their symptoms and seeking the assistance they need for the best possible quality of life, because they feel embarrassed or incompetent. Such attitudes are likely to be deeply entrenched, and it is a remarkable feature of this report that such issues are explained succinctly. How stigma in society might have changed with time is indeed interesting. Although Figure 2.1 is an oversimplification – for example, it does not refer to any preventative interventions for dementia – it does highlight the progress that has been made.

In Goffman's (1963) seminal work, the term *stigma* is used to refer to 'an attribute that is deeply discrediting within a social interaction' (p.13). Individuals possessing such an attribute are different from others in ways that are shameful and undesirable. The stigmatised individual is reduced 'from a whole and usual person to a tainted, discounted one' (Goffman, 1963, p.12). Stigmas are typically the attributes that, when observed by a majority group member, may lead to labelling, stereotyping, social separation, loss of status, and discrimination (see, for example, Link and Phelan, 2001).

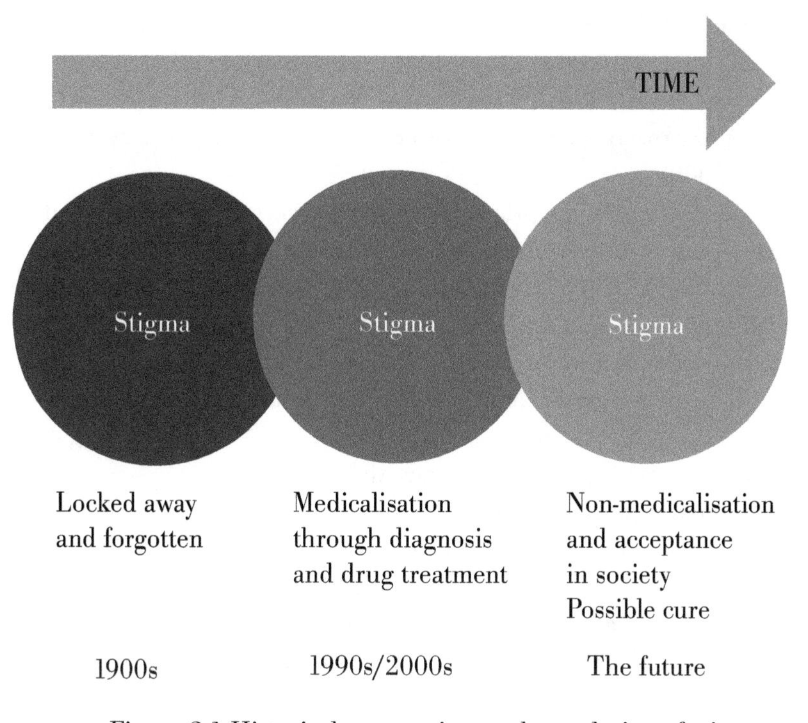

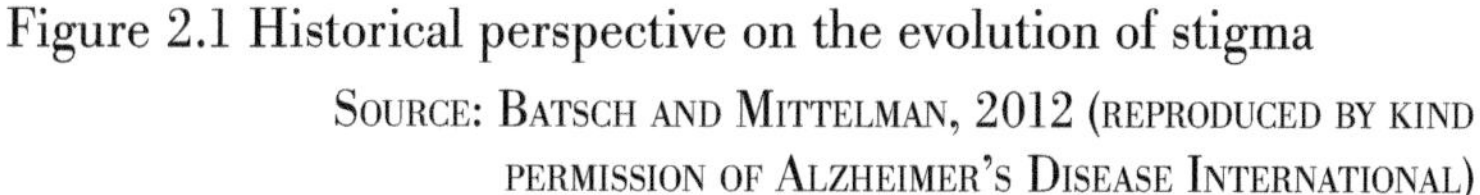

Figure 2.1 Historical perspective on the evolution of stigma

Source: Batsch and Mittelman, 2012 (reproduced by kind permission of Alzheimer's Disease International)

Labelling and stereotyping involve the recognition of differences and the assignment of social salience to those differences. In the context of illness, labelling is the recognition that a person with a particular diagnosis differs from the norm in ways that have social significance. Stereotyping is the assignment of negative attributions to these socially salient differences (i.e. the perception that the differences are undesirable). Separation occurs when the reactions of others to these differences lead to a pronounced sense of 'otherness' (i.e. the individual's personal awareness that others are treating him or her differently due to some personal attribute) (Green *et al.*, 2005).

Prejudice refers to emotional reactions to a stereotyped person, and discrimination refers to behaviours that are associated with prejudice, including avoidance, coercion and segregation. Discrimination means any distinction, exclusion or preference that has the effect of nullifying or impairing equal enjoyment of rights (World Health Organization, 2002). Status loss and discrimination occur when stigma interferes with an individual's ability to participate fully in the networks of his or her community. In these circumstances of 'enacted stigma', there is most likely a power differential favouring those without the trait over those who have it (Green *et al.*, 2005). Age discrimination is an additional factor since dementia is often an illness of later life, and that age discrimination accentuates the role of stigma; this has been called 'double jeopardy' (Benbow and Reynolds, 2000).

In addition to public stigma, people with certain diagnostic labels may also experience an internalisation of the stereotypes held by the general public (Corrigan, 2007). This internalisation may deter individuals from seeking treatment and social services, even when the opportunities are available, simply to avoid the stigma associated with that label. Indeed, initial evidence already suggests that the stigma of dementia has been associated with delays in or lack of accurate diagnosis and treatment, potentially negatively impacting on disease progression and management (Koch and Iliffe, 2010).

Burgener and colleagues (2013) reported on perceived stigma in persons with dementia. The authors observed that social rejection was associated with anxiety, behavioural symptoms, health and activity participation. Internalised shame was associated with anxiety, personal control, health, self-esteem, social support understanding and assistance, and activity participation. The stigma tends 'to spread from the stigmatized individual to his close connexions' (Goffman, 1963, p.43), in parallel with the concept of 'discrimination by association' to be found in various legal jurisdictions. Furthermore, individuals may choose not to seek professional help as a means of protecting themselves from yet further perceived embarrassment and feelings of inferiority or incompetence (Nadler, 1990). Secondary stigma influences how staff working in dementia services are undervalued in comparison with staff working in other areas of health and social care. This is evidenced by work showing that the social workforce is less qualified and less likely to be working towards any qualifications (Hussein and Manthorpe, 2011). Phillipson and colleagues (2011) presented results from a comprehensive study to explore stigma towards dementia in Australia. Through an online survey, they found that people with dementia were not expected to have meaningful conversation (50.8%) and can have poor personal hygiene (14.3%).

Framing the narrative

Stigma and the media are, of course, intensely interrelated.

Negative public images, stereotypes and terms associated with dementia can all potentially lead to stigmatisation. Fear linked to dementia encourages a reluctance by some members of the public to engage with those who have a dementia, and so the messages from the media and the large charities carry with them a huge burden of responsibility. It is important to note that the terrifying accounts are not just confined to newspaper headlines with the words 'timebomb', 'explosion' and 'flood'. However, self-identity in older persons 'suffering from dementia' and how the narrative is framed inevitably takes on a new significance (Cohen-Mansfield, Golander and Arnheim, 2000).

Caddell and Clare (2010), in a meticulous examination of personhood in 33 papers obtained using their selection criteria, identified that various qualitative approaches have been employed in various ways to investigate the self in dementia, but the majority of these studies suggest that the self is being preserved in people with dementia, although some studies highlight the losses that may be experienced. Personhood is a remarkably interesting field, and I introduced the impact of Kitwood's work first in Chapter 6 of my book *Living Well with Dementia* (Rahman, 2014). It will be interesting to pursue, as English policy progresses, the extent to which enthusiasts about personhood share the same enthusiasm for person-centred care.

As Hannah Zeilig (2014, p.259) observes, 'cultural metaphors' for dementia pervade a number of formats of the media, including film, TV and political speeches: 'Metaphors, then, are not simply a device of our language. They also influence the way in which we perceive our worlds and therefore the way we explain and live in them.'

Works such as Sontag's *Illness as Metaphor* (1978) are not simply an intellectual curiosity. The various metaphors help to frame the narrative, and, indeed, potentially bias the public perception of dementia. It is claimed (e.g. Lane, McLachlan and Philip, 2013) that the use of military metaphor to describe illness dates back to at least the seventeenth century when John Donne described his illness as 'a cannon shot' and 'a siege'. That military metaphors in framing the narrative can cause more damage than good has become very apparent, though, in the contemporary academic press.

It is now acknowledged that the military metaphors suggest a sense of 'urgency', even suggesting that, societally, at best we have been slow to understand the immediate 'threat' or at worst 'complacent' in doing something about it. The 'fighting approach' does suggest 'a call to action', and the fact that 'Fight Alzheimer's: Save Australia' is the tagline of Alzheimer's Australia (2014) necessitates the question as to what the action should be. Lane and colleagues (2013, p.282) – helpfully – raise the notion that the fighting metaphor may be a failure of expectation management: 'Additionally, fighting metaphors may leave some individuals feeling they have "lost" as the disease progresses, an unnecessary burden for someone facing illness and disability.'

The prevalence of dementias is described in such dramatic terms as an 'epidemic' and a 'crisis' (Mandell and Green, 2011). There is a strange cognitive dissonance in the use of the word 'epidemic'; indeed, recent evidence from the Medical Research Council Cognitive Function and Ageing Study (MRC CFAS) suggests that later-born populations in England have a lower risk of prevalent dementia than those born earlier in the past century (Matthews *et al.*, 2013). The word 'dementia' is often used interchangeably with Alzheimer's disease, which still comprises one of the most common causes of dementia worldwide and is the most well-known condition. The construct itself of 'Alzheimer's disease' has been well explored (George, Whitehouse and Ballenger, 2011).

'Framing the narrative' as a concept originated in the field of social psychology (Bartlett, 1932). In communication science, framing in its broadest sense refers to the manner in which the media and the public decide to represent a particular topic or issue (Reese, 2001). The analysis of Van Gorp and Vercruysse (2012) produces examples of framing which will be familiar to many people who have been reading about dementia in the popular press or perusing public Twitter accounts on dementia. One of the common narratives is of dementia as a 'travelling companion', 'whom you meet out of the blue and who accompanies you to the end of your journey' (Van Gorp and Vercruysse, 2012, p.1277). According to Van Gorp and Vercruysse (2012), dementia is a meeting at an unpredictable moment, a meeting that you somehow have to learn to deal with, but dementia can cross the path of anyone.

Framing has thus become a powerful way for social movements to mobilise their ideas (Benford and Snow, 2000). As reviewed by Benford and Snow (2000), the concept of frame as used in the study of social movements is derived primarily from the work of Goffman (1974).

'Suffering'

There are in fact about a hundred different types of dementia, not all of which present predominantly with significant memory problems. Some can present in a 'hidden' way, much like any disability. Some persons with dementia have marked changes in behaviour and personality (with normal cognition). There has been active debate about the extent to which medical intervention can ever 'eliminate' suffering (George *et al.*, 2011).

In experimental psychology, suffering and pleasure are respectively the negative and positive effects, or hedonic tones or valences, that psychologists often identify as basic in our emotional lives. The evolutionary role of physical and mental suffering, through natural selection, is considered to be quite primitive in nature: it warns of threats, motivates coping (fight or flight, escape), and reinforces negatively certain behaviours (punishment). The brain areas involved in someone's perception of suffering using this reductionist approach might be identifiable. Shany-Ur and colleagues (2014) have recently thrown some light on the neural substrates underlying self-awareness in neurological disease in their paper published in the journal *Brain*. Whilst not a paper on how much persons with dementia feel they suffer per se, the paper does identify the brain areas which might be implicated in overestimating or underestimating one's performance in cognitive tasks, which possibly might be related to one's awareness of one's own symptoms.

But who's to say that what you measure in a brain scanner is the same as a person's perception of suffering? And if the disease process alters the parts of the brain involved in the perception of suffering, have such individuals lost an ability to perceive suffering?

Campaigning for social change: Dementia Alliance International

The finding that not all people living with dementia perceive the experience as a 'negative one' has attracted much interest recently. For example, Wendy Hulko recently commented:

> ...practitioners should not operate from the assumption that dementia is universally experienced as negative and be cautious about treating dementia as a problem if, by all indications, it is not problematic for the person who is living with it on a daily basis. (Hulko, 2009, p.140)

As summarised by Tom Kitwood (1997, p.8), personhood is a 'standing or status that is bestowed upon one human being, by others, in the context of relationship and social being. It implies recognition, respect and trust.' In a highly influential article a decade later, Ruth Bartlett and Deborah O'Connor (2007) proposed something very significant. They argued that personhood is essentially an apolitical concept concerned with psychosocial issues and therefore it may be too limiting, whereas the notion of citizenship can be used in cognate disciplines to promote the status of discriminated groups of people still further, to that of people with power entitled to the same from life as everyone else.

Bartlett and O'Connor (2007) provide a very useful analysis comparing personhood and modern citizenship across a number of different attributes, including conferment of status, position of self and level of entitlement. From their analysis, there are clearly important distinctions.

And yet the shift in emphasis to a person with rights – such as the right to a fair trial or the right to privacy – is highly significant in political terms, and takes the narrative from simply 'involving' people with dementia. The narrative therefore undergoes a frame shift from a 'person *with dementia*, to *person* with dementia' (Kitwood, 1997, p.7). Interestingly, Bartlett and O'Connor (2007) argue that, because personhood is essentially an apolitical concept primarily concerned with psychological and health matters such as love, morality, spirituality and wellbeing, it does not really provide the language for discussing people's situation in terms of power (as opposed to psychosocial) relations. The issue of who holds the power in the social movement then becomes a critical one. In the analysis by Behuniak (2010), it is conceded that power is a complex term that encompasses multiple definitions and perspectives, and yet its dominant formulation has been that of forcefulness and how this is used over individuals.

Behuniak goes on to cite that power as a force has been characterised as influence (French and Raven, 1959), as effectiveness (Josefowitz, 1980) and as acceptance of authority (Barnard, 1938).

The really important question therefore is: How can people living with dementia lead? A really important steer for this came from the Joseph Rowntree Foundation in a report by Toby Williamson called 'A stronger collective voice for people with dementia' (Williamson, 2012). The Dementia Engagement and Empowerment Project (DEEP) aimed to explore, support, promote and celebrate groups and projects led by or actively involving people with dementia across the UK that were influencing services and policies, and affecting the lives of people with dementia.

Ruth Bartlett found that keeping a diary has the potential to be used much more widely in patients living with dementia (2011). In her opinion, the main advantage of this method is that, unlike interviews, the diarist, rather than the researcher, is ultimately in control of how and when data are collected. Bartlett argues that diaries encourage participants to record thoughts and feelings as and when they occur and wherever they feel most comfortable; the diary therefore has the potential to compensate for short-term memory problems associated with dementia, plus it could help to minimise 'respondent burden' traditionally associated with interview-based studies involving people with dementia (Cottrell and Schulz, 1993).

Dementia Alliance International (DAI) is the first global group for people with dementia where membership is comprised exclusively of people with dementia. DAI was established in January 2014 to promote education and awareness about dementia, in order to eradicate stigma and discrimination, and to improve the quality of the lives of people with dementia. DAI advocates for the voice and needs of people with dementia, and provides a global forum, 'aiming to unite all people with dementia around the world to stand up and speak out' (Dementia Alliance International, 2014, p.1).

The internet now offers incredible opportunities for organising social movements that would be too large or too difficult for a single person to undertake. In typical crowdsourcing applications, large numbers of people add to the global value of content, measurements or solutions by individually making small contributions. Such a system can succeed if it attracts a large enough group of motivated participants, such as Wikipedia, Flickr and YouTube. Friendsourcing attempts to synthesise social information in a social context: it is the 'use of motivations and incentives over a user's social network to collect information or produce a desired outcome, using as a guide what members of the network themselves consider to be important' (Bernstein *et al.*, 2010, p.2).

Batsch and Mittelman (2012), in their Alzheimer's Disease International World Alzheimer Report called *Overcoming the Stigma of Dementia*, remark that local regulations and education have a role to play in tackling discrimination. Beard and colleagues (2009) had previously offered practical suggestions for concrete help including environmental adaptations and cognitive aids. The intriguing aspect now is that even the narrative of 'involvement' is being reframed. This was indeed warned about by Beresford (2002) who suggested service-user involvement has emerged out of two different rationales for participation – one consumerist, the other democratic. The former claims that greater efficiency, efficacy and effectiveness will result from appropriately placed service-user feedback mechanisms. The democratic approach, often framed in a rights discourse, views user participation as a form of self-advocacy. The history of mental health activism can be dated far further back, to 1620, when inmates at the Bedlam asylum petitioned for their rights (Weinstein, 2010). That the DAI finds itself attracting the attention of large charities, Big Pharma and social enterprises promoting living well with dementia is not altogether surprising therefore, even despite its relatively young existence.

Conclusion

Persons living well with dementia and their friends and family cannot tell whether they are going to be the imminent beneficiaries of global initiatives to reduce stigma, prejudice and discrimination. In the alternative, they have unwittingly found themselves as bit parts following someone else's script.

In reality, people living with dementia are not simply defined by the label 'dementia'. A person with dementia might be Asian, might be bisexual, or might have had prior intellectual difficulties – or all three. Stigma in relation to dementia tends to be studied in the complete absence of the rest of the make-up of a person, and this underlying assumption has very rarely been mentioned by so-called 'experts' in stigma.

Chapter 3 looks at the diversity of people trying to live better with dementia.

References

Alzheimer's Australia (2014) Fight Alzheimer's: Save Australia. Available at www.fightdementia.org.au (accessed 6 December 2014).

Barnard, C. (1938) The Functions of the Executive. Cambridge, MA: Harvard University Press.

Bartlett, F.C. (1932) Remembering: A Study in Experimental and Social Psychology. Cambridge: Cambridge University Press.

Bartlett, R. (2011) Realities Toolkit #18: using diaries in research with people with dementia. Available at www.socialsciences.manchester.ac.uk/medialibrary/morgancentre/toolkits/18-toolkit-using-diaries.pdf (accessed 6 December 2014).

Bartlett, R. and O'Connor, D.O. (2007) From personhood to citizenship: broadening the lens for dementia practice and research. Journal of Aging Studies, 21, 107–18.

Batsch, N.L. and Mittelman, M. (2012) World Alzheimer Report: Overcoming the Stigma of Dementia. Executive Summary. London: Alzheimer's Disease International. Available at https://www.alz.co.uk/research/WorldAlzheimerReport2012.pdf (accessed 22 May 2015).

Beard, R.L., Knauss, J. and Moyer, D. (2009) Managing disability and enjoying life: how we reframe dementia through personal narratives. Journal of Aging Studies, 23, 227–35.

Behuniak, S.M. (2010) Toward a political model of dementia: power as compassionate care. Journal of Aging Studies, 24, 231–40.

Benbow, S.M. and Reynolds, D. (2000) Challenging the stigma of Alzheimer's disease. Hospital Medicine, 61, 174–7.

Benford, R.D. and Snow, D.A. (2000) Framing processes and social movements: an overview and assessment. Annual Review of Sociology, 26, 611–39.

Beresford, P. (2002) User involvement in research and evaluation: liberation or regulation? Social Policy and Society, 1, 2, 95–105.

Bernstein, M.S., Tan, D., Smith, G., Czerwinski, M. and Horvitz, E. (2010) Personalization via friendsourcing. Transactions on Computer Human Interaction, 17, 2, 6.

Burgener, S.C., Buckwalter, K., Perkhounkova, Y. and Liu, M.F. (2013) The effects of perceived stigma on quality of life outcomes in persons with early-stage dementia: longitudinal findings: Part 2. Dementia (London) [Epub ahead of print].

Caddell, L.S. and Clare, L. (2010) The impact of dementia on self and identity: a systematic review. Clinical Psychology Review, 30, 113–26.

Cohen-Mansfield, J., Golander, H. and Arnheim, G. (2000) Self-identity in older persons suffering from dementia: preliminary results. Social Science and Medicine, 51, 381–94.

Corrigan, P.W. (2007) How clinical diagnosis might exacerbate the stigma of mental illness. Social Work, 52, 31–9.

Cottrell, V. and Schulz, R. (1993) The perspective of the patient with Alzheimer's disease: a neglected dimension of dementia research. Gerontologist, 33, 2, 205–11.

Dementia Alliance International (2014) Introducing Dementia Alliance International (DAI). Available at www.dementiaallianceinternational.org/wp-content/uploads/2014/03/DAI-Newsletter-01_2014.pdf (accessed 6 December 2014).
French, J. and Raven, B. (1959) The Basis of Social Power. In D. Cartwright (ed.) Studies in Social Power. Ann Arbor, MI: Institute of Social Research.
Garand, L., Lingler, J.H., Conner, K.O. and Dew, M.A. (2009) Diagnostic labels, stigma, and participation in research related to dementia and mild cognitive impairment. Research in Gerontological Nursing, 2, 2, 112–21.
George, D.R., Whitehouse, P.J. and Ballenger, J. (2011) The evolving classification of dementia: placing the DSM-V in a meaningful historical and cultural context and pondering the future of 'Alzheimer's'. Culture, Medicine, and Psychiatry, 35, 3, 417–35.
Goffman, E. (1963) Stigma: Notes on the Management of Spoiled Identity. Englewood Cliffs, NJ: Prentice Hall.
Goffman, E. (1974) Frame Analysis: An Essay on the Organisation of the Experience. New York, NY: Harper Colophon.
Green, S., Davis, C., Karshmer, E., Marsh, P. and Straight, B. (2005) Living stigma: the impact of labeling, stereotyping, separation, status loss, and discrimination in the lives of individuals with disabilities and their families. Sociological Inquiry, 75, 197–215.
Hulko, W. (2009) From 'not a big deal' to 'hellish': experiences of older people with dementia. Journal of Aging Studies, 23, 131–44.
Hussein, S. and Manthorpe, J. (2011) The dementia social care workforce in England: secondary analysis of a national workforce dataset. Aging and Mental Health, 16, 1, 110–18.
Josefowitz, N. (1980) Paths to Power. Reading, MA: Addison-Wesley.
Kitwood, T. (1997) Dementia Reconsidered: The Person Comes First. Buckingham: Open University Press.
Koch, T. and Iliffe, S. (2010) Rapid appraisal of barriers to the diagnosis and management of patients with dementia in primary care: a systematic review. BMC Family Practice, 11, 1–8.
Lane, H.P., McLachlan, S. and Philip, J. (2013) Commentary: the war against dementia: are we battle weary yet? Age and Ageing, 42, 3, 281–3.
Link, B.G. and Phelan, J.C. (2001) Conceptualizing stigma. Annual Review of Sociology, 27, 363–85.
Mandell, A.M. and Green, R.C. (2011) Alzheimer's Disease. In A.E. Budson and N.W. Kowall (eds) The Handbook of Alzheimer's Disease and Other Dementias. Chichester: Wiley-Blackwell.
Matthews, F.E., Arthur, A., Barnes, L.E., Bond, J. *et al.* (Medical Research Council Cognitive Function and Ageing Collaboration) (2013) A two-decade comparison of prevalence of dementia in individuals aged 65 years and older from three geographical areas of England: results of the Cognitive Function and Ageing Study I and II. Lancet, 26, 382, 9902, 1405–12.
Nadler, A. (1990) Help-Seeking Behavior: Psychological Costs and Instrumental Benefits. In M.S. Clark (ed.) Prosocial Behavior: Review of Personality and Social Psychology, Vol. 12. Thousand Oaks, CA: Sage.
Phillipson, L., Magee, C., Jones, S.C., Reis, S. and Skladzien, E. (2011) Dementia, stigma and intentions to help-seek: a pilot study of Australian adults 40 to 65 years, 14th National Conference, Alzheimer's Australia.
Rahman, S. (2014) Living Well with Dementia: The Importance of the Person and the Environment for Wellbeing. Oxford: Radcliffe Health.
Reese, S.D. (2001) Introduction. In S.D. Reese, O.H. Gandy and A.E. Grant (eds) Framing Public Life: Perspectives on Media and Our Understanding of the Social World. Mahwah, NJ: Erlbaum.
Shany-Ur, T., Lin, N., Rosen, H.J., Sollberger, M., Miller, B.L. and Rankin, K.P. (2014) Self awareness in neurodegenerative disease relies on neural structures mediating reward driven attention. Brain [Epub ahead of print].

Sontag, S. (1978) Illness as Metaphor. New York, NY: Farrar, Straus and Giroux.

Van Gorp, B. and Vercruysse, T. (2012) Frames and counter-frames giving meaning to dementia: a framing analysis of media content. Social Science and Medicine, 74, 8, 1274–81.

Weinstein, J. (ed.) (2010) Mental Health, Service User Involvement and Recovery. London: Jessica Kingsley Publishers.

Wessely, S. (2005) Book: Sartorius on Stigma. Lancet, 366, 196.

Williamson, T. (2012) A stronger collective voice for people with dementia. Available at www.jrf.org.uk/publications/stronger-collective-voice (accessed 6 December 2014).

World Health Organization (2002) Reducing stigma and discrimination against older people with mental disorders: a technical consensus statement. WHO/MSD/MBD/02.3. Available at http://whqlibdoc.who.int/hq/2002/WHO_MSD_MBD_02.3.pdf (accessed 5 February 2015).

Zeilig, H. (2014) Dementia as a cultural metaphor. Gerontologist, 54, 2, 258–67.

Chapter 3

CULTURE AND DIVERSITY IN LIVING BETTER WITH DEMENTIA

'A nation's culture resides in the hearts and in the soul of its people.'

Mahatma Gandhi (1869–1948)

Introduction

Culture and diversity are crucial components in understanding the context of people trying to live better with dementia. Adverse perspectives can unfortunately include stigma and prejudice (see Chapter 2). Culture depends on our interconnectedness as persons, and we all have different backgrounds. Fundamentally, personhood will be heavily influenced by the social setting. (I gave a detailed account of personhood in Chapter 6 of my first book, *Living Well with Dementia* (Rahman, 2014).) This chapter will look at various communities, including black, Asian and minority ethnic (BAME) communities, lesbian, gay, bisexual and transgender (LGBT) communities, and persons with intellectual difficulties. The analysis overall tends to make simplifying assumptions in order to make it manageable, but it is germane to the entire reason of why it is important for all persons to be included in service provision and research. For any topic in service provision, local culture has a huge effect.

Two trends in contemporary Europe are the subject of widespread discussion – and often anxiety. The first is the increasing diversity of our population, and the second is the ageing of that population. Anxieties about diversity are frequently framed as a cultural threat to Europe's identity or way of life, while anxieties about an ageing population are more regularly framed in economic terms, or about the viability of Europe's economic model in an increasingly competitive world (Lievesley/Runnymede Centre for Policy on Ageing, 2010). Professor Alistair Burns and colleagues (2010) have observed transcultural influences in dementia care in the form of a psychosocial interventional study. Differences in carers' attitudes have also been reported. Clearly, more research is needed for wellbeing (Day and Francisco, 2013).

Caruana has attempted to document the core characteristics of effective healing programmes that have applicability across the range of different programmes identified in these searches (Wanganeen, 2008). There, arguably, should be a holistic and multi-disciplinary approach that addresses mental, physical, emotional and spiritual needs through a focus on familial and community interconnectedness as well as connections to the environment and the spiritual realm (see, for example, Aboriginal and Torres Strait Islander Healing Foundation Development Team, 2009). A large number of longitudinal studies of population-based ageing cohorts are in progress internationally, but the insights from these studies into the risk and protective factors for cognitive ageing and conditions such as mild cognitive impairment and dementia have been inconsistent.

Some of the problems confounding this research can be reduced by harmonising and pooling data across studies. COSMIC (Cohort Studies of Memory in an International Consortium) aims to harmonise data from international cohort studies of cognitive ageing, in order to better understand the determinants of cognitive ageing and neurocognitive disorders. Longitudinal studies of cognitive ageing and dementia with at least 500 individuals aged 60 years or over are eligible and invited to be members of COSMIC (Sachdev *et al.*, 2013). COSMIC may in time identify risk and protective factors and biomarkers of cognitive ageing and dementia in diverse ethnic and sociocultural groups.

Race is sometimes taken as a proxy for culture, but currently data indicate that not all African Americans share the same cultural beliefs to the same extent (Rovner, Casten and Harris, 2013). After exploring how the term 'diversity' is used, it could be proposed that an organisation that successfully promotes diversity will take account of age, disability, gender, sexual orientation, social class, religion and faith and 'race' issues (Butt, 2006).

Diversity, furthermore, has become an important focus in commissioning for dementia services. A recent commissioning pack makes it clear that specific attention should be given to disadvantaged groups to ensure equality of access and that services are sensitive and appropriate to particular needs. In relation to dementia, groups who require particular attention include:

- people with learning disabilities
- people with early-onset dementia
- people from BAME communities
- carers.

Each specification in the commissioning pack asks that, at a local level, commissioners consider specific issues of equality of access that are relevant to their community (Department of Health, 2011). This chapter will provide a basic overview of the diagnosis and post-diagnosis groups of people in three categories: BAME, LGBT and intellectual difficulties.

BAME

Introduction to BAME communities

It is interesting first to consider the international picture. Dementia is under-diagnosed to a greater extent among ethnic minorities in the age group 60 years and older, but is over-diagnosed in the age group younger than 60 years. Several factors may contribute to this pattern, including cultural differences in help-seeking behaviour and problems in navigating the healthcare system. From linking the Danish hospital registers with the Danish Civil Registration System, it is now believed that dementia is under-diagnosed and under-treated to a greater extent among ethnic minorities than in the native population (Nielsen *et al.*, 2011).

Ethnic minorities make up approximately 8% of the overall population in the UK. Out of that number, approximately 11% of the Asian, 15% of the black and 3% of the Chinese populations were between 60 and 74 years of age (Evandrou, 2000). Dementia tends to be misunderstood and highly stigmatised in many UK BAME communities. There are now organisations that have developed good practice in working with BAME communities, but there needs to be a more developed structure to share the learning from good practice (Truswell, 2013). The number of people with dementia from BAME groups is expected to rise significantly as the BAME population ages: the number is expected to grow to nearly 50,000 by 2026 and to more than 172,000 people by 2051 (All-Party

Parliamentary Group on Dementia, 2013). There are increasing indications that the prevalence of dementia in black African-Caribbean and South Asian UK populations is greater than the white UK population, and that the age of onset is lower for black African-Caribbean groups than the white UK population (Truswell, 2013; Turner *et al.*, 2012). Since these groups are also more likely to experience high blood pressure, it is suggested that the increased risk of vascular dementia contributes to increased prevalence (Bhattacharyya, Benbow and Kar, 2012).

It is thought that 6.1% of all people with dementia among BAME groups have early-onset dementia, compared with only 2.2% for the UK population as a whole, reflecting the younger age profile of BAME communities (Dementia UK, 2007). South Asian and black African-Caribbean populations represent the largest ethnic minority groups in the UK, yet the evidence on dementia care in these communities is profoundly limited (Milne and Chryssanthopoulou, 2005). A study by Knapp and Prince (2007) also suggests that although BAME communities tend to have a relatively young age profile at present, this will change as a consequence of immigration patterns in the latter part of the twentieth century, leading to significantly higher numbers of members from these communities with dementia. Furthermore, it is warned that mental health services are not well equipped to meet the needs of BAME elders and their families (Lievesley, 2010). African-Caribbean and South Asian communities represent the largest BAME communities in the UK, and yet the evidence base regarding dementia care in these communities is, surprisingly, limited. People from BAME communities comprise 15% of the English population and 39% of the London population (National Audit Office, 2007). The majority of BAME people live in London, the Midlands and the North West of England. Most BAME people with dementia have African-Caribbean and South Asian backgrounds because these are the BAME communities with the highest proportion of older people. Numbers of older people from black, Asian and minority ethnic groups are increasing rapidly in the UK, but more epidemiological research is required to clarify dementia prevalence and risk among black, Asian and minority ethnic groups.

Although they access primary care at a similar rate to the indigenous population, people from BAME communities are less likely to access mental health services (Livingston *et al.*, 2001). The available evidence suggests that people from BAME groups have higher rates of psychiatric admissions than the general population. Research also suggests that people from BAME groups stay in hospital for longer and have a higher tendency than the general population to be secluded (Department of Health, 2011).

The All-Party Parliamentary Group on Dementia and BAME diversity

In December 2012 the All-Party Parliamentary Group (APPG) on Dementia, led by Baroness Sally Greengross, announced that it would undertake an inquiry into services and support for people living with dementia in the UK within minority ethnic groups.

In particular, the APPG considered the following questions:

» What are the factors, if any, which stop people from BAME communities seeking early help/intervention and/or getting a diagnosis? How can these factors be overcome?

» How can we improve diagnostic tools and the diagnostic experience for people from BAME communities?

» How do BAME individuals and families experience living with dementia?

» What services might BAME individuals and families be looking for?

» What are the best ways to reach BAME communities?

» What challenges might be encountered when developing and providing tailored services to people with dementia from minority groups? How can these be overcome?

» Which organisations and individuals, at local and national level, are best placed to lead this work?

The APPG made a series of recommendations, which are summarised in Box 3.1.

Box 3.1 Recommendations of the All-Party Parliamentary Group on Dementia

Recommendation 1: Raise awareness

Recommendation 2: Undertake preventative work and tackle modifiable risk factors

Recommendation 3: Ensure local areas are aware of the need to support people with dementia from BAME groups in their communities

Recommendation 4: Share good practice in commissioning and support

Recommendation 5: Improve access to high-quality services for people with dementia from BAME communities

Recommendation 6: Alzheimer's Society programmes

Recommendation 7: Improve staff knowledge and skills

Source: All-Party Parliamentary Group on Dementia, 2013 (pp.12–14) (reproduced by kind permission of the Secretariat of the All-Party Group on Dementia for the UK parliament)

Attitudes

Low *et al.* (2010) conducted a study to investigate recognition, attitudes and causal beliefs regarding dementia in Italian, Greek and Chinese Australians in comparison with third-generation Australians. Third-generation participants (85%) were more likely to recognise dementia symptoms in a vignette in comparison with Italian (61%), Greek (58%) and Chinese (72%) participants. Overall, the racial and ethnic minority groups had more negative attitudes about persons with dementia.

Different communities may have differing views and attitudes about whether they wish these services to be culturally specific or mixed (Moriarty, Sharif and Robinson, 2011). In the past, organisations responsible for planning and delivering services have reported that they know very little about the numbers of BAME people with dementia in their area. The most recent Carers' Strategy guidance identifies a need for services to reach out to carers from BAME communities and to develop information and advice services that are accessible to all carers (HM Government, 2010).

Delays in diagnosis

Cultural and social differences may be a barrier for some ethnic communities accessing health and social care services, such as the stigma or lack of understanding of mental health problems. There is, for example, no word for dementia in five South Asian languages.

People of South Asian origin in the United Kingdom may recognise symptoms associated with dementia but not conceptualise these as part of an illness even when they are severe (Department of Health, 2011).

Some research shows that African Americans and Hispanics experience longer delays in dementia diagnosis than do 'whites'. Findings from Schrauf and

Iris (2011) suggest that long pathways have been marked by a shift away from diagnosis-seeking behaviour (44.5%) towards the family's taking over of key daily tasks (55.5%). The authors suggest that Hispanic and African American carers effectively provide some sort of 'scaffolding' for the patient. Furthermore, the normalisation of symptoms as 'just old-age' (Krull, 2005) coupled with the under-diagnosis of the disease (Valcour, Masaki and Curb, 2000) may well leave many individuals who in fact have dementia of the Alzheimer type (but no diagnosis) under the research radar. The number of people from ethnic minorities with dementia, and their proportion of the population as a whole, is set to rise sharply with the ageing of ethnic minority populations (Department of Health, 2009).

Cognitive tests developed in one ethnic group may not be appropriate for use in another ethnic group because they are influenced by a range of factors including culture, education, language, literacy skills, numeracy skills and sensory impairments. There is a need to develop instruments which account for the influence of these factors. In a multi-centre study, the 10/66 Dementia Research Group interviewed 2885 people aged 60 years and older in 25 centres, mostly universities, in India, China and South East Asia, Latin America and the Caribbean, and Africa. Their algorithm is a sound basis for culturally and educationally sensitive dementia diagnosis in clinical and population-based research, supported by translations of its constituent measures into most languages used in the developing world (Prince, 2009; Prince *et al.*, 2003).

The arguments on cost savings from early diagnosis of dementia used by Banerjee and Wittenberg (2009) for the general population can be applied to the economic case for targeting information and resources to support early diagnosis and intervention in dementia for BAME communities.

Do some ethnic groups have an earlier age of onset?

In a study by Adelman and colleagues (2011), a total of 218 people of African-Caribbean country of birth and 218 white UK-born people aged ≥ 60 years were recruited from five general practices in North London; those who screened positive for cognitive impairment using a culturally valid instrument were offered a standardised diagnostic interview. These authors found that there is an increased prevalence of dementia in older people of African-Caribbean country of birth in the UK and at younger ages than in the indigenous white population (Adelman *et al.*, 2011).

Cultural diversity in caregiving

The experience of giving and receiving care usually occurs in the context of a long-standing relationship which predates the onset of dementia and continues to evolve as the illness progresses (Ablitt, Jones and Muers, 2009). Evidence from the literature continues to highlight that a number of carers from BAME communities had culturally based perceptions of dementia (Johl, Patterson and Pearson, 2014). In an exhaustive review of racial, ethnic and cultural differences in dementia caregiving, a number of useful observations have been made. For example, it is suggested that black carers were more likely to be an adult child, friend or other family member; white carers were more likely to be a spouse; and white carers were more likely to be married, older, more highly educated and to report higher incomes than black carers (O'Connell and Gibson, 1997).

A wide range of symptoms led carers to seek help from healthcare services. These included early symptoms of dementia of the Alzheimer type such as forgetfulness, as well as later neuropsychiatric symptoms such as wandering, aggression or paranoia. In some studies, carers cited critical events that led to the realisation that there was a problem and hence to seeking help. Examples given included chronic and acute disorientation to time and place (Hispanic Latino carers; Neary and Mahoney, 2005), 'crisis point' being reached (British South Asian carers; Lawrence *et al.*, 2008) and noticing 'behavioural changes' (Asian American carers; Zhan, 2004). Mukadam, Cooper and Livingston (2011) conducted a systematic review of qualitative and quantitative studies that explored pathways to dementia specialist care in minority ethnic groups, and found that there are significant barriers to help seeking for dementia in minority ethnic groups.

Research on dementia caregiving is guided largely by the Stress and Coping Model of Lazarus and Folkman (1984) or its topical counterpart, the Carer Stress Process Model developed by Pearlin and colleagues (1990). Race/ethnicity is often included as a control variable in these models, but this unidimensional measure does not adequately reflect or explain the role of ethnic or cultural values in the caregiving process (Knight *et al.*, 2000). Robert W. Schrauf and Madelyn Iris (2011) suggest that Hispanic and African American carers effectively provide a kind of 'scaffolding' for the patient, which may in fact be adaptive rather than dysfunctional. In 2003, a review found about half of older people met the criteria for dementia without GP awareness or dementia documentation in their medical record (Boustani *et al.*, 2003). The issue of late diagnosis is particularly true for people from culturally and linguistically diverse (CALD) backgrounds. It is well documented that this group of older people often presents to health professionals at a much later stage to seek help for diagnosis, and when family and the person with dementia do present for assistance, it is often in 'crisis mode' (Cheng *et al.*, 2009).

However, even when diagnosis is made, access to medications and health care by people from CALD backgrounds is also limited (Cooper *et al.*, 2010).

Limited research is available on access to Cognitive Dementia and Memory Services (CDAMS) for people with dementia from CALD communities. A recent systematic review indicated that little research is currently available on dementia service use among people from CALD backgrounds (Cooper *et al.*, 2010).

A very helpful study was conducted to determine the barriers and enablers to accessing CDAMS for people with dementia and their families of Chinese and Vietnamese backgrounds (Haralambous *et al.*, 2014). Consultations with community members, community workers and health professionals were conducted using the 'Cultural Exchange Model' framework.

An important element of the model was action research which covered planning, taking action, evaluation and reflection (Andrews *et al.*, 2009). For carers, barriers to accessing services included the complexity of the health system, lack of time, travel required to get to services, language barriers, interpreters and lack of knowledge of services. Similarly, community workers and health professionals identified language, interpreters and community perceptions as key barriers to service access.

Asian communities

One of the most consistent observations is a relative lack of knowledge and understanding of dementia in the Asian community. Such individuals are not reported as conceptualising the illness as an organic disease or treatable illness. Asian languages do not have an equivalent word for dementia. There is an almost universal negative perception of dementia; in its early stages, it is often regarded as a 'normal' part of ageing. This perception, coupled with the lack of knowledge about treatment and services, acts as a powerful barrier to both users and carers seeking support. An excellent review of these issues is provided by the Meri Yaadai Dementia Team (2010). Asian people place great emphasis on the importance of being self-sufficient, portraying an image of wellbeing, and 'hiding' mental health problems.

A further helpful overview is provided by Seabrooke and Milne (2004). A lack of willingness amongst many Asian persons and their families to acknowledge dementia, coupled with the perceived pressures of the average GP workload, undermines the facilitation of early diagnosis. Additionally, there are often language problems, and standard 'tests' may not be culturally appropriate. Specific barriers to service usage amongst Asians have been reported to include lack of knowledge about dementia and services, cultural differences, communication and language difficulties, fear of breach of confidentiality and stigma. South Asian persons with dementia are under-represented in UK health and social care services (Cooper *et al.*, 2010). Despite this, vascular dementia is more common in the UK among Asian and black African-Caribbean people than the majority white population (Richards *et al.*, 2000). One explanation for this is the higher rate of cardio-risk factors for diabetes (Ahtiluoto *et al.*, 2010) and hypertension (Oveisgharan and Hachinski, 2010) in these cultural groups.

Another contribution has been a report of a study to explore perceptions of ageing, dementia and ageing-associated mental health difficulties amongst British people of Punjabi Indian origin (La Fontaine *et al.*, 2007). Among the Punjabi-speaking older Sikh community, where there is a particular stigma attached to the disease, this leads to isolation among people living with dementia and puts additional strain on families. A groundbreaking West Yorkshire scheme to turn Sikh 'gurdwaras' (temples) into dementia-friendly spaces, making them the first port of call for support, has attracted interest from across the country, with considerable positive media coverage (Lambert, 2014).

LGBT communities living well with dementia

The experiences of gay and lesbian people in health and social care contexts and the ways in which they navigate the disclosure of their sexuality to service providers has only recently begun to attract research attention (Cant and Taket, 2007). The transition from living at home to moving into residential care may be particularly challenging for older people from the LGBT community. Older people from this community are fearful of the attitudes and potential prejudice of staff, other residents and their family. Some older people choose not to disclose their sexuality within the home, which has a detrimental effect on their wellbeing and quality of life (Department of Health, 2011). Sensitive and individually tailored transmission of information to patients and carers is recommended as a moral and legal obligation (Koch and Iliffe, 2010; Werner, Karnieli-Miller and Eidelman, 2013). Back in November 2013, the Dementia Engagement and Empowerment Project (DEEP) held a meeting to generate ideas and knowledge to ensure that there are LGBT voices within DEEP (Innovations in Dementia, 2014). The meeting was hosted by Sue Westwood, and speakers included trainer and consultant Sally Knocker and Liz Price from Hull University.

Recent findings suggest a lack of information and continued support following a diagnosis (Stokes, Combes and Stokes, 2014). The experiences of gay men and lesbian women at the health and social care interface have been characterised by homophobia (irrational fear of, or aversion to, gay or lesbian people) and heterosexism (the heterocentric assumption that all people are heterosexual and that heterosexuality is the only permissible sexuality) (Rose and Platzer, 1993). Indeed, previous research has indicated that many carer support groups are implicitly limited to a heterosexual framework (Moore, 2002). Further evidence suggests that a diagnosis does not always help the person and their family to understand and make sense of their experiences (Paton *et al.*, 2004). Difficulty understanding the condition may be linked to the finding that many dementia carers find it difficult to access quality information pre- and post-diagnosis (Chenoweth and Spencer, 1986). Carers report only limited explanations of the meaning or consequences of the condition (Aneshensel *et al.*, 1995). Apart from the expressed desire for more psychological support, one-third of the respondents also highlighted the need for more organised social activities for older lesbians, gays, bisexuals and transgendered people (Cantor, Brennan and Shippy, 2004).

Sally Knocker (2012) reports having had opportunities to bring her into contact 'with hundreds of older gay people, including facilitating workshops for individuals contemplating "coming out", being the first lesbian Carers' Contact for the Alzheimer's Society, and working as a volunteer with London Lesbian and Gay Switchboard' (Knocker, 2012, p.3).

Elizabeth Price (2010) reports on findings from a qualitative study, undertaken in England, that explored the experiences of 21 gay men and lesbian women who care, or cared, for a person with dementia. The results demonstrate the ways in which carers mediated disclosures of their sexualities to health and social care service providers and, for some, their wider support network. For older gay and lesbian people, the prospect of requiring health and social care services causes increasingly well-documented anxiety (Hubbard and Rossington, 1995). A critical issue for respondents in the study from Brotman and colleagues (2007), for example, was the fear of having to come out to service providers or, worse, of having to forcibly return to the closet.

Most social care services such as day centres have LGBT older people among their users, but they are often 'invisible' (Manthorpe and Moriarty, 2014). King and colleagues (2008) have recommended routine inclusion of sexual orientation in data collection. This is because there is often no attempt to distinguish care services for this group from those of heterosexual people or to investigate access and experiences. However, LGBT users and carers may not wish to expose themselves to possible negative reactions by asserting themselves and appearing to be different (Price, 2008).

Persons with intellectual difficulties diagnosed with a dementia

For an excellent introduction to intellectual disability and dementia, please refer to *Intellectual Disability and Dementia* by Karen Watchman (2014). In this text, recognised experts from the UK, Ireland, Canada, Australia and Holland discuss good practice and the way forward in relation to assessment, diagnosis, interventions, staff knowledge and training, care pathways, service design, measuring outcomes and the experiences of individuals, families and carers.

In recent years, policy and practice have focused on supporting people with intellectual disabilities to live in community settings rather than large institutions (Department of Health, 1992). There have been significant improvements in the mean life expectancy of people with intellectual disabilities from as little as an estimated 18.5 years in the 1930s to 59 years in the 1970s to 66 years in the 1990s (Braddock, 1999). The life expectancy of those with a more severe level of disability, however, remains reduced compared with the general population, as does the mean life expectancy of people with Down's syndrome, which has been estimated at 55 years (Holland *et al.*, 2000). Prevalence rates for dementia in people with learning disabilities are at least twice as high as in the general population (Patel, Goldberg and Moss, 1993). People with Down's syndrome are at particular risk of developing dementia (Hutchinson, 1999). As life expectancy increases for people with learning disabilities, the impact of dementia on people with learning disabilities and their families, carers and services is becoming more apparent. Psychological services for learning disabilities are receiving an increasing number of referrals requesting dementia assessment (Kirk, Hick and Laraway, 2006).

Risk factors regarding the development of dementia in people living with Down's syndrome have been reviewed by Bush and Beail (2004). Diagnosis of dementia in people with learning disabilities can be complex (Wilkinson and Janicki, 2002). Evidence is needed of progressive deterioration in an individual's level of functioning (Aylward *et al.*, 1997) and such deterioration can be difficult to detect in people with learning disabilities. But a strong focus in service provision must actively seek out ways of improving wellbeing for persons with intellectual disabilities who develop dementia. Sunny Kalsy-Lillico (2014) has helpfully reviewed the psychosocial models of dementia, and summarised a cogent framework for psychosocial interventions in this field, including behaviour-oriented, emotion-oriented, cognition-oriented and stimulation-oriented. There has also been a renewed focus in enabling persons with intellectual disabilities and dementia to live well at home in a community, with supportive housemates and family (Udell, 2014). These recent developments draw into sharp focus the potential strengths of a tailored approach of dementia-friendly communities, celebrating diversity.

It can be hard to obtain an accurate baseline or measure of change in cognitive functioning. As long ago as 2001, good practice guidance from the Foundation for People with Learning Disabilities (Turk, Dodd and Christmas, 2001) recommended that every service for people with learning disabilities should set up a register of adults with Down's syndrome, conduct a baseline assessment of cognitive and adaptive functioning before the age of 30 years, develop specialist skills in this area, offer training to other professionals, front-line staff and carers, and seek high-quality coordination between agencies. Despite this, the availability of screening and treatment across the UK is inequitable. Janicki and Dalton (1999) referred to a person with a learning disability and dementia remaining in their own home environment, with adaptations, after a diagnosis of dementia as 'ageing in place'. This refers to a move to, or creation of, a dementia-specific environment for people with an intellectual disability. More than 80% of people with Down's syndrome and dementia develop seizures (Lai and Williams, 1989). Older people with Down's syndrome (over 45 years) are more likely to have seizures than younger people. Those authors argue that, within the policy and practice context of aiming to support residents to 'age in place', support for staff in care home settings is a crucial aspect of ensuring that such an approach is effective and provides a coordinated approach to planning, resourcing and support (Wilkinson, Kerr and Cunningham, 2005).

Conclusion

It is evident that not only do we need to identify sources of diversity in communities, but we need to be able to characterise their main features. This is essential so that health and social care systems, in all jurisdictions, are able to tailor diagnostic and post-diagnostic processes accordingly. This 'one glove does not fit all' is no simple ask, especially when you consider that there are countless countries with different aims of strategy, different demands and, most significantly, differing extents of comprehensiveness and universality in provision of care and support for living better with dementia. Notwithstanding that, there is a lot more that unites us than divides us in the global policy. It is also abundantly clear that nation states benefit from national dementia policies. Chapter 4 hopes to provide an overview of the global picture for dementia, with particular focus on promoting living better with dementia.

References

Ablitt, A., Jones, G.V. and Muers, J. (2009) Living with dementia: a systematic review of the influence of relationship factors. Aging and Mental Health, 13, 4, 497–511.

Aboriginal and Torres Strait Islander Healing Foundation Development Team (2009) Voices from the Campfires: Establishing the Aboriginal and Torres Strait Islander Healing Foundation. Canberra, Australia: Department of Families, Housing, Community Services and Indigenous Affairs.

Adelman, S., Blanchard, M., Rait, G., Leavey, G. and Livingston, G. (2011) Prevalence of dementia in African Caribbean compared with UK-born white older people: two-stage cross-sectional study. British Journal of Psychiatry, 199, 2, 119–25.

Ahtiluoto, S., Polvikoski, T., Peltonen, M., Solomon, A. *et al.* (2010) Diabetes, Alzheimer disease, and vascular dementia: a population-based neuropathologic study. Neurology, 75, 13, 1195–202.

All-Party Parliamentary Group on Dementia (2013) Dementia does not discriminate: the experiences of black, Asian and minority ethnic communities. Available at www.alzheimers.org.uk/site/scripts/download.php?fileID=1857 (accessed 6 December 2014).

Andrews, S., Robinson, A., Churchill, B., Haines, T. *et al.* (2009) Facilitating best practice falls prevention through an action research approach. Paper presented at the 42nd National Conference of the Australian Association of Gerontology, Canberra, Australia.

Aneshensel, C., Pearlin, L.I., Mullan, J.T., Zarit, S.H. and Whitlatch, C.J. (1995) Profiles in Caregiving: The Unexpected Career. San Diego, CA: Academic Press.

Aylward, E.H., Burt, D.B., Thorpe, L.U., Lai, F. and Dalton, A. (1997) Diagnosis of dementia in individuals with intellectual disability. Journal of Intellectual Disability Research, 41, 2, 152–64.

Banerjee, S. and Wittenberg, R. (2009) Clinical and cost effectiveness of services for early diagnosis and intervention in dementia. Available at http://ec.europa.eu/health/ph_information/dissemination/diseases/docs/dementia_cost_en.pdf (accessed 6 December 2014).

Bhattacharyya, S., Benbow, S.M. and Kar, N. (2012) Unmet service needs of ethnic elders with dementia in United Kingdom. Indian Journal of Gerontology, 26, 1, 242–58.

Boustani, M., Peterson, B., Hanson, L., Harris, R. and Lohr, K.N. (2003) Screening for dementia in primary care: a summary of the evidence for the U.S. Preventive Services Task Force. Annals of Internal Medicine, 138, 927–37.

Braddock, D. (1999) Ageing and developmental disabilities: demographic and policy issues affecting American families. Mental Retardation, 37, 155–61.

Brotman, S., Ryan, B., Collins, S., Chamberland, L. *et al.* (2007) Coming out to care: caregivers of gay and lesbian seniors in Canada. Gerontologist, 47, 4, 490–503.

Burns, A., Mittelman, M., Cole, C., Morris, J. *et al.* (2010) Transcultural influences in dementia care: observations from a psychosocial intervention study. Dementia and Geriatric Cognitive Disorders, 30, 5, 417–23.

Bush, A. and Beail, N. (2004) Risk factors for dementia in people with Down's syndrome: issues in assessment and diagnosis. American Journal on Mental Retardation, 109, 83–97.

Butt, J. (2006) Are we there yet? Identifying the characteristics of social care organisations that successfully promote diversity. Social Care Institute for Excellence Race Equality Discussion Paper. Bristol: SCIE.

Cant, B. and Taket, A. (2007) Lesbian and gay experiences of primary care in one borough in North London, UK. Diversity in Health and Social Care, 4, 271–9.

Cantor, M., Brennan, M. and Shippy, A. (2004) Caregiving among Older Lesbian, Gay, Bisexual, and Transgender New Yorkers. New York, NY: National Gay and Lesbian Task Force Policy Institute.

Cheng, A., Cruysmans, B., Draper, B., Hayward-Wright, N. *et al.* (2009) Report on Strategic Directions in CALD Dementia Research in Australia. Sydney: Dementia Collaborative Research Centres, University of New South Wales.

Chenoweth, B. and Spencer, B. (1986) Dementia: the experience of family caregivers. Gerontologist, 26, 267–72.

Cooper, C., Tandy, A.R., Balamurali, T.B. and Livingston, G. (2010) A systematic review and meta-analysis of ethnic differences in use of dementia treatment, care, and research. American Journal of Geriatric Psychiatry, 18, 193–203.

Day, A. and Francisco, A. (2013) Social and emotional wellbeing in indigenous Australians: identifying promising interventions. Australian and New Zealand Journal of Public Health, 37, 4, 350–5.

Dementia UK (2007) A report into the prevalence and cost of dementia prepared by the Personal Social Services Research Unit (PSSRU) at the London School of Economics and the Institute of Psychiatry at King's College London, for the Alzheimer's Society.

Department of Health (1992) Guidelines for Health Services for People with Learning Disabilities. London: Department of Health.

Department of Health (2009) Equality Impact Assessment: Living Well with Dementia National Dementia Strategy. Available at www.gov.uk/government/publications/living-well-with-dementia-a-national-dementia-strategy (accessed 6 December 2014).

Department of Health (2011) National Dementia Strategy: Equalities Action plan. Available at www.gov.uk/government/uploads/system/uploads/attachment_data/file/215522/dh_128525.pdf (accessed 6 December 2014).

Evandrou, M. (2000) Social inequalities in later life: the socio-economic position of older people from ethnic minority groups in Britain. Population Trends, 101, 32–9.

Haralambous, B., Dow, B., Tinney, J., Lin, X. *et al.* (2014) Help seeking in older Asian people with dementia in Melbourne: using the Cultural Exchange Model to explore barriers and enablers. Journal of Cross-Cultural Gerontology, 29, 1, 69–86.

HM Government (2010) Recognised, valued and supported: next steps for the Carers' Strategy. London: The Stationery Office. Available at www.gov.uk/government/uploads/system/uploads/attachment_data/file/213804/dh_122393.pdf (accessed 6 December 2014).

Holland, A.J., Hon, J., Huppert, F.A. and Stevens, F. (2000) Incidence and course of dementia in people with Down's syndrome: findings from a population-based study. Journal of Intellectual Disability Research, 44, 138–46.

Hubbard, R. and Rossington, J. (1995) As We Grow Older: A Study of the Housing and Support Needs of Older Lesbians and Gay Men. London: Polari Housing Association.

Hutchinson, N. (1999) Association between Down's syndrome and Alzheimer's disease: a review of the literature. Journal of Learning Disabilities for Nursing, Health and Social Care, 3, 4, 194–203.

Innovations in Dementia (2014) February 2014, Newsletter No. 71. Available at www.innovationsindementia.org.uk/Newletter/InnovationsInDementia_BrainWaves_February2014.pdf (accessed 5 February 2014).

Janicki, M.P. and Dalton, A. (eds) (1999) Dementia, Aging and Intellectual Disabilities: A Handbook. Philadelphia, PA: Brunner/Mazel.

Johl, N., Patterson, T. and Pearson, L. (2014) What do we know about the attitudes, experiences and needs of black and minority ethnic carers of people with dementia in the United Kingdom? A systematic review of empirical research findings. Dementia (London), pii: 1471301214534424 [Epub ahead of print].

Kalsy-Lillico, S. (2014) Living Life with Dementia: Enhancing Psychological Wellbeing. In K. Watchman (ed.) Intellectual Disability and Dementia: Research into Practice. London: Jessica Kingsley Publishers.

King, M., Semlyen, J., Tai, S.S., Killaspy, H. *et al.* (2008) A systematic review of mental disorder, suicide, and deliberate self harm in lesbian, gay and bisexual people. BMC Psychiatry, 8, 70.

Kirk, L.J., Hick, R. and Laraway, A. (2006) Assessing dementia in people with learning disabilities: the relationship between two screening measures. Journal of Intellectual Disabilities, 10, 4, 357–64.

Knapp, M. and Prince, M. (2007) Dementia UK (A Report to the Alzheimer's Society on the Prevalence and Economic Cost of Dementia in the UK Produced by King's College London and London School of Economics). London: Alzheimer's Society.

Knight, B.G., Silverstein, M., McCallum, T.J. and Fox, L.S. (2000) A sociocultural stress and coping model for mental health outcomes among African American caregivers in southern California. Journals of Gerontology Series B: Psychological Sciences and Social Sciences, 55, 3, 142–50.

Knocker, S. (2012) Perspectives on ageing: lesbians, gay men and bisexuals. York: Joseph Rowntree Foundation. Available at www.jrf.org.uk/sites/files/jrf/ageing-lesbians-bisexuals-gay-men-summary.pdf (accessed 16 February 2015).

Koch, T. and Iliffe, S. (2010) Rapid appraisal of barriers to the diagnosis and management of patients with dementia in primary care: a systematic review. BMC Family Practice, 11, 54–9.

Krull, A.C. (2005) First signs and normalizations: caregiver routes to the diagnosis of Alzheimer's disease. Journal of Aging Studies, 19, 407–17.

La Fontaine, J., Ahuja, J., Bradbury, N.M., Phillips, S. and Oyebode, J.R. (2007) Understanding dementia amongst people in minority ethnic and cultural groups. Journal of Advanced Nursing, 60, 6, 605–14.

Lai, F. and Williams, R.S. (1989) A prospective study of Alzheimer's disease in Down's syndrome. Archives of Neurology, 46, 849–53.

Lambert, A. (2014) Sikh temple shows how to become dementia-friendly, The Telegraph, 5 May 2014. Available at www.telegraph.co.uk/health/10808058/Sikh-temple-shows-how-to-become-dementia-friendly.html (accessed 6 December 2014).

Lawrence, V., Murray, J., Samsi, K. and Banerjee, S. (2008) Attitudes and support needs of black Caribbean, South Asian and white British carers of people with dementia in the UK. British Journal of Psychiatry, 193, 3, 240–6.

Lazarus, R.S. and Folkman, S. (1984) Stress, Appraisal, and Coping. New York, NY: Springer.

Lievesley, N. (2010) The Future Ageing of the Ethnic Minority Population of England and Wales. London: Runnymede Trust.

Lievesley, N./Runnymede Centre for Policy on Ageing (2010) Older BME People and Financial Inclusion Report: The Future Ageing of the Ethnic Minority Population of England and Wales. London: Runnymede. Available at www.runnymedetrust.org/uploads/publications/pdfs/TheFutureAgeingOfTheEthnicMinorityPopulation-ForWebJuly2010.pdf (accessed 6 December 2014).

Livingston, G., Leavey, G., Kitchen, G., Manela, M., Sembhi, S. and Katona, C. (2001) Mental health of migrant elders – the Islington study. British Journal of Psychiatry, 179, 361–6.

Low, L.F., Anstey, K.J., Lackersteen, S.M., Camit, M. *et al.* (2010) Recognition, attitudes and causal beliefs regarding dementia in Italian, Greek and Chinese Australians. Dementia and Geriatric Cognitive Disorders, 30, 6, 499–508.

Manthorpe, J. and Moriarty, J. (2014) Examining day centre provision for older people in the UK using the Equality Act 2010: findings of a scoping review. Health and Social Care in the Community, 22, 4, 352–60.

Meri Yaadai Dementia Team (2010) Caring for Dementia: exploring good practice on supporting South Asian carers through access to culturally competent service provision. Available at www.meriyaadain.co.uk/pdfs/publications/Dementiaguide2011ENGLISH19may11.pdf (accessed 6 December 2014).

Milne, A. and Chryssanthopoulou, C. (2005) Dementia care-giving in black and Asian populations: reviewing and refining the research agenda. Journal of Community and Applied Social Psychology, 15, 5, 319–37.

Moore, W.R. (2002) Lesbian and gay elders: connecting care providers through a telephone support group. Journal of Gay and Lesbian Social Services, 14, 3, 23–41.

Moriarty, J., Sharif, N. and Robinson, J. (2011) SCIE Research Briefing 35: black and minority ethnic people with dementia and their access to support and services. Available at www.scie.org.uk/publications/briefings/briefing35 (accessed 6 December 2014).

Mukadam, N., Cooper, C. and Livingston, G. (2011) A systematic review of ethnicity and pathways to care in dementia. International Journal of Geriatric Psychiatry, 26, 1, 12–20.

National Audit Office (2007) Improving Services and Support for People with Dementia. London: The Stationery Office.

Neary, S.R. and Mahoney, D.F. (2005) Dementia caregiving: the experiences of Hispanic/Latino caregivers. Journal of Transcultural Nursing, 16, 2, 163–70.

Nielsen, T.R., Vogel, A., Phung, T.K., Gade, A. and Waldemar, G. (2011) Over- and under-diagnosis of dementia in ethnic minorities: a nationwide register-based study. International Journal of Geriatric Psychiatry, 26, 11, 1128–35.

O'Connell, C.M. and Gibson, G.D. (1997) Racial, ethnic, and cultural differences in dementia caregiving: review and analysis. Gerontologist, 37, 3, 355–64.

Oveisgharan, S. and Hachinski, V. (2010) Hypertension, executive dysfunction, and progression to dementia: the Canadian study of health and aging. Archives of Neurology, 67, 187–92.

Patel, P., Goldberg, D. and Moss, S. (1993) Psychiatric morbidity in older people with moderate and severe learning disability. II: the prevalence study. British Journal of Psychiatry, 163, 481–91.

Paton, J., Johnson, K., Katona, C. and Livingston, G. (2004) What causes problems in Alzheimer's disease: attributions by caregivers. A qualitative study. International Journal of Geriatric Psychiatry, 19, 527–32.

Pearlin, L.I., Mullan, J.T., Semple, S.J. and Skaff, M.M. (1990) Caregiving and stress process: an overview of concepts and their measures. Gerontologist, 30, 5, 583–94.

Price, E. (2008) Pride or prejudice? Gay men, lesbians and dementia. British Journal of Social Work, 38, 1337–52.

Price, E. (2010) Coming out to care: gay and lesbian carers' experiences of dementia services. Health and Social Care in the Community, 18, 2, 160–8.

Prince, M. (2009) The 10/66 Dementia Research Group – 10 years on. Indian Journal of Psychiatry, 51, Suppl. 1, S8–15.

Prince, M., Acosta, D., Chiu, H., Scazufca, M. and Varghese, M. (2003) 10/66 Dementia Research Group. Dementia diagnosis in developing countries: a cross-cultural validation study. Lancet, 361, 9361, 909–17.

Rahman, S. (2014) Living Well with Dementia: The Importance of the Person and the Environment for Wellbeing. Oxford: Radcliffe Health.

Richards, M., Brayne, C., Dening, T., Abas, M. *et al.* (2000) Cognitive function in UK community-dwelling African Caribbean and white elders: a pilot study. International Journal of Geriatric Psychiatry, 15, 7, 621–30.

Rose, P. and Platzer, H. (1993) Confronting prejudice. Nursing Times, 89, 31, 52–4.

Rovner, B.W., Casten, R.J. and Harris, L.F. (2013) Cultural diversity and views on Alzheimer disease in older African Americans. Alzheimer Disease and Associated Disorders, 27, 2, 133–7.

Sachdev, P.S., Lipnicki, D.M., Kochan, N.A., Crawford, J.D. et al. (Cohort Studies of Memory in an International Consortium) (2013) An international consortium to identify risk and protective factors and biomarkers of cognitive ageing and dementia in diverse ethnic and sociocultural groups. BMC Neurology, 13, 165.

Schrauf, R.W. and Iris, M. (2011) A direct comparison of popular models of normal memory loss and Alzheimer's disease in samples of African Americans, Mexican Americans, and refugees and immigrants from the former Soviet Union. Journal of the American Geriatrics Society, 59, 4, 628–36.

Seabrooke, B. and Milne, A. (2004) Culture and Care in Dementia: A Study of the Asian Community in North West Kent. Northfleet, Kent: Alzheimer's and Dementia Support Services. Available at www.mentalhealth.org.uk/content/assets/PDF/publications/culture_care_dementia.pdf (accessed 5 February 2015).

Stokes, L.A., Combes, H. and Stokes, G. (2014) Understanding the dementia diagnosis: the impact on the caregiving experience. Dementia (London), 13, 1, 59–78.

Truswell, D. (2013) Black and Minority Ethnic Communities and Dementia: Where Are We Now? (Race Equality Foundation Briefing Paper 30). Available at www.raceequalityfoundation.org.uk/resources/downloads/black-and-minority-ethnic-communities-and-dementia-where-are-we-now (accessed 6 December 2014).

Turk, V., Dodd, K. and Christmas, M. (2001) Down's Syndrome and Dementia: Briefing for Commissioners. London: Foundation for People with Learning Disabilities.

Turner, D., Salway, S., Chowbey, P. and Mir, G. (2012) Mini case study book: real world examples of using evidence to improve health services for minority ethnic people. Sheffield: Sheffield Hallam University/Centre for Health and Social Care Research. Available at http://clahrc-sy.nihr.ac.uk/images/health%20inequalities/resources/EEiC_mini_case_study_book.pdf (accessed 10 February 2015).

Udell, L. (2014) Belief in a Place Called Home: Reflections on Twenty Years of Dementia Specific Service Provision. In K. Watchman (ed.) Intellectual Disability and Dementia: Research into Practice. London: Jessica Kingsley Publishers.

Valcour, V.G., Masaki, K.H. and Curb, J.D. (2000) The detection of dementia in the primary care setting. Archives of Internal Medicine, 160, 2964–8.

Wanganeen, R. (2008) Grief and Loss. In A. Day, M. Nakata and K. Howells (eds) Indigenous Men and Anger: Understanding and Responding to Violence. Annandale, Australia: Federation Press.

Watchman, K. (2014) Intellectual Disability and Dementia: Research into Practice. London: Jessica Kingsley Publishers.

Werner, P., Karnieli-Miller, O. and Eidelman, S. (2013) Current knowledge and future directions about the disclosure of dementia: a systematic review of the first decade of the 21st century. Alzheimer's and Dementia, 9, 2, e74–88.

Wilkinson, H. and Janicki, M.P. (Edinburgh Working Group on Dementia Care Practices) (2002) The Edinburgh Principles with accompanying guidelines and recommendations. Journal of Intellectual Disability Research, 46, 3, 279–84.

Wilkinson, H., Kerr, D. and Cunningham, H. (2005) Equipping staff to support people with an intellectual disability and dementia in care home settings. Dementia: The International Journal of Social Research, 4, 3, 387–400.

Zhan, L. (2004) Caring for family members with Alzheimer's disease: perspectives from Chinese American caregivers. Journal of Gerontological Nursing, 30, 8, 19–29.

Chapter 4

GLOBAL STRATEGIES FOR LIVING BETTER WITH DEMENTIA

'The world is a book, and those who do not travel read only a page.'

St Augustine of Hippo (354–430)

Introduction

Fox and Petersen (2013, p.1969) remarked, concerning the G8 Dementia Summit, 'The G8 Dementia Summit needs to be the beginning rather than the end of the conversation.' But the enthusiasm to include people living with dementia in that conversation has been mindblowingly disappointing. And the narrative sadly has continued to be dominated by Pharma. Heller and Heller (2013) observe that a more detailed reading of a National Institute for Health and Care Excellence (NICE) (2001) report on donepezil, a cholinesterase inhibitor, and associated commentaries might be necessary for us to gain a balanced view of the effectiveness of these new medications and to put the claims of the drug manufacturers into perspective.

A perfectly reasonable hope, of course, is that future projections of numbers of people with dementia may be modified substantially by preventive interventions (lowering incidence), improvements in treatment and care (prolonging survival) and disease-modifying interventions (preventing or slowing progression). All countries need to commission nationally representative surveys that are repeated regularly to monitor trends (Prince *et al.*, 2013). Likewise, it is a laudable aim to focus in a targeted way on timely diagnosis, and intervention and research (into causes, cure and care) are likely to be of major value in personal, societal, political and economic terms (Banerjee, 2012). For a very helpful contemporaneous account of the 'big picture', including accounts of particular countries including Japan, Nigeria and Peru, and a discussion of trickier aspects such as outreach of dementia policy for remote and rural areas, the reader is strongly urged to refer to *Dementia: A Global Approach* (Krishnamoorthy, Prince and Cummings, 2010).

There are general problems with current projections of dementia prevalence anyway (Norton, Matthews and Brayne, 2013). It is unclear whether changes in the treatment of other conditions may impact on the prevalence of dementia. For example, increased post-stroke survival may lead to increases in dementia incidence, but there is also some evidence suggesting statins may have some preventative implications for dementia (e.g. McGuinness *et al.*, 2009). And it is clear that there has to be an emphasis on research on living better with dementia other than pure pharmaceutical and cellular approaches, and that this should ideally be reflected in any national dementia research strategy. For example, interventions aimed at maintaining independence or wellbeing need to target different activities of daily living across different dementia stages and perhaps also tailor interventions to the context of different countries. These findings then contribute to the development of non-pharmaceutical interventions and governmental pledges to promote independence in dementia (Giebel *et al.*, 2014). There is also further work to be done as to where is the best location to make the dementia diagnosis – for example, whether it is primary or secondary care (Wimo *et al.*, 2013).

Development of national policies

There are a great number of faultlines in dementia policy, a reflection of the numerous stakeholders within the policy sphere. For example, Innes and Manthorpe (2013, p.683) provide that: 'In some debates policy and practice are set within a mental illness framework; in others dementia is seen as a disease related to later life, in yet others it is discussed as a long-term condition or as an element of frailty.' There have been general concerns about a possible schism between 'rhetoric' and 'reality' in dementia policies (Venturato, Moyle and Steel, 2011).

In 2013, an excellent document was published by Bupa and Alzheimer's Disease International (ADI), entitled 'Improving dementia care worldwide: ideas and advice on implementing a National Dementia Plan'. As is correctly acknowledged in this report, 'stigma, denial and inadequate financial resources remain key barriers to proper treatment and care' (Pot and Petrea, 2013, p.7). This is indeed consistent with previous work from the ADI. In their World

Alzheimer Report 2012 ('Overcoming the stigma of dementia'), the ADI drew attention to people with dementia 'often isolated, or hidden, because of stigma or the possibility of negative reactions from neighbours and relatives to behavioural and psychological symptoms' (Alzheimer's Disease International, 2012, p.2). The authors of that report further add that 'the idea that nothing can be done to help people with dementia often leads to hopelessness and frustration' (p.2).

'Improving dementia care worldwide: ideas and advice on developing and implementing a National Dementia Plan' (Pot and Petrea, 2013) offers various points for guidance on content, development and implementation. Box 4.1 provides an overview of these points.

Box 4.1 Guidance points on best practice 'content', 'development' and 'implementation' from 'Improving dementia care worldwide: ideas and advice on developing and implementing a National Dementia Plan'

Content

* Improve awareness and education
* Improve (early) diagnosis and treatment
* Improve support available at home
* Strengthen support available to family carers
* Improve residential/institutional care
* Better integrate care pathways and the coordination of care
* Improve training for healthcare professionals
* Monitor progress
* Commitment to research
* Recognise the role of innovative technologies

Development

* Agree a clear evidence base
* Build a broad base of engaged people

* Commit to draft the National Dementia Plan in a collaborative way
* Set a timeframe, including key milestones
* Agree resource, roles and responsibilities
* Set up a system for monitoring and evaluation
* Execute a high-profile launch

Implementation

* Recognition of dementia as a public health priority
* Leadership at a national level
* People engagement
* Involvement of all key stakeholders
* Introducing a 'system of care' and a 'case management' approach
* Committing funding
* Effective monitoring, evaluation and update

Source: Pot and Petrea, 2013 (p.8) (reproduced by kind permission of Alzheimer's Disease International)

It is described in the report that each domestic national plan has a different emphasis. For example, it states what while France focuses on 'legislation, regulations and standard setting', the UK has a different emphasis on 'consumer participation'. The report settles on a number of issues which should form part of any national dementia policy, and it is very difficult to disagree with any of them.

Critical issues in the content of national dementia policies

Below are the issues which the report has identified. I would like to discuss each of them briefly in the context of an international 'direction of travel'. There are wider areas of specialism which the national policies might have as pervasive issues, such as end-of-life care and ethical considerations.

1. Improve awareness and education

Increasing awareness can be achieved through a number of valid approaches. England, of course, has the highly ambitious Dementia Friends campaign, aiming for one million Dementia Friends who have understood five key facts about the dementias (see Chapter 1).

As Wortmann (2013, p.3) notes, 'A promising concept in this area is the creation of dementia friendly communities, which have been developed in several countries in Europe and in Japan. Part of awareness and education are educational programs that aim at a basic understanding of dementia among large groups of the population, which has started in South Korea and Japan and recently was taken over in the UK.' A success of this policy has also been to embrace diversity. For example, Blackstock and colleagues (2006) note from their experiences in rural Scotland that experience of dementia in rural communities, characterised by low populations surrounded by large rural spaces, is a prerequisite for improving service provision.

2. Improve (early) diagnosis and treatment

Since the introduction of the National Dementia Strategy in England, there has been a significant increase in dementia diagnosis rates (Mukadam *et al.*, 2014). It is impossible to deny that the prevalence rates for dementia vary relatively little from country to country, at least among high-income countries.

Previous estimates of dementia burden, based on smaller datasets, might have underestimated the burden of dementia in China (Chan *et al.*, 2013). That prevalence rates can vary means also that policy has to be vigilant about addressing any modifiable risk factors for dementia. For example, one interesting finding of the descriptive studies on dementia is that rates of dementia, including dementia of the Alzheimer type, have been reported to be relatively high for African Americans (Hendrie *et al.*, 2006). In Europe, there are three ongoing multi-domain interventional randomised controlled trials that focus on the optimal management of vascular risk factors and vascular diseases. It is hoped that these studies will, eventually, provide new insights into prevention of cognitive impairment and dementia (Mangialasche *et al.*, 2012).

Investigation of topics that relate to the role of culture in the recognition, diagnosis and treatment of age-related cognitive impairment and dementia is important and timely (Ferraro *et al.*, 2002; Manly, 2006). Despite the growing evidence on dementia risk reduction, half of current Australian adults are apparently unaware of the potential of dementia risk-reduction activities. Some Australians associate mental activity with reduced risk, but very few are aware of the important link between vascular risk factors and dementia (Australian Department of Health, 2013).

It is generally accepted, however, that there are slightly lower prevalence rates of dementia in less developed regions and this has important implications for research (10/66 Dementia Research Group, 2000). Despite this probability, the huge numbers of people in less developed regions mean that dementia is still likely to be an important issue (McCabe, 2006). The experience in Kerala is very interesting. The symptoms of dementia are not seen as such but are assumed to be part of normal ageing. The first step carers take is to contact their doctor looking for a diagnosis and treatment. Carers may try different doctors, specialists and other practitioners such as *Āyurvedic* practitioners. McCabe (2006) discovered from her research that there is a stigma associated with what is perceived as a mental disorder and families may conceal people with dementia. It was reported that some carers do not cope well and that they do not seek appropriate help at the appropriate time.

The semantics of what type of dementia diagnosis occurs clearly does matter hugely. The term 'early' has been thrown into confusion, in that an early diagnosis could in theory be for someone with a strong genetic risk of dementia or a series of lifestyle habits but who is yet to exhibit symptoms consistent with dementia, such as profound problems in short-term learning and memory. Culture is defined as a 'set of behavioural norms, meanings, and values or reference points utilised by members of a particular society to construct their unique view of the world, and ascertain their identity' (Alarcón, 2009, p.133), and how this can impact upon a timely diagnosis can be underestimated. Therefore, attention has rightly focused on not missing out on the timely diagnosis because of cultural influences. Prince and colleagues (2011) reported that the cognitive and informant scales of the Community Screening Instrument for Dementia could be considerably abbreviated (to seven and six items respectively), while seemingly retaining the excellent culture-fair screening properties of its parent instrument.

3. Improve support available at home

There is a long history of wishing to improve support at home. Dementia contributes 11.2% of years lived with disability in people aged 60 years and older; more than stroke (9.5%), musculoskeletal disorders (8.9%), cardiovascular disease (5.0%) and all forms of cancer (2.4%) (Ferri *et al.*, 2005).

The 'disability movement' has had a profound effect on the organisation and delivery of care services, particularly for younger people with disabilities. Lobbying and campaigning has led to a profound shift in perceptions about people with disabilities; no longer were they seen as dependent 'patients', but as individuals who can promote 'no decision about us without us' (Oliver, 1990, cited in O'Dwyer, 2013, p.234). I will be returning to this potent theme in Chapter 13 on human rights and equality perspectives on dementia-friendly communities, and their importance as enforceable legal rights to promote an individual's dignity and autonomy. There is growing acknowledgement of dementia as a disability and that reasonable adjustments are mandated to allow people living with dementia to achieve a good quality of life. The global instrument that binds all jurisdictions is the United Nations Convention on the Rights of Disabled People (HM Government, 2010).

4. Strengthen support available to family carers

With an estimate of 41,470 people with dementia, the total baseline annual cost was found to be more than €1.69 billion, 48% of which was attributable to the opportunity cost of informal care provided by family and friends and 43% to residential care (Connolly *et al.*, 2014).

Due to the impact of demographic ageing in the coming decades and the expected increase in the number of people with dementia, family carers and the general health and social care system will come under increasing pressure to provide adequate levels of care. That family carers need support is a strong policy message internationally. For example, it is considered that service providers should formulate support services that are appropriate to address the care needs of persons with dementia and family carers for older Chinese citizens in Hong Kong (Chung, 2006). The quality of life of family carers directly impacts on the quality of life of people living with dementia.

5. Improve residential/institutional care

McCormack (2003) has been instrumental in developing an operational model of person-centred care and has emphasised the need for carers to be able to particularise the care recipient's unique sense of personhood through an understanding of the care recipient's 'authentic values'. Indeed, there has latterly been a focus on the use of biographical knowledge (Kellett *et al.*, 2010) and tasks (Edvardsson, Fetherstonhaugh and Nay, 2010).

The general consensus is that national plans have been useful in 'filling the gaps' in policy. There has been some concern about whether Greece has suffered in its management of behavioural and psychological symptoms due to a lack of a national dementia plan (Azermai *et al.*, 2013). Residential or institutional care remains a complicated area of policy globally, and is affected by particular health systems of particular jurisdictions including the degree to which social care is provided by the State. Presenting regimented activities can diminish personhood inadvertently, and an analysis of activities in English policy is already underway (I discussed leisure activities in Chapter 7 of *Living Well with Dementia* (Rahman, 2014)).

By the 1980s, the focus on consumerism throughout the Western world was engrained; people defined their individual identity through the choices they made as consumers (Gilleard and Higgs, 2005). For example, the contemporary conceptualisation of person-centred care in the Irish Standards adopts 'a consumer-driven approach, portraying residential care as hotel-style accommodation and residents as discerning consumers with agency' (O'Dwyer, 2013, p.240). The challenge, of course, is how this is rationalised with policy drives in other jurisdictions. For example, the Australian national dementia strategy stresses access and equity to dementia information, support and care for all people with dementia and their carers and families, regardless of their location or cultural background (Australian Health Ministers' Conference, 2006).

6. Better integrate care pathways and the coordination of care

Large differences exist in the organisation and functions of different healthcare systems, including in the relative weighting of private and public healthcare resource allocation (Commonwealth Fund, 2013).

An example of health and social care working closely is provided by Scotland. The aim of Alzheimer Scotland's 8 Pillar Model of Community Support (Alzheimer Scotland, 2012; Centre for Welfare Reform, 2013) is to enable health and social care to work together closely in providing a continuous service of seamless care, for both the individual with a diagnosis of dementia and their family/carers within the community, during the moderate to severe stages of their illness.

The 8 pillars are described in Box 4.2.

Box 4.2 8 Pillar Model of Community Support

The 8 Pillars are:

* Pillar 1: The Dementia Practice Coordinator (to coordinate the 8 Pillars)
* Pillar 2: Therapeutic interventions to tackle the symptoms of the illness
* Pillar 3: General health care and treatment
* Pillar 4: Mental health care and treatment
* Pillar 5: Personalised support
* Pillar 6: Support for carers
* Pillar 7: Environment
* Pillar 8: Community connections

Source: Alzheimer Scotland, 2012 (p.8) (reproduced by kind permission of Alzheimer Scotland)

Some countries operate health insurance systems. It is noted that, with the exception of the US, all developed countries have universal coverage for their own citizens through their primary insurance programmes (Ellis, Chen and Luscombe, 2014). Various jurisdictions have seen a change from a purely biomedical model positioning dementia as an 'incurable illness' to a model emphasising living well. Through a structural reform, put into practice in 1992, all Swedish long-term medical care of older people in residential care, nursing homes and group living units became a municipal responsibility; this organisational change implied a politically marked ideological shift from medical-based health care to social care work with practically no element of medical care (Emilsson, 2012). A common 'complaint' is that persons who have received a diagnosis of dementia and their friends and family feel utterly lost in the system, waiting for follow-up. Care and support coordination is clearly needed for integrated or 'whole-person care' systems. In Leeds, in England, the success of an integrated service for dementia care has been thought to have reflected the willingness of primary care, social and voluntary agencies in Leeds to cooperate to provide early support for dementia patients and their carers in the community (Kümpers *et al.*, 2005).

The national policy in the Netherlands is characterised by the development of dementia case managers who can work as healthcare providers, social care workers, public officers, elderly advisers (*ouderenadviseur*) or elderly consultants (*consultatiebureaus ouderen*) (Nakanishi and Nakashima, 2014). In France, several measures have been developed to bridge the lack of coordination, including the Local Centre for Information and Coordination (Centre Locaux d'Information et de Coordination) and the gerontology networks (Nakanishi and Nakashima, 2014).

7. Improve training for healthcare professionals

The training needs of the workforce must be served properly to deliver the core competences of dementia care. This might include doctors long after they have left university. For example, Hallberg and colleagues (2014) recently reported on a study of professional care providers in dementia care in eight European countries and their training and involvement in the early dementia stage and in home care. Professionals specifically trained in dementia care are not common. When the All-Party Parliamentary Group (APPG) on Dementia reviewed the progress of the English dementia strategy in 2014, one of their key recommendations was that every clinical commissioning group (CCG) and local authority should appoint a 'Dementia Lead' with specific responsibility to ensure high-quality dementia services.

Healthcare professionals will inevitably work in a number of settings, including hospitals, GP surgeries and residential care, for example. Whatever the setting of a healthcare professional, the principles of giving priority to personhood are widely applicable. Quality of care – and, indeed, quality of life – for people living with dementia in long-term care is often underpinned by philosophies of care, such as person-centred care and relationship-centred care. The translation of these philosophies into practice is influenced by a range of individual and organisational features, including the context in which such care occurs (Venturato *et al.*, 2011).

8. Monitor progress

Progress on the impact of dementia care and support on individuals living with dementia needs to be monitored, and any problems identified and acted upon. Also, it is essential that lessons are learnt from each five-year period of the English dementia policy, and to examine with an open mind what worked well and what did not work so well.

9. Commitment to research

Some jurisdictions commit to research more than others. For example, Norway focuses on research as a key area in its dementia plan. In June 2010, Scotland reported that the Scottish Dementia Clinical Research Network in the Scottish National Dementia Strategy had been established with more than £1 million of Scottish Government money (Scottish Government, 2010). Across all jurisdictions, it is critical that research is not only concerned with involving members of the public, including those with possible dementia, in drug trials. The lack of emphasis on research monies going into living well with dementia is not only staggering, but quite unacceptable.

10. Recognise the role of innovative technologies

It has been a big emphasis of policy to take proper account of innovative technologies that might improve the wellbeing of people with dementia and their carers.

Developing the national plan for dementia

There is no doubt that any policy has to be firmly positioned in the current evidence base. For example, the policy on the use of antipsychotics in dementia needs to take account of the current prescribing habits of medical doctors.

The Ware Invitational Summit in 2012 had the aim of linking science with care and engaging the participation of patients, families, scientists, pharmaceutical companies, regulatory agencies and advocacy organisations (Naylor *et al.*, 2012). However, the evidence base is not without different opinions. For example, the claim that 'biomarkers have become essential tools in drug development, both for enriching study populations with subjects likely to respond to the drug and for monitoring response to treatment' (Naylor *et al.*, 2012, p.447), might be hotly contested by some.

Pot and Petrea (2013) outline best practice recommendations in their Bupa/ADI report. Recommendations 2 and 3, relating to development, call for 'building a broad base of engaged people' and to 'commit to draft the national dementia plan in a collaborative way' (p.8). Other points are operational in the delivery of the national plan which are entirely sensible.

The 'sticking point' remain recommendations 2 and 3. People living well with dementia are increasingly expressing disenchantment about being used in a tokenistic way to 'rubber stamp' decisions made by authorities about dementia.

The lack of representation from people living well with dementia and carers on the World Dementia Council caused consternation from relevant parties, such as Dementia Alliance International. There is clearly much work still to be done here in bringing about a change in organisational culture from all stakeholders. Indeed, one of the key recommendations from the APPG on Dementia in England (2014, p.12) proposes that there is a need for a 'major culture shift to improve the status and morale, both perceived and experienced, in care work to ensure it is an attractive and fulfilling career choice'.

I feel that many people of all countries will not be convinced by political leaders being the figureheads of their domestic policies. I think they will instead 'buy into' policy represented by people with dementia themselves, or carers, as such an approach may appear more authentic. Otherwise, a dangerous 'democratic deficit' could emerge.

Implementing the national plan for dementia

Dementia is set to become one of the key health and social care challenges of the twenty-first century and is attracting global policy attention, mainly arising from concern about increases in the number of people with dementia, particularly in developed countries (Innes and Manthorpe, 2013). The case for dementia being a public health priority is overwhelming. In the next few decades, the global burden of dementia will shift to poorer countries, particularly rapidly developing middle-income countries that are members of the G20, but not the G8 (Alzheimer's Disease International, 2013).

Dementia costs in developing countries are estimated to be US$73 billion annually, but care demands social protection, which seems scarce in these regions (Kalaria *et al.*, 2008). Jurisdictions inevitably vary about the future 'cost' of dementia. For example, across Australia, dementia prevalence is currently expected to grow by around 254% between 2011 and 2050 (Alzheimer's Australia, 2011a). There is an economic case as well as a moral one for an approach that encourages living better with dementia. For example, regarding non-pharmacological treatments, cognitive stimulation therapy, tailored activity programmes and occupational therapy were found to be more cost-effective than usual care (Knapp, Iemmi and Romeo, 2012).

It is becoming increasingly clear that the 'involvement of all key stakeholders' (recommendation 4 of the Pot and Petrea 2013 report, relating to implementation) can affect the overall flavour of the national dementia policy. For example, it is described that the 'War on Dementia' plan in South Korea was jointly developed by neurology/psychiatry associations, the Ministry of Health and Welfare, nurses' associations and Alzheimer's Association Korea (Alzheimer's Australia, 2011b). The lack of prominent opinions of people living well with dementia in the earlier stages of the condition therefore has the potential to bias the overall policy towards the later stages of dementia. It has therefore been suggested that the Korean model is overly medical and does not address the social supports required for individuals with dementia and their families (Alzheimer's Australia, 2011b). In contrast, in the report 'Living Longer, Living Better' (Commonwealth of Australia, 2012), it is argued that the ageing of Australia's population is a profound social shift which requires an equally profound shift in society's mindset about ageing. Australia has drifted towards a more holistic view of dementia care. The framework depicted in Figure 4.1, for example, puts the person living with dementia at the hub of the community at large (including awareness and acceptance), care and support networks, including family.

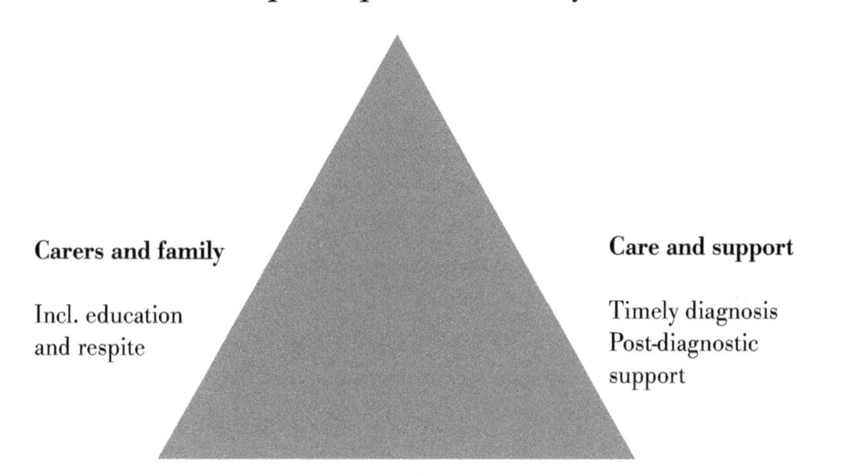

Figure 4.1 A holistic model for living positively with dementia
Source: Adapted from Australian Health Ministers' Conference, 2006 (p.3)

Some jurisdictions clearly already have more experience in introducing a proactive system of care that is well coordinated, and which involves an active case-management approach. For example, the Dutch Dementia Strategy stressed the importance of a coordinated approach to care. Health Care Insurance (Zorgverzekeraars Nederland), Alzheimer Netherlands and the Ministry of Health worked together on the Coordinated Dementia Care Programme (*ketenzorg dementie*), the aim of which was to produce a demand-led, coordinated care programme, to ensure the integration of services (Nakanishi and Nakashima, 2014).

There is no doubt that all parts of the health and social care systems need proper funding. Under recommendation 6 of the Pot and Petrea (2013) report, relating to implementation, it is stated that proper funding must be given to:

» prevention and early detection

» health care

» social care

» other issues such as monitoring and continual improvement.

The parts of the system are heavily reliant on one another. For example, it has been a historic and enduring problem that patients of the National Health Service have not often been discharged to social care in a timely fashion. So cuts in social care will inevitably impact on the operational management of the NHS; this is one of the issues that 'whole-person care' in England would mitigate against.

Conclusion

Clearly, global policies in dementia comprise 'work in progress'. There is considerable harmony, but strategising dementia policies needs clarity in thinking about the risks and uncertainties which can blow a country's dementia strategy off course. Within a country, there might be political, social, economic, technological, environmental and legal issues which might push the dementia policy in one direction. However, superimposed on this, globalisation without barriers might assist in the free movement of capital for funding of dementia policies. Resource allocation from the State to fund cures from global companies hugely distorts policy. A good example of this is the 'cure versus care' schism which lurks in the background of young-onset dementia policy, notably in developed countries. That is the topic of Chapter 5.

References

10/66 Dementia Research Group (2000) Methodological issues for population-based research into dementia in developing countries. International Journal of Geriatric Psychiatry, 15, 21–30.

Alarcón, R.D. (2009) Culture, cultural factors and psychiatric diagnosis: review and projections. World Psychiatry, 8, 3, 131–9.

All-Party Parliamentary Group (APPG) on Dementia (2014) Building on the National Dementia Strategy: change, progress and priorities. Available at www.alzheimers.org.uk/site/scripts/download.php?fileID=2249 (accessed 6 December 2014).

Alzheimer Scotland (2012) Delivering Integrated Dementia Care: The 8 Pillar Model of Community Support. Edinburgh: Alzheimer Scotland.

Alzheimer's Australia (2011a) Dementia across Australia: 2011–2050. Available at https://fightdementia.org.au/sites/default/files/20111014_Nat_Access_DemAcrossAust.pdf (accessed 6 December 2014).

Alzheimer's Australia (2011b) National Strategies to Address Dementia. Available at https://fightdementia.org.au/sites/default/files/20111410_Paper_25_low_v2.pdf (accessed 6 December 2014).

Alzheimer's Disease International (2012) World Alzheimer Report 2012: overcoming the stigma of dementia. Available at www.alz.co.uk/research/WorldAlzheimerReport2012ExecutiveSummary.pdf (accessed 6 December 2014).

Alzheimer's Disease International (2013) Policy Brief for Heads of Government: The Global Impact of Dementia 2013–2050. Available at www.alz.co.uk/research/GlobalImpactDementia2013.pdf (accessed 6 December 2014).

Australian Department of Health (2013) Consultation Paper National Framework for Action on Dementia 2014–2018. Available at www.dss.gov.au/our-responsibilities/ageing-and-aged-care/consumers-families-and-carers/dementia/national-framework-for-action-on-dementia-2014-2018 (accessed 6 December 2014).

Australian Health Ministers' Conference (2006) National Framework for Action on Dementia 2006–2010 (Australian National Dementia Strategy). Available at www.nhmrc.gov.au/_files_nhmrc/file/grants/apply/strategic/dementia_attachmenta.pdf (accessed 6 December 2014).

Azermai, M., Kane, J., Liperoti, R., Tsolaki, M. *et al.* (2013) The same patient in various European countries. Management of behavioural and psychological symptoms of dementia: Belgium, Greece, Italy, United Kingdom. European Geriatric Medicine, 4, 50–8.

Banerjee, S. (2012) The macroeconomics of dementia: will the world economy get Alzheimer's disease? Archives of Medical Research, 43, 8, 705–9.

Blackstock, K.L., Innes, A., Cox, S., Smith, D. and Mason, A. (2006) Living with dementia in rural and remote Scotland: diverse experiences of people with dementia and their carers. Journal of Rural Studies, 22, 161–76.

Centre for Welfare Reform (2013) The 8 pillar model of community support. A report in association with Alzheimer Scotland (author: Lisa Monaghan). Available at www.centreforwelfarereform.org/uploads/attachment/382/delivering-integrated-dementia-care-the-8-pillars-model-of-community-support.pdf (accessed 6 December 2014).

Chan, K.Y., Wang, W., Wu, J.J., Liu, L. *et al.* Global Health Epidemiology Reference Group (GHERG) (2013) Epidemiology of Alzheimer's disease and other forms of dementia in China, 1990–2010: a systematic review and analysis. Lancet, 381, 9882, 2016–23.

Chung, J.C. (2006) Care needs assessment of older Chinese individuals with dementia in Hong Kong. Aging and Mental Health, 10, 6, 631–7.

Commonwealth Fund (2013) International profiles of health care systems, 2013. Australia, Canada, Denmark, England, France, Germany, Italy, Japan, the Netherlands, New Zealand, Norway, Sweden, Switzerland, and the United States. Available at www.commonwealthfund.org/~/media/files/publications/fund-report/2013/nov/1717_thomson_intl_profiles_hlt_care_sys_2013_v2.pdf (accessed 6 December 2014).

Commonwealth of Australia (2012) Living Longer. Living Better. Available at www.flexiliving.org.au/files/2012/07/D0769-Living-Longer-Living-Better-SCREEN-070512.pdf (accessed 14 May 2015).

Connolly, S., Gillespie, P., O'Shea, E., Cahill, S. and Pierce, M. (2014) Estimating the economic and social costs of dementia in Ireland. Dementia (London), 13, 1, 5–22.

Edvardsson, D., Fetherstonhaugh, D. and Nay, R. (2010) Promoting a continuation of self and normality: person-centred care as described by people with dementia, their family members and aged care staff. Journal of Clinical Nursing, 19, 17–18, 2611–18.

Ellis, R.P., Chen, T. and Luscombe, C.E. (2014) Comparisons of Health Insurance Systems in Developed Countries. In A. Culyer (ed.) Encyclopedia of Health Economics. London: Elsevier Press. Available at www.bu.edu/law/faculty/scholarship/documents/EllisPaper.pdf (accessed 6 December 2014).

Emilsson, U.M. (2012) The staff's view on dementia and the care in three cultures: a qualitative study in France, Portugal and Sweden. Dementia, 11, 1, 31–47.

Ferraro, F.R., Bercier, B.J., Holm, J. and McDonald, J.D. (2002) Preliminary Normative Data from a Brief Neuropsychological Test Battery in a Sample of Native American Elderly. In L. Bieliauskas (series ed.) and F.R. Ferraro (vol. ed.) Minority and Cross-Cultural Aspects of Neuropsychological Assessment: Studies on Neuropsychology, Development, and Cognition. Lisse: Swets & Zeitlinger.

Ferri, C.P., Prince, M., Brayne, C., Brodaty, H. *et al.* Alzheimer's Disease International (2005) Global prevalence of dementia: a Delphi consensus study. Lancet, 366, 9503, 2112–17.

Fox, N.C. and Petersen, R.C. (2013) The G8 Dementia Research Summit – a starter for eight? Lancet, 382, 9909, 1968–9.

Giebel, C.M., Sutcliffe, C., Stolt, M., Karlsson, S. *et al.* (2014) Deterioration of basic activities of daily living and their impact on quality of life across different cognitive stages of dementia: a European study. International Psychogeriatrics, 26, 8, 1283–93.

Gilleard, C. and Higgs, P. (2005) Contexts of Ageing: Class, Cohort and Community. Cambridge, MA: Polity Press.

Hallberg, I.R., Cabrera, E., Jolley, D., Raamat, K. *et al.* (2014) Professional care providers in dementia care in eight European countries: their training and involvement in early dementia stage and in home care. Dementia (London), pii: 1471301214548520 [Epub ahead of print].

Heller, T. and Heller, L. (2003) First among equals? Does drug treatment for dementia claim more than its fair share of resources? Dementia, 2, 7–19.

Hendrie, H.C., Murrell, J., Gao, S., Unverzagt, F.W., Ogunniyi, A. and Hall, K.S. (2006) International studies in dementia with particular emphasis on populations of African origin. Alzheimer Disease and Associated Disorders, 20, 3, Suppl. 2, S42–6.

HM Government (2010) Creating a fairer and more equal society: United Nations Convention on the Rights of Disabled People. Available at www.gov.uk/government/policies/creating-a-fairer-and-more-equal-society/supporting-pages/united-nations-convention-on-the-rights-of-disabled-people (accessed 6 December 2014).

Innes, A. and Manthorpe, J. (2013) Developing theoretical understandings of dementia and their application to dementia care policy in the UK. Dementia (London), 12, 6, 682–96.

Kalaria, R.N., Maestre, G.E., Arizaga, R., Friedland, R.P. *et al.* World Federation of Neurology Dementia Research Group (2008) Alzheimer's disease and vascular dementia in developing countries: prevalence, management, and risk factors. Lancet Neurology, 7, 9, 812–26.

Kellett, U., Moyle, W., McAllister, M., King, C. and Gallagher, F. (2010) Life stories and biography: a means of connecting family and staff to people with dementia. Journal of Clinical Nursing, 19, 11–12, 1707–15.

Knapp, M., Iemmi, V. and Romeo, R. (2012) Dementia care costs and outcomes: a systematic review. International Journal of Geriatric Psychiatry, 28, 6, 551–61.

Krishnamoorthy, E.K., Prince, M.J. and Cummings, J.L. (2010) Dementia: A Global Approach. Cambridge: Cambridge University Press.

Kümpers, S., Mur, I., Maarse, H. and van Raak, A. (2005) A comparative study of dementia care in England and the Netherlands using neo-institutionalist perspectives. Qualitative Health Research, 15, 9, 1199–230.

Mangialasche, F., Kivipelto, M., Solomon, A. and Fratilioni, L. (2012) Dementia prevention: current epidemiological evidence and future perspective. Alzheimer's Research and Therapy, 4, 1, 6.

Manly, J.J. (2006) Cultural Issues. In D.K. Attix and K.A. Welsh-Bohmer (eds) Geriatric Neuropsychology. New York, NY: Guilford Press.
McCabe, L.F. (2006) The cultural and political context of the lives of people with dementia in Kerala, India. Dementia, 5, 1, 117–36.
McCormack, B. (2003) A conceptual framework for person-centred practice with older people. International Journal of Nursing Practice, 9, 3, 202–20.
McGuinness, B., Craig, D., Bullock, R. and Passmore, P. (2009) Statins for the prevention of dementia. Cochrane Database of Systematic Reviews, 2, CD003160.
Mukadam, N., Livingston, G., Rantell, K. and Rickman, S. (2014) Diagnostic rates and treatment of dementia before and after launch of a national dementia policy: an observational study using English national databases. BMJ Open, 4, 1, e004119.
Nakanishi, M. and Nakashima, T. (2014) Features of the Japanese national dementia strategy in comparison with international dementia policies: how should a national dementia policy interact with the public health and social-care systems? Alzheimer's and Dementia, 10, 4, 468–76.
National Institute for Health and Care Excellence (2001) Guidance on the Use of Donepezil, Rivastigmine and Galantamine for the Treatment of Alzheimer's Disease. Technology Appraisal Guidance No. 19. London: NICE.
Naylor, M.D., Karlawish, J.H., Arnold, S.E., Khachaturian, A.S. *et al.* (2012) Advancing Alzheimer's disease diagnosis, treatment, and care: recommendations from the Ware Invitational Summit. Alzheimer's and Dementia, 8, 5, 445–52.
Norton, S., Matthews, F.E. and Brayne, C. (2013) A commentary on studies presenting projections of the future prevalence of dementia. BMC Public Health, 13, 1.
O'Dwyer, C. (2013) Official conceptualizations of person-centered care: which person counts? Journal of Aging Studies, 227, 3, 233–42.
Oliver, M. (1990) The Politics of Disablement: A Sociological Approach. New York, NY: St. Martin's Press.
Pot, A.M. and Petrea, I. (Bupa/ADI report) (2013) Improving dementia care worldwide: ideas and advice on developing and implementing a National Dementia Plan. London: Bupa/ADI. Available at www.alz.co.uk/sites/default/files/pdfs/global-dementia-plan-report-ENGLISH.pdf (accessed 25 February 2015).
Prince, M., Acosta, D., Ferri, C.P., Guerra, M. *et al.* (2011) A brief dementia screener suitable for use by non-specialists in resource poor settings: the cross-cultural derivation and validation of the brief Community Screening Instrument for Dementia. International Journal of Geriatric Psychiatry, 26, 9, 899–907.
Prince, M., Bryce, R., Albanese, E., Wimo, A., Ribeiro, W. and Ferri, C.P. (2013) The global prevalence of dementia: a systematic review and metaanalysis. Alzheimer's and Dementia, 9, 1, 63–75.
Rahman, S. (2014) Living Well with Dementia: The Importance of the Person and the Environment for Wellbeing. Oxford: Radcliffe Health.
Scottish Government (2010) Scotland's National Dementia Strategy, June 2010. Available at www.scotland.gov.uk/Resource/Doc/324377/0104420.pdf (accessed 10 February 2014).
Venturato, L., Moyle, W. and Steel, A. (2011) Exploring the gap between rhetoric and reality in dementia care in Australia: could practice documents help bridge the great divide? Dementia (London), 12, 2, 251–67.
Wimo, A., Jönsson, L., Bond, J., Prince, M. and Winblad, B./Alzheimer Disease International (2013) The worldwide economic impact of dementia 2010. Alzheimer's and Dementia, 9, 1, 1–11.
Wortmann, M. (2013) Importance of national plans for Alzheimer's disease and dementia. Alzheimer's Research and Therapy, 5, 5, 40.

Chapter 5

WHAT MIGHT LIVING BETTER WITH YOUNG-ONSET DEMENTIA MEAN?

'When your friends begin to flatter you on how young you look, it's a sure sign you're getting old.'

Mark Twain (1835–1919)

Introduction

Claudia Chaufan and colleagues contributed a truly outstanding piece, 'Medical ideology as a double-edged sword: the politics of cure and care in the making of Alzheimer's disease', which, although focused on one type of dementia and not confined to any age bracket, made some pertinent observations on the 'cure versus care' debate. They draw attention to the 'curable, biomedical entity' nature of dementia. Various societal trends, prominent in the Reagan US administration, such as the 'nuclear family' and the notion that costs of cure are becoming increasingly unaffordable in the context of a drive for 'small government', are reviewed elegantly by Chaufan and colleagues (2012).

And this is watching the division between YOD (young-onset dementia) and LOD (late-onset dementia) from a distance still. Of course, this has all to do with a malign influence on the overall discussion, which can euphemistically be described as complicated. I have no doubt that Beth Britton is essentially correct in her perspective 'Cure versus care – let's not fight about it' (Britton, 2013), but the various strands of the arguments are important and ultimately rooted in what policy decisions our governments make on our behalf, presumably on a legitimate democratic basis. That ultimately gives governments a licence to operate in making complex decisions about resource allocation that are particularly relevant to young-onset dementia.

'Cure versus care' in dementia and the question of resource allocation

In an article provocatively titled 'We are a long way from an Alzheimer's cure', Howard Gleckman (2014) concluded:

> In the meantime, let's acknowledge the painful reality: We are making only slow, incremental progress in the war against Alzheimer's and other dementias. We are far from prevention or cure. For now, we should increase our focus on living with dementia and caring for those with this condition.

But one cannot but worry about the way in which the issues are being presented. There is no doubt that dementia presents a massive societal issue. Large multinational drug companies will need to recoup their direct costs in research and development, marketing and intellectual property *inter alia*, and make distributed profits available as dividends, but close scrutiny is needed concerning the extent to which the public subsidises the business plans of private entities.

There is a relative lack of focused research looking at resource allocation in 'cure versus care' for dementia. Considering how easy it was for G7 countries to convene a summit and legacy events, this omission is striking. We can attempt to begin to glean clues from the resource allocation discussion in palliative care which has run in parallel. As described by Haycox (2009), the issues of quantity of life (years added) and quality of life come up, but there is a lack of formal analysis looking at how much benefit is accrued from every pound spent.

Genetics, 'big data' and personalised medicine

The fact that there are real individuals at the heart of a policy strand summarised as 'young-onset dementia' is all too easily forgotten, especially by people who prefer to construct 'policy by spreadsheet'.

It is relatively uncommon for a dementia to be down to a single gene, but it can happen. And certainly, even if there might not be 'cure' for today or tomorrow, identification of precise genetic abnormalities might provide scope for genetic counselling. Markus (2012) argues that many monogenic forms of stroke are untreatable, and therefore specialised genetic counselling is important before mutation testing.

'Big data' refers to information that is too large, varied or high-speed for traditional methods of storage, processing and analytics. For example, one application of mining large datasets that has been particularly productive in the research community is the search for genome-wide associations (Genomic Data Sharing (GDS)). GDS relies on analysis of DNA segments across vast patient populations to search for DNA variants associated with a particular disease. To date, GDS analyses have identified a handful of promising genetic associations with Alzheimer's disease, including APOE ε4.

As the McKinsey Centre for Business Technology (2012, p.32) states in an interesting document called 'Perspectives on digital business', 'Large hospital chains, national insurers, and drug manufacturers, by contrast, stand to gain substantially through the pooling and more effective analysis of data.' Vast collections of genomic data obviously represent a goldmine for health providers around the world. Meltzer (2013) reviews correctly that personalised medicine has been the subject of increased basic and clinical research interest and funding. Meltzer describes how a knowledge of the genetic and molecular basis of clinical heterogeneity should make it possible to more reliably predict the likely outcomes of alternative approaches to treatment for specific individuals and therefore what course of action is likely to be best for any given patient. Knowledge of personal genetic traits might allow accurate prediction of those individuals who are most likely to experience adverse events through medication (Markus, 2012). Both 'big data' and 'personalised medicine', being couched in the language of bringing value to operational processes in corporate strategy, tend to lose the precise cost-effectiveness arguments at an accounting level. The *Guardian* piece entitled 'New NHS boss: service must become world leader in personalised medicine' from 4 June 2014 may be a taste of things to come (Campbell, 2014).

Frontotemporal dementia (FTD) is the second most common cause of dementia in individuals younger than 65 years (Ratnavalli *et al.*, 2002). It is a progressive neurodegenerative disorder characteristically defined by behavioural changes, executive dysfunction and language deficits. The behavioural variant of FTD (bvFTD) is characterised in its earliest stages by a progressive, insidious change in behaviour and personality, considered to reflect underlying problems in the ventromedial prefrontal cortex (Rahman *et al.*, 1999). FTD has a strong genetic background in some individuals, as supported by positive family history in up to 40% of cases, higher than that reported in other neurodegenerative disorders, and by the identification of causative genes related to the disease (Seelaar *et al.*, 2011). It is proposed that genetic background might affect disease outcomes and rate of survival, modulating the onset and the progression of the pathological process when disease is overt (Premi *et al.*, 2012).

Given the consolidated role of genetic loading in FTD, the likely effect of environment has almost been neglected. Only recently, it has been reported that modifiable factors (i.e. education and occupation) might act as proxies for reserve capacity in FTD. Patients with a high level of education and occupation can recruit an alternative neural network to cope better with cognitive functions (see, for example, Borroni *et al.*, 2009; Spreng *et al.*, 2011). But the search for treatments for particular types of dementia based on their underlying genes and genetic products is arguably not an unreasonable one. A good example is provided by the Horizon Scanning Centre of the National Institute for Health Research of NHS England in September 2013: leuco-methylthioninium, which is a 'tau protein aggregation inhibitor'. The clinical trials for this are under way. The medication, at the time of writing, may or may not work safely.

Introduction to the current young-onset dementia policy

The UK National Service Framework for Older People states that there should be specialist services for younger people with dementia (Department of Health, 2001), while the National Service Framework for Long-term Neurological Conditions advises that there should be a person-centred service, early recognition, prompt diagnosis, treatment and early rehabilitation (Department of Health, 2005). It can be argued that there should be greater clarity in service provision: as mooted by Tolhurst, Bhattacharyya and Kingston (2014), 'the definition "young onset dementia" may have independent effects, with the availability of specialist age-specific services reinforcing this definition and the absence of such services potentially attenuating the influence of this age-related definition' (p.198). The authors helpfully suggest that a more rounded view of personhood and young-onset dementia might develop. The learning curve for young-onset dementia will surely be very steep. Armari, Jarmolowicz and Panegyres (2013) recently argued that the perceived concerns of patients with YOD differ from those of the carer, and that continued person involvement is essential in ensuring a tailored approach to young people with dementia.

Emerging research also supports the need to focus studies specifically on younger people with dementia, as they have been found to represent an important and unique psychosocial and medical position (e.g. Luscombe, Brodaty and Freeth, 1998). Service provision has tended to focus on the person living with dementia and their primary carers. However, many of the young people living with a parent with YOD can have emotional problems themselves, problems at school and conflict with the parent with YOD, said to be more common if the father is affected (Luscombe *et al.*, 1998). Moreover, these young people can feel isolated and are often ill equipped for the caring role they find themselves in (Brodaty and Donkin, 2009). A recent report looking at caring responsibilities of young carers (Cass *et al.*, 2011) across a broad range of situations, not specific to YOD, has emphasised the association with young carers' mental and physical health and its deterioration over time, particularly as young carers move into adulthood.

Young-onset dementia is conventionally thought to include patients with onset before 65 years of age. This cutoff point is indicative of a sociological partition in terms of employment and retirement age, but this age has no specific biological significance and there is a range of disease features across this arbitrary divide (Rossor *et al.*, 2010): Alzheimer's disease, vascular disease, frontotemporal dementia and dementia with Lewy bodies are the most common diseases that cause dementia both in the elderly and in younger patients, although not in those who are younger than 35 years (Kelley, Boeve and Josephs, 2008). The highest prevalences of young-onset dementia have been identified as Alzheimer's disease, vascular dementia and frontotemporal dementia (21.7, 10.9 and 9.3 per 100,000 respectively) (Sampson, Warren and Rossor, 2004).

As comprehensively reviewed by Kuruppu and Matthews (2013), the differential diagnosis of young-onset dementia is extensive and includes early-onset forms of adult neurodegenerative conditions including Alzheimer's disease, vascular dementia, frontotemporal dementia, Lewy body dementias, Huntington's disease and prion disease. Late-onset forms of childhood neurodegenerative conditions may also present as young-onset dementia. Potentially reversible aetiologies are important too.

There are concerns that this important group of people has been mistreated in research and service provision, by either being ignored completely or being erroneously sampled together with older age groups (Clemerson, Walsh and Isaac, 2013). The actual definition of dementia is the first obstacle that must be addressed for people with young-onset dementia. This is dementia that happens at a younger age, and many dementias have special presentations in the younger age group. From a cognitive neurological perspective, Rossor and colleagues (2010) report that young-onset dementia will present an important challenge in the future.

Indeed, Alois Alzheimer's first patient was only 51 years old at the time of presentation and for the next 50 years 'Alzheimer's disease' was referred to as a presenile dementia. It was the work of Blessed and colleagues that led to the recognition of the importance of the disease in the elderly (Blessed, Tomlinson and Roth, 1968). These findings led to the view that the disease was the same regardless of age, and the term 'Alzheimer's disease' has since been used to include all ages. The reader is encouraged to review Burns, Tomlinson and Mann (1997) in this regard. Professor German Berrios of the University of Cambridge (1997), from the perspective of a history of psychiatry, has correctly described how in the eighteenth century dementia was not defined as a distinct condition, nor was it associated with any particular age group.

As Hughes (1995) has discussed, services for older people are generally viewed as low status and low priority, are unpopular with staff and attract minimal investment. The meaning of ageing in people with young-onset dementia of the Alzheimer type can be viewed as a positive or negative experience (Rozario and DeRienzis, 2009) and can serve to maintain a sense of youthful self or to explain biological decline.

The delay in diagnosis for persons developing young-onset dementia

Delay in diagnosis appears to instil uncertainty and confusion for young people, as tests take place and new hypotheses are expressed regarding possible diagnoses. I will return to the general topic of risk and uncertainty in my conclusion (Chapter 18).

The diagnosis of the younger-onset dementias in any individual can take a protracted length of time. Lack of diagnosis, or misdiagnosis, was described as having financial implications for the family, and a diagnosis appeared to be important to acquire the correct support from health or social services. Diagnosis is particularly problematic when young patients have a history of psychiatric disorders, given the frequency of neuropsychiatric characteristics in the course of YOD, which often overshadows cognitive deficits (Beattie *et al.*, 2002; Werner, Stein-Shvachman and Korczyn, 2009). Misdiagnosis is common in this age group, and has been reported in 30% to 50% of patients with YOD (Werner *et al.*, 2009). These figures have often been attributed to poor clinician understanding of the disease and its symptomatic progression (Beattie *et al.*, 2002). Luscombe and colleagues (1998) revealed that 71% of YOD carers reported that obtaining an accurate and early diagnosis was problematic and had several trickling effects including increased financial burden and psychosocial strain upon carers and children. This is further highlighted in this study, with both patients and carers revealing 'early recognition and referral' as the principal area needing improvement, which supports the World Alzheimer's Report findings (Alzheimer's Disease International, 2011).

There is a considerable delay in the diagnosis of YOD compared with LOD (Kelley *et al.*, 2008). On average, it is not until two to three years after the onset of symptoms that YOD is diagnosed, and it is indeed conceded that younger people are an overlooked population for research, policy and practice attention (Harris and Keady, 2004). In part, this delay is explained by patients and family members not considering the possibility of dementia at a young age, which delays seeking medical advice. There is very little literature that considers both personhood and young-onset dementia. A systematic review paper considers the impact of dementia on self and identity (Caddell and Clare, 2010), but no mention is made of any distinctive factors presented by YOD which might have an impact upon the person with the condition.

Even when subject to evaluation, YOD is often misdiagnosed for a variety of reasons. Clinicians, who are more familiar with LOD, are less likely to consider a diagnosis of dementia in young patients. Also, YOD has a broader differential diagnosis compared to LOD (Mendez, 2006). Although dementia of the Alzheimer type is the most common cause of YOD, it accounts for only 34% of YOD, compared with approximately 80% of LOD. Another reason for misdiagnosis in YOD is the often prominent psychiatric manifestations and affected non-memory cognitive domains (Mendez, 2006). Changes in personality, behaviour and cognition are often deemed referable to mood disorders such as depression or anxiety. Signs and symptoms that suggest a psychiatric rather than neurodegenerative diagnosis include abrupt onset, identifiable emotional precipitant and lack of progression over time. Periodic clinical reassessment also helps clarify this distinction (Sampson *et al.*, 2004).

Overall impact on individual and partner

Once the diagnosis does finally arrive, many people feel a sense of having been 'written off'.

Celebrated blogger, speaker and advocate living with a dementia Kate Swaffer speaks of this most elegantly in a construct that she has articulated as 'prescribed disengagement':

> There is no other illness I know of where the medical and health care providers tell you to give up. To me, this is a ridiculous and negative

> prescription... It is time all people with dementia and their families stood up for better advice and services that enhance well being. (Swaffer, 2014)

While a diagnosis of dementia at any age has the potential to have a disruptive and devastating effect on the life of the individual and their partner, the experience of dementia in a younger person may be more difficult for the individual and their partner to accept (Tindall and Manthorpe, 1997). The impact of dementia for younger people is also exacerbated by the nature of some of the disease processes involved, in that there is an increased risk of genetic transmission and consequent need for counselling (Whalley, 1997). McNess and Baran (1996) identify the following factors as being important in the experience of younger people:

- boredom and lack of meaningful occupation
- feelings of frustration that they are unable to continue to pursue previous interests
- having to give up driving and the associated feelings of loss of independence
- having a lack of 'money in my pocket'
- flat affect and low self-esteem.

Coping with a diagnosis of young-onset dementia

Clemerson *et al.* (2013) found that the experience of living and coping with YOD of the Alzheimer type was strongly situated within an individual's social context. Most significantly, participants felt too young to develop the disease and felt out of time with age-related psychological tasks.

According to Clemerson and colleagues (Clemerson *et al.*, 2013), the main 'superordinate' themes are:

1. *Disruption of the life cycle.* Experiences of feeling 'too young', including associated premature ageing and death, contributed to the life-cycle disruption alongside the sub-theme of 'losing adult competencies'.
2. *Identity.* A strong theme of identity emerged for all participants reported in this study.
3. *Social orientation.* A shared phenomenon of feeling isolated or disconnected from others emerged in Clemerson *et al.*'s paper, and this notion is strongly reinforced elsewhere in the literature.

4. *Agency.* A common phenomenon reported for many participants was a sense of powerlessness and loss of agency – a sense that they are no longer in control of their own minds, actions, future and overall experience of living with dementia of the Alzheimer type. This is inevitably going to lead to a sense of low mood consistent with the mood disorder literature.

In relation to the identity theme, it is not uncommon for the receipt of the diagnosis of young-onset dementia to be intimately enmeshed with the effects of dignity. For example, Johannessen and Möller (2013, p.413) report:

> The core category fighting for dignity covered the two subcategories intrapsychic challenges and social challenges and describes the informants' experiences of the process of being diagnosed with dementia, and their experiences of living with the disorder knowing that there can be no recovery, along with the informants' experiences of society's and other people's attitudes towards the disorder and what this means for the informants.

Inability to work, and stigma

The decrease in ability to perform at work can cause depression (Fossey and Baker, 1995).

Williams (1995) and Tindall and Manthorpe (1997) cite a number of reports in which younger people with dementia often have more insight into their condition, and are more frustrated by it, particularly as the diagnosis of dementia in younger people is more unexpected than a similar diagnosis in older age (Tindall and Manthorpe, 1997). Indeed, the workplace environment and old colleagues are potentially as significant as the job itself, as described by Johannessen and Möller (2013).

There is greater realisation that workplace engagement might be prioritised better. For example, Robertson and colleagues (2013) recently described an innovative demonstration programme called 'Side by Side' which was initiated to assess the feasibility of supported workplace engagement for people with YOD.

Social isolation

The effect on social isolation has been particularly well described by Johannessen and Möller:

> The dementia disease had affected the informants' lives in various ways. The informants said they were losing opportunities for participation in previous activities, because of their memory loss, communication difficulties, lack of initiative and difficulties with public transport on their own. They also had difficulties maintaining old friendships and making new friends. (Johannessen and Möller, 2013, p.417)

The finding that disconnection from others created a sense of powerlessness mirrors the experience of living with chronic conditions such as diabetes in younger people (e.g. Schur, Gamsu and Barley, 1999). Radley (1994) suggests isolation may be a response to living with illness in a world of health. This was consistent with the discomfort at being 'ill' expressed by some. Furthermore, the use of control as a coping strategy is supported in the literature on chronic pain (Bates and Rankin-Hill, 1994), breast cancer (Taylor, 1983), asthma (Adams, Phil and Jones, 1997) and diabetes (Kelleher, 1988) in adulthood.

Impact on carers

Lockeridge and Simpson (2013) investigated the coping strategies of carers of persons who had received a diagnosis of YOD.

Four major themes became evident:

- 'This is not happening': the use of denial as a coping strategy
- 'Let's not have any more of this demeaning [treatment]'
- 'I've had to fight every inch': struggling to maintain control of events and emotions
- 'What will become of me?'

(Lockeridge and Simpson, 2013, p.635)

Comparisons with existing literature are made and implications for clinical practice are considered. Despite the high levels of admission of younger people with dementia to continuing care services, Newens, Foster and Kay (1995) report that the majority of younger people are still cared for at home up to five years after their diagnosis. Furthermore, it is reported that younger carers report experiencing higher levels of psychological distress compared with carers of older people with dementia (Freyne *et al.*, 1999), and can experience greater difficulty coping with the often accompanying challenging behaviour (Arai *et al.*, 2007).

While deficiencies in YOD management can only be remedied with the insight and experience of service users, the integration of patient and carer perspective in the development of our understanding of the disease, its management and appropriate services has historically been largely absent (Beattie *et al.*, 2002).

Similarly, there are arguments made for the differences in carers' experiences. Several studies have reported high stress levels amongst carers of younger people with dementia (e.g. Harvey *et al.*, 1996; Keady and Nolan, 1997; Sperlinger and Furst, 1994; Williams, 1995). Keady and Nolan (1997) suggest that the higher levels of stress among carers of younger people with dementia are due to the more extensive range of disturbed behaviour in this group. Harvey *et al.* (1996) more specifically found that carer distress and burden were higher in relation to couples who had a prior poor marital relationship and where non-cognitive symptoms were present. Indeed, a noteworthy cross-sectional analysis (Kaiser and Panegyres, 2006) showed that the diagnosis of YOD has a significant impact on spouses, characterised by concerns of dependency, fear and increased depression, especially in the spouses of patients with frontotemporal lobar degeneration.

Keady and Nolan (1997) note that carers often feel trapped in their role. Several studies have found that financial problems are significant (Keady and Nolan, 1997; Sperlinger and Furst, 1994), with Delany and Rosenvinge (1995) reporting that more than 50% of carers had to give up their job or reduce their hours of work. These identified differences between younger and older people with dementia have formed a basis for the argument that specialised services should be available to younger people with dementia. The field of care and support, encouragingly, for YOD is fast developing, thanks to yet another EU initiative on dementia. The EU project 'Rhapsody' intends to analyse the health and social care systems and infrastructures in six European countries that are available to the severely burdened yet underserved group of people with YOD.

Conclusion

Ultimately what seems to have happened is a fundamental breakdown of trust between the public and those 'in power'.

Elegant stage-managed events such as #G7dementia have clearly been less about having a respectful dialogue about what the current challenges in care and cure are, including for the young-onset dementia community. Carefully packaged memes such as 'cure for today, care for tomorrow' are a complete fallacy, in that efforts for a cure for today have been substantially unsuccessful, and a feeling of disdain for care has engulfed certain economies driven by a passion for a small State. There is a virtually absent literature on resource allocation on 'cure versus care' in young-onset dementia, which distorts the whole field to begin with.

Research into living well with dementia is marginalised by large charities which are fixated on cure, certain types of care and prevention.

The case for 'big data' and personalised medicine is in danger of being completely mis-sold in the context without a transparent discussion of the costs needed to deliver this 'added value'. All of this is incredibly sad, and stressful, for people with young-onset dementia who do not just want 'communities' to be 'friendly' towards them; they want to face a future, perhaps in a job, living with their diagnosis, but still with friends or family, and without stigma and discrimination.

As such, an aberrant flaw in 'big data' is not going to cause an acute admission to a NHS Foundation Trust. Delirium superimposed on a person trying to live better with dementia might, however. And the health and social care systems need to be able to cope with persons arriving in the Emergency Room with delirium.

Chapter 6 considers delirium, closely associated in English policy with dementia.

References

Adams, S., Phil, R. and Jones, A. (1997) Medication, chronic illness and identity: the perspective of people with asthma. Social Science and Medicine, 45, 189–201.

Alzheimer's Disease International (2011) World Alzheimer's Report 2011: The Benefits of Early Diagnosis and Intervention. London: ADI. Available at www.alz.co.uk/research/world-report-2011 (accessed 6 December 2014).

Arai, A., Matsumoto, T., Ikeda, M. and Arai, Y. (2007) Do family caregivers perceive more difficulty when they look after patients with early onset dementia compared with late onset dementia? International Journal of Geriatric Psychiatry, 22, 1255–61.

Armari, E., Jarmolowicz, A. and Panegyres, P.K. (2013) The needs of patients with early onset dementia. American Journal of Alzheimer's Disease and Other Dementias, 28, 1, 42–6.

Bates, M.S. and Rankin-Hill, L. (1994) Control, culture and chronic pain. Social Science and Medicine, 39, 629–45.

Beattie, A.M., Daker-White, G., Gilliard, J. and Means, R. (2002) Younger people in dementia: a review of service needs, service provision and models of good practice. Aging and Mental Health, 6, 3, 205–12.

Berrios, G.E. (1997) Dementia during the seventeenth and eighteenth centuries: a conceptual history. Psychological Medicine, 17, 829–37.

Blessed, G., Tomlinson, B.E. and Roth, M. (1968) The association between quantitative measures of dementia and of senile change in the cerebral grey matter of elderly subjects. British Journal of Psychiatry, 114, 797–811.

Borroni, B., Premi, E., Agosti, C., Alberici, A. *et al.* (2009) Revisiting brain reserve hypothesis in frontotemporal dementia: evidence from a brain perfusion study. Dementia and Geriatric Cognition Disorders, 28, 130–5.

Britton, B. (2013) Cure versus care – let's not fight about it. Huffington Post, 28 December. Available at www.huffingtonpost.co.uk/beth-britton/dementia-cure_b_4511265.html (accessed 6 December 2014).

Brodaty, H. and Donkin, M. (2009) Family caregivers of people with dementia. Dialogues in Clinical Neuroscience, 11, 217–28.

Burns, A., Tomlinson, B.E. and Mann, D.M. (1997) Observations on the brains of demented old people. B.E. Tomlinson, G. Blessed and M. Roth, Journal of the Neurological Sciences (1970) 11, 205–42 and Observations on the brains of non-demented old people. B.E. Tomlinson, G. Blessed and M. Roth, Journal of Neurological Sciences (1968) 7, 331–56. International Journal of Geriatric Psychiatry, 12, 8, 785–90.

Caddell, L. and Clare, L. (2010) The impact of dementia on self and identity: a systematic review. Clinical Psychology Review, 30, 1, 113–26.

Campbell, D. (2014) New NHS boss: service must become world leader in personalised medicine. The Guardian, 4 June. Available at www.theguardian.com/society/2014/jun/04/nhs-boss-world-leader-personalised-medicine (accessed 6 December 2014).

Cass, B., Brennan, D., Thomson, C., Hill, T. *et al.* (2011) Young carers: social policy impacts of the caring responsibilities of children and young adults. Report prepared for ARC Linkage Partners, October 2011. Available online at www.youngcarers.ie/userfiles/file/UsefulReports/Young_Carers_Report_Final_October_2011_w_cover_page.pdf (accessed 10 February 2015).

Chaufan, C., Hollister, B., Nazareno, J. and Fox, P. (2012) Medical ideology as a double-edged sword: the politics of cure and care in the making of Alzheimer's disease. Social Science and Medicine, 74, 5, 788–95.

Clemerson, G., Walsh, S. and Isaac, C. (2013) Towards living well with young onset dementia: an exploration of coping from the perspective of those diagnosed. Dementia (London), 13, 4, 451–66.

Delany, N. and Rosenvinge, H. (1995) Presenile dementia: sufferers, carers and services. International Journal of Geriatric Psychiatry, 10, 7, 597–601.

Department of Health (2001) National Service Framework for Older People (DH publication number 23633). London: Department of Health.

Department of Health (2005) National Service Framework for Long-term Neurological Conditions (DH publication number 265109). London: Department of Health. Available at www.gov.uk/government/uploads/system/uploads/attachment_data/file/198033/National_Service_Framework_for_Older_People.pdf (accessed 10 February 2015).

EU 'Rhapsody Project'. Research to Assess Policies and Strategies for Dementia in the Young. Available at www.rhapsody-project.eu (accessed 6 December 2014).

Fossey, J. and Baker, M. (1995) Different needs demand different services. Journal of Dementia Care, 3, 6, 22–3.

Freyne, A., Kidd, N., Cohen, R. and Lawlor, B.A. (1999) Burden in carers of dementia patients: higher levels in carers of younger sufferers. International Journal of Geriatric Psychiatry, 14, 784–8.

Genomic Data Sharing (GDS) (n.d.). Available at http://gds.nih.gov (accessed 6 December 2014).

Gleckman, H. (2014) We are a long way from an Alzheimer's cure. Forbes, 23 July. Available at www.forbes.com/sites/howardgleckman/2014/07/23/we-are-a-long-way-from-an-alzheimers-cure (accessed 10 February 2015).

Harris, P.G. and Keady, J. (2004) Living with early onset dementia: exploring the experience and developing evidence-based guidelines for practice. Alzheimer's Care Today, 5, 2, 111–22.

Harvey, R.J., Roques, P., Fox, N.C. and Rossor, M.N. (1996) Services for younger sufferers of Alzheimer's disease. British Journal of Psychiatry, 168, 384–5.

Haycox, A. (2009) Optimizing decision making and resource allocation in palliative care. Journal of Pain and Symptom Management, 38, 1, 45–53.

Horizon Scanning Centre (2013) Leuco-methylthioninium (LMTX) for behavioural variant frontotemporal dementia – first line. NIHR HSC ID: 8239. NIHR Horizon Scanning Centre, University of Birmingham.

Hughes, B. (1995) Older People and Community Care. Buckingham: Open University Press.

Johannessen, A. and Möller, A. (2013) Experiences of persons with early-onset dementia in everyday life: a qualitative study. Dementia (London), 12, 4, 410–24.

Kaiser, S. and Panegyres, P.K. (2006) The psychosocial impact of young onset dementia on spouses. American Journal of Alzheimer's Disease and Other Dementias, 21, 6, 398–402.

Keady, J. and Nolan, M. (1997) Raising the profile of younger people with dementia. Mental Health Nursing, 17, 2, 7–10.

Kelleher, D. (1988) Diabetes. London: Tavistock.

Kelley, B.J., Boeve, B.F. and Josephs, K.A. (2008) Young-onset dementia: demographic and etiologic characteristics of 235 patients. Archives of Neurology, 65, 1502–8.

Kuruppu, D.K. and Matthews, B.R. (2013) Young-onset dementia. Seminars in Neurology, 33, 4, 365–85.

Lockeridge, S. and Simpson, J. (2013) The experience of caring for a partner with young onset dementia: how younger carers cope. Dementia (London), 12, 5, 635–51.

Luscombe, G., Brodaty, H. and Freeth, S. (1998) Younger people with dementia: diagnostic issues, effects on carers and use of services. International Journal of Geriatric Psychiatry, 13, 323–30.

Markus, H.S. (2012) Stroke genetics: prospects for personalized medicine. BMC Medicine, 27, 10, 113.

McKinsey Centre for Business Technology (2012) Perspectives on digital business. McKinsey & Company.

McNess, G. and Baran, M. (1996) Addressing the needs of younger people with dementia and their spouses: what can be achieved when service providers collaborate. Paper presented to the Alzheimer's Association of Australia, 6th Annual Conference, 1–5.

Meltzer, D.O. (2013) Opportunities in the economics of personalized health care and prevention. Forum for Health Economics and Policy, 16, 2, 47–56.

Mendez, M. (2006) The accurate diagnosis of early-onset dementia. International Journal of Psychiatry in Medicine, 36, 4, 401–12.

National Institute for Health Research (2013) Horizon Scanning Centre: leuco-methylthioninium (LMTX) for behavioural variant frontotemporal dementia – first line. Available at www.hsc.nihr.ac.uk/topics/leuco-methylthioninium-lmtx-for-behavioural-varian (accessed 14 May 2015).

Newens, A.J., Foster, D.P. and Kay, D.W. (1995) Dependency and community care in presenile Alzheimer's disease. British Journal of Psychiatry, 166, 777–82.

Premi, E., Garibotto, V., Alberici, A., Paghera, B. *et al.* (2012) Nature versus nurture in frontotemporal lobar degeneration: the interaction of genetic background and education on brain damage. Dementia and Geriatric Cognitive Disorders, 33, 6, 372–8.

Radley, A. (1994) Making Sense of Illness: The Social Psychology of Health and Disease. London: Sage.

Rahman, S., Sahakian, B.J., Hodges, J.R., Rogers, R.D. and Robbins, T.W. (1999) Specific cognitive deficits in mild frontal variant frontotemporal dementia. Brain, 122, 8, 1469–93.

Ratnavalli, E., Brayne, C., Dawson, K. and Hodges, J.R. (2002) The prevalence of frontotemporal dementia. Neurology, 58, 11, 1615–21.

Robertson, J., Evans, D. and Horsnell, T. (2013) Side by Side: a workplace engagement program for people with younger onset dementia. Dementia (London), 12, 5, 666–74.

Rossor, M.N., Fox, N.C., Mummery, C.J., Schott, J.M. and Warren, J.D. (2010) The diagnosis of young-onset dementia. Lancet Neurology, 9, 8, 793–806.

Rozario, P.A. and DeRienzis, D. (2009) So forget how old I am! Examining age identities in the face of chronic conditions. Sociology of Health and Illness, 31, 540–53.

Sampson, E.L., Warren, J.D. and Rossor, M.N. (2004) [Review.] Young onset dementia. Postgraduate Medical Journal, 80, 941, 125–39.

Schur, H.V., Gamsu, D.S. and Barley, V.M. (1999) The young person's perspective on living and coping with diabetes. Journal of Health Psychology, 4, 223–36.

Seelaar, H., Rohrer, J.D., Pijnenburg, Y.A., Fox, N.C. and van Swieten, J.C. (2011) Clinical, genetic and pathological heterogeneity of frontotemporal dementia: a review. Journal of Neurology, Neurosurgery and Psychiatry, 82, 476–86.

Sperlinger, D. and Furst, M. (1994) The service experiences of people with presenile dementia: a study of carers in one London borough. International Journal of Geriatric Psychiatry, 9, 47–50.

Spreng, R.N., Drzezga, A., Diehl-Schmid, J., Kurz, A., Levine, B. and Perneczky, R. (2011) Relationship between occupation attributes and brain metabolism in frontotemporal dementia. Neuropsychologia, 49, 3699–703.

Swaffer, K. (2014) Re-investing in life after a diagnosis of dementia [blog]. Available at http://kateswaffer.com/2014/01/20/re-investing-in-life-after-a-diagnosis-of-dementia (accessed 6 December 2014).

Taylor, S.E. (1983) Adjustment to threatening events: a theory of cognitive adaptation. American Psychologist, 38, 1161–73.

Tindall, L. and Manthorpe, J. (1997) Early onset dementia: a case of ill-timing. Journal of Mental Health, 6, 3, 237–49.

Tolhurst, E., Bhattacharyya, S. and Kingston, P. (2014) Young onset dementia: the impact of emergent age-based factors upon personhood. Dementia (London), 13, 2, 193–206.

Werner, P., Stein-Shvachman, I. and Korczyn, A.D. (2009) Early onset dementia: clinical and social aspects. International Psychogeriatrics, 21, 4, 631–6.

Whalley, L. (1997) Early Onset Dementia. In S. Hunter (ed.) Dementia: Challenges and New Directions. Research Highlights in Social Work No. 31. London: Jessica Kingsley Publishers.

Williams, D.D.R. (1995) Services for younger sufferers of Alzheimer's disease. British Journal of Psychiatry, 166, 699–700.

Chapter 6

DELIRIUM AND LIVING BETTER WITH DEMENTIA

'I pause to record that I feel in extraordinary form. Delirium perhaps.'

Samuel Beckett, *Malone Dies* (1956)

Introduction

The word 'delirium' comes from the Latin *delirare*. In its Latin form, the word means to become 'crazy' or 'to rave'. Delirium has many synonyms, which include acute brain failure, acute organic brain syndrome, acute confusional state and postoperative psychosis. However, delirium is now the preferred term (Gill and Mayou, 2012; Saxena and Lawley, 2009). There would appear to be several reasons. MacLullich and Hall (2011) report that patients rarely speak of their experiences of delirium, perhaps because of embarrassment or bewilderment; and, currently, there are no specific charities or patient advocacy groups.

It is generally thought that dementia fractionates into different subtypes, with work on phenomenology mostly for psychomotor activity; classifications of hyperactive type (15–29%), hypoactive type (19–43%), mixed type (43–52%) and no psychomotor disturbance (0–14%) have been proposed in the elderly (O'Keeffe, 1999). Accordingly, some feel that there is still a need to improve understanding of the pathophysiology of delirium and the efficacy of specific drug therapy in delirium subtypes, with the subtext that these complexities may not successfully be encapsulated in a single clinical guideline (Tahir, Morgan and

Eeles, 2011). Despite an enhanced spotlight on scrutiny, it is striking that one of the most obvious questions remains unanswered: 'How common is delirium and what are its adverse outcomes in people in long term care?' (National Institute for Health and Care Excellence, 2010).

The past decade has witnessed considerable advances in our understanding of how to prevent and manage delirium. Despite its clinical importance, there is little documentation regarding delirium prevalence and physician detection rates within the emergency setting (Barron and Holmes, 2013). In a recent paper, Wong and colleagues (2010) systematically review the evidence on the accuracy of bedside instruments in diagnosing delirium in adults in hospital inpatients. Following operations for hip fracture in the elderly, delirium is common, with the incidence varying between 16 and 62% (O'Keeffe and Chonchurhair, 1994).

The emergence of the European Delirium Association and the American Delirium Society can foster and support research while advocating improved delirium care (O'Hanlon *et al.*, 2014). Much delirium is undetected or misdiagnosed in acute hospitals (Barron and Holmes, 2013). Delirium is a serious neuropsychiatric syndrome, with considerable heterogeneity, characterised by acute and fluctuating inattention, other cognitive deficits and alterations in level of consciousness (American Psychiatric Association, 2000). Core features include disturbance of consciousness, disturbance of cognition, rapid onset, fluctuating course and external causation (the syndrome can be attributed to an independently diagnosable cerebral or systemic disease or disorder) (National Institute for Health and Care Excellence, 2010).

Delirium is often experienced in the light of significant co-morbidity. With treatment of the illness, some individuals recover from delirium, while for others the symptoms persist. It is not understood why some individuals improve but others do not (Dasgupta and Hillier, 2010). Delirium affects 11–30% of hospitalised older patients (Siddiqi, House and Holmes, 2006). It has been suggested that delirium represents a marker for increased risk of dementia, but the mechanism for this at present is uncertain (Rockwood *et al.*, 1999). Two possibilities for this might be that delirium is a form of 'aberrant brain repair' (Davies, 1994) or a sub-clinical form of dementia (Persson and Skoog, 1992). I will be returning to co-morbidity in two major ways in the rest of my book: first, Chapter 10 on whole-person care and, second, my conclusion in Chapter 18.

The overall literature suggests some common predisposing factors for delirium, listed in Box 6.1.

Box 6.1 Possible predisposing factors for delirium

* Alcohol misuse
* Co-morbidity
* Cognitive decline
* Decreased oral intake (dehydration, malnutrition)
* Demographic characteristics (> 65 years)
* Environmental disturbances
* History of stroke
* History of surgery, 'insults' or trauma
* Infection
* Polypharmacy
* Previous episode of delirium
* Sensory impairment
* Sleep deprivation

Source: Adapted from Hein et al., 2014; Hölttä et al., 2014; Laurila et al., 2008; Inouye, Westendorp and Saczynski, 2014; Saxena and Lawley, 2009

Delirium is independently associated with several adverse outcomes, including elevated costs, increased length of stay, long-term cognitive and functional decline, increased risk of institutionalisation, higher mortality, reduced functional independence, and patient and carer distress (Trzepacz, Meagher and Leonard, 2010; Witlox *et al.*, 2010). Ward, Perera and Stewart (2014) demonstrated a substantially raised mortality in people with delirium seen in routine mental health care, and defined subgroups at particularly high risk, but the obvious key question remains what can be done to prevent this increased risk of mortality. Remedial action, such as explanatory information to patients and their families, may reduce distress and psychological morbidity (Partridge *et al.*, 2013). Recognition of delirium will inevitably improve outcomes, most people agree (e.g. Inouye *et al.*, 2001). For these reasons, detection is important. It is possible that the lack of detection of delirium may be, in part, due to problems with training in clinical practice in screening tests (see, for example, Young and Arseven, 2010). Routine delirium screening could improve delirium detection, but it remains unclear as to which screening tool is most suitable.

A wide range of neuropsychiatric symptoms distinguish delirium from dementia. Spatial span forward is disproportionately diminished in delirium, suggesting usefulness as a differentiating screening test (Meagher *et al.*, 2010). So it is therefore unsurprising that attention has really focused on not missing cases of delirium. 'Subsyndromal delirium' has an increasing relevance in the medical literature, but there had been until recently only three studies in hospitalised elderly patients (Velilla *et al.*, 2012). Patients with core symptoms of delirium not reaching full syndromal criteria (subsyndromal delirium) experience outcomes similar to those for the full syndromal illness (Marcantonio *et al.*, 2005; Meagher and Leonard, 2008). Previously, it had been reported that up to two-thirds of ICU delirium cases are missed if a validated screening tool is not used. Several scales were found by Morandi and colleagues (2013) in their sampling of members of the European Delirium Association. The most popular instrument used to assess delirium is the Confusion Assessment Method (CAM) (52%).

The notion of 'delirium readiness' emerged a long time ago (Henry and Mann, 1965). The National Institute for Health and Care Excellence (2010) helpfully identify risk factors for delirium in their guidance. In their review, NHS Evidence (National Institute for Health and Care Excellence, 2012) found that there had been no change in their advice that specific groups of medications may be potential risk factors for development of delirium, but they did concede that evidence is currently limited and further research is required. In an older person undergoing acute medical admission, polypharmacy, poor vision, low albumin and having a urinary catheter indicate vulnerability to developing delirium (Ahmed, Leurent and Sampson, 2014). One thing is pretty certain, though. Delirium risk is closely linked to pharmacological factors that include polypharmacy in general, sudden withdrawal of certain classes of drugs and administration of particular deliriogenic agent classes, with anticholinergic agents, benzodiazepines and opioid medications consistently implicated across clinical populations (Clegg and Young, 2011). Clinical guidelines to manage delirium are provided by the British Geriatrics Society (2006). It is emphasised by Saxena and Lawley (2009) that nursing supportive measures include maintaining the patient's airway, volume status through the correction and prevention of dehydration, ensuring adequate nutrition, providing skin care to prevent sores, and mobilisation to prevent deep vein thrombosis and pulmonary embolism.

CQUIN: the Commissioning for Quality and Innovation framework

A high proportion of older people in acute hospital settings have dementia, with one study suggesting that incidence may be as high as 42.4% (Sampson *et al.*, 2009).

The Department of Health has increased the emphasis on earlier detection of dementia among patients aged over 75 admitted to hospital in an emergency in England. The Department of Health has estimated that only 42% of those living in England with likely dementia have a formal diagnosis, and has expressed its commitment to achieving better and more timely diagnosis rates (Department of Health, 2013).

The introduction of a Commissioning for Quality and Innovation (CQUIN) payment provides an incentive for NHS Trusts to screen patients for memory problems on admission. The key aim of the CQUIN framework for 2014/15 is to support improvements in the quality of services and the creation of new, improved patterns of care (NHS England, 2014). It is argued that primary care practitioners often feel unable to manage or diagnose dementia, with limited awareness of the National Dementia Strategy (Department of Health, 2009) and with significant numbers of dementia-related admissions to acute hospitals referred via general practitioners (National Audit Office, 2010). One major 'positive' of this initiative, it is argued, is that it is reported that people with dementia have felt more valued by the system.

According to Kristensen, McDonald and Sutton (2013), local design was intended to offer flexibility to local priorities and generate local enthusiasm, while retaining good design properties of focusing on outcomes and processes with a clear link to quality, using established indicators where possible. But the authors concluded:

> Balancing the policy goal of localism with the objective of improving patient outcomes leads us to conclude that a somewhat firmer national framework would be preferable to a fully locally designed framework. (p.38)

CQUIN is, nonetheless, intended to complement the approach to the NHS payment system, providing a coherent set of national rules. This approach was consistent with the conclusions from NHS England's review of incentives, rewards and sanctions, based on the principle of a national default position, but with freedom, support and encouragement for genuine innovation (NHS England, 2014). NHS England was firmly committed to supporting the full implementation of the recommendations set out in 'Innovation, Health and Wealth: Accelerating Adoption and Diffusion in the NHS' (NHS England, 2011). Specifically, providers will be required, as part of their NHS Standard Contract, to agree an action plan for innovation during 2014–15. Full details of the contractual requirements in this respect can be found in the NHS Standard Contract 2014–15 and supporting guidance.

In summary, the goal of the CQUIN for delirium and dementia was to incentivise the identification of patients with dementia and delirium, alone and in combination with their other medical conditions, to prompt appropriate referral and follow-up after they leave hospital and to ensure that hospitals deliver high-quality care to people with dementia and support their carers.

The relationship between delirium and subsequent cognitive decline

It is hypothesised that delirium can accelerate the trajectory of cognitive decline in patients with dementia of the Alzheimer type. It has indeed been found that a significant acceleration in the slope of cognitive decline occurs following an episode of delirium, and suggests that future randomised intervention studies to determine whether prevention of delirium might ameliorate or delay cognitive decline in patients with dementia of the Alzheimer type would be useful (Fong *et al.*, 2009). This might be somehow related to the issue of 'cognitive reserve'. In his most recent review, Stern (2012) articulates two models of reserve pertaining to neurocognitive functioning: brain and cognitive. 'Brain reserve' refers to structural aspects of the brain, and cognitive reserve relates to how cognitive tasks are initiated and coordinated, involving access to complex cognitive networks. I will refer to this again in my Conclusion (Chapter 18).

Mills, Minhas and Robotham (2014) have indeed argued, in the reality of clinical practice, that many patients on an elderly care ward admitted acutely, who have not been diagnosed with dementia formally, may in fact be showing the early signs of memory difficulties. Ahmed and colleagues (2014) very helpfully conducted a meta-analysis of relevant data to ascertain the risk factors for incident delirium among older people in acute hospital medical units. Eleven articles met their inclusion criteria and were included for review. The commonest factors significantly associated with delirium were dementia, older age, co-morbid illness, severity of medical illness, infection, 'high-risk' medication use, diminished activities of daily living, immobility, sensory impairment, urinary catheterisation, urea and electrolyte imbalance, and malnutrition delirium.

National Institute for Health and Care Excellence and delirium

The National Institute for Health and Care Excellence (NICE) recommendations are based on systematic reviews of best available evidence and explicit consideration of cost-effectiveness. When minimal evidence is available, recommendations are based on the experience of the Guideline Development Group and their opinion of what constitutes good practice (Young *et al.*, 2010). Several potential benefits of guidelines have been noted, including benefits to patients through improved health outcomes on an individual level, along with shaping public policy at a 'macro level' (Bush *et al.*, 2014). NICE suggests screening for possible delirium based on four risk factors: age 65 or over, dementia, presentation with hip fracture and severity of illness (Young *et al.*, 2010).

However, these recommendations were developed from studies of a wide range of clinical populations recruited from surgical, intensive care and general medical settings. Furthermore, due to a relative current lack of large, multi-centre trials in this field, it would have been prudent for NICE to have relaxed the strict exclusion criteria of any randomised controlled trial with fewer than 20 patients in each arm and integrated the results of smaller, yet significant, studies (Tahir *et al.*, 2011). It is important to recognise that delirium risk factors may differ between medical and surgical patients where the latter are exposed to iatrogenic factors such as anaesthetic agents or surgical procedures (Ahmed *et al.*, 2014). Other predictive models for delirium in older people with general medical admission include a wider range of factors such as malnutrition, use of a urinary catheter and physical restraints (Inouye and Charpentier, 1996). Weiner (2012) indeed identified that patients who had developed delirium maintained a more rapid rate of cognitive deterioration throughout a five-year period following hospitalisation.

There are still substantial uncertainties over best practice in delirium care. The European Delirium Association (EDA) conducted a survey of its members and other interested parties on various aspects of delirium care. The invitation to participate in the online survey was distributed among the EDA membership. The survey covered assessment, treatment of hyperactive and hypoactive delirium, and organisational management. The results have been reported by Morandi and colleagues (2013). A total of 200 responses were collected.

The NICE guidelines (National Institute for Health and Care Excellence, 2010) provided recommendations on non-pharmacological and pharmacological interventions for delirium treatment, without differentiating between the hyperactive and hypoactive form. The guidelines suggested that there should first be a non-pharmacological approach, identifying and managing underlying causes, providing reorientation and involving family and carers. These guidelines, furthermore, reported information only on extrapyramidal signs as side effects of antipsychotics, but there is no mention of the cardiac effects and the need for electrocardiogram monitoring. A recent study has found that haloperidol, risperidone, aripiprazole and olanzapine were equally effective in the management of delirium; however, they differed in terms of their side-effect profile (Boettger, Jenewein and Breitbart, 2014).

Interestingly, the NICE guidelines did not mention follow-up after an episode of delirium, although an association between delirium, cognitive impairment and worsening dementia has been reported (Davis *et al.*, 2012; Girard *et al.*, 2010). In their cohort of responders from the European Delirium Association, Morandi and colleagues (2013) found different approaches but, most importantly, 60% of responders follow up patients after an episode of delirium, and, even more interestingly, in almost 7% of the cases there are dedicated delirium follow-up clinics. The importance of referring patients with cognitive impairment/dementia to a memory clinic has been shown previously (Morgan *et al.*, 2009). Intriguingly, Davis and colleagues (2012) report that dementia following delirium may not be as strongly linked with classical dementia neuropathological markers as dementia in those without a history of delirium; clearly further work is needed in this area.

Prophylaxis of delirium

Reducing delirium is important because of the considerable distress it causes and the poor outcomes associated with it, such as increased admissions to hospital, falls, mortality and costs to the National Health Service (Heaven *et al.*, 2014). In a recent study by Hein and colleagues (2014), polypharmacy is an independent risk factor for delirium in a population of elderly patients after emergency admission. Pharmacological delirium prevention currently seems promising.

Improving delirium care and financial incentives

International interest in using financial incentives to improve quality of care is growing (McDonald *et al.*, 2007). One of the ways health systems worldwide strive to improve quality in health care is by the use of 'pay for performance', linking quality targets to provider revenues. The impact of financial incentives designed at a policy level is influenced by the understanding of costs and benefits at the local operational level (Abma *et al.*, 2014). In 2004 general practitioners in the United Kingdom were given substantial financial incentives to meet a range of clinical and organisational targets, known as the quality and outcomes framework (Roland, 2004).

McDonald and colleagues (2007) found that nurses expressed more concern than doctors about changes to their clinical practice but also appreciated being given responsibility for delivering on targets in particular disease areas; most doctors did not question the quality targets that existed at the time or the implications of the targets for their own clinical autonomy. This is generally consistent with the current wider literature. Incentives might result in diminished provider professionalism, neglect of patients for whom quality targets are perceived to be more difficult to achieve, and widening of health inequalities (McDonald *et al.*, 2007). Doctors might also focus on the conditions linked to incentives and neglect other conditions, or, where certain activities are incentivised within the management of a particular condition, might neglect other activities for patients with that condition (Doran *et al.*, 2011).

Living better after delirium

In contrast to the available studies linking a history of delirium to cognitive decline, there is an overall paucity of research prospectively studying long-term outcomes in people who experience an episode of delirium (Kalaria and Mukaetova-Ladinska, 2012). An important implication of recent research is that the traditional concept of delirium as a highly reversible condition may not be borne out in practice, where many patients experience persistent illness and/or longer-term cognitive impairment (MacLullich *et al.*, 2009).

Efforts are restricted by a lack of clarity as to what represents recovery in delirium, and in real-world practice many delirious patients are discharged to post-acute facilities and nursing homes before full resolution of symptoms (Marcantonio *et al.*, 2005). Subjects with delirium were more likely to experience one or more complications than subjects with no delirium (73% vs 41%). Within 30 days of post-acute admission, subjects with delirium were more than twice as likely to be rehospitalised (30% vs 13%), and less than half as likely to be discharged to the community (30% vs 73%), than subjects without delirium. Distress is particularly linked to the experience of psychosis and psychomotor disturbance (Breitbart, Gibson and Tremblay, 2002). The psychological aftermath of delirium is under-studied, but around 50% of patients can recall the episode and in many cases are still distressed by their recollections six months later (O'Malley *et al.*, 2008). Follow-up visits can facilitate post-delirium adjustment by allowing for discussion of the meaning of delirium and planning of how to minimise future risk (e.g. by addressing risk factors such as medication exposure and sensory impairments) (O'Hanlon *et al.*, 2014).

The mechanisms underlying the association between delirium and dementia are under-researched in humans. Post-mortem studies have raised the intriguing possibility that the processes linking delirium and dementia may not be mediated by classical dementia pathology (Davis *et al.*, 2012); these findings are the first to demonstrate in a true population study that delirium is a strong risk factor for incident dementia and cognitive decline in the oldest-old. It is likely that inflammatory pathways are important given the evidence from animal studies (Cunningham *et al.*, 2009). Chronic neurodegeneration results in microglial activation, but the contribution of inflammation to the progress of neurodegeneration remains unclear. It is becoming increasingly apparent that infections and other systemic inflammatory conditions do increase the risk of dementia of the Alzheimer type and accelerate the progression of established dementia (Cunningham, 2011; Cunningham *et al.*, 2009).

Patients with co-morbid conditions characterised by progressive supranuclear palsy and dementia of the Alzheimer type may exhibit prominent bouts of delirium along with emotional and personality changes (Sakamoto *et al.*, 2009). Gore and colleagues (2014) have observed that delirium and dementia of Lewy body (DLB) type share a number of features, and they hypothesise on a number of converging sources, including from neuroimaging, that delirium may, in some cases, represent early or 'prodromal' DLB. In the study by Vardy and colleagues (2014), 25% of DLB cases had at least one reported episode of suspected delirium, compared with 7% of the cases of dementia of the Alzheimer type. For the DLB cases who had a prior suspected delirium, 23% had more than one episode compared with 14% of the dementia of the Alzheimer-type group. These authors suggested that delirium may lead to a higher risk of DLB as opposed to other forms of dementia, or delirium may, at least in some cases, represent the early stages of DLB.

Delirium is also a frequent occurrence after stroke – episodes being diagnosed in 20% of ischaemic stroke patients aged 55–85 years and associated with dementia at three months in approximately half of those affected, with age and severity of stroke injury leading to increased long-term mortality in patients who have experienced delirium (Melkas *et al.*, 2011). Postoperative cognitive impairment associated with delirium may be transient, but persistent cognitive decline (beyond three months after surgical treatments) has also been demonstrated in a number of studies (Hovens *et al.*, 2012). Furthermore, delirium superimposed on dementia (DSD) may warrant especial attention. Morandi and colleagues (2014) undertook a study to examine association between DSD and related adverse outcomes at discharge from rehabilitation and at one-year follow-up in older in-patients undergoing rehabilitation, and found that DSD is a strong predictor of functional dependence, institutionalisation and mortality in older patients admitted to a rehabilitation setting, leading them to suggest that strategies to detect DSD routinely in practice should be developed and DSD should be included in prognostic models of health care. However, it is felt that, currently, the evidence base on tools for detection of DSD is limited, although some existing tools show some promise (Morandi *et al.*, 2012). Despite the fact that delirium in people with dementia is common, serious and costly, there is yet to be a convincing body of published reports on the use of the electronic medical record in any jurisdiction for delirium detection and management (Fick *et al.*, 2011).

This particular policy strand is definitely one to watch.

Conclusion

As Professor Alistair Burns, England's clinical lead for dementia, has repeatedly emphasised, with others, a person given a diagnosis of dementia is never given that diagnosis on his or her own. That person is not an island but exists in a community, in the nearest vicinity of which are close friends and family. It is, perhaps, too simplistic to think that the person who has received a diagnosis exists in a 'dyadic' relationship with a carer or a 'triadic' one with a professional included. A person with dementia is likely to rely on care and support from a changing ecosystem of individuals at different junctures in his or her personal 'journey' (a term which many dislike). The dynamic nature of care and support networks might be a more productive way of conceptualising the immediate dementia-friendly community of a person living with dementia. The relative strengths of ties and links between these actors and the person living with dementia is likely, in computational connective terms, to affect the output. And what might the output be? One form of output is clearly the quality of life of the person with dementia. But, more concretely, that output might be the personalised care plan so crucial to the function of whole-person care.

I would like to consider, first, in Chapter 7, care and support networks.

References

Abma, I., Jayanti, A., Bayer, S., Mitra, S. and Barlow, J. (2014) Perceptions and experiences of financial incentives: a qualitative study of dialysis care in England. BMJ Open, 4, 2, e004249.

Ahmed, S., Leurent, B. and Sampson, E.L. (2014) Risk factors for incident delirium among older people in acute hospital medical units: a systematic review and meta-analysis. Age and Ageing, 43, 3, 326–33.

American Psychiatric Association (2000) Diagnostic and Statistical Manual of Mental Disorders, 4th edition. Washington, DC: American Psychiatric Association.

Barron, E.A. and Holmes, J. (2013) Delirium within the emergency care setting, occurrence and detection: a systematic review. Emergency Medicine Journal, 30, 4, 263–8.

Boettger, S., Jenewein, J. and Breitbart, W. (2014) Haloperidol, risperidone, olanzapine and aripiprazole in the management of delirium: a comparison of efficacy, safety, and side effects. Palliative Support Care, 5, 1–7 [Epub ahead of print].

Breitbart, W., Gibson, C. and Tremblay, A. (2002) The delirium experience: delirium recall and delirium-related distress in hospitalized patients with cancer, their spouses/caregivers, and their nurses. Psychosomatics, 43, 183–94.

British Geriatrics Society (2006) Guidelines for the prevention, diagnosis and management of delirium in older people in hospital. Available at www.bgs.org.uk/index.php/clinicalguides/170-clinguidedeliriumtreatment (accessed 10 February 2015).

Bush, S.H., Bruera, E., Lawlor, P.G., Kanji, S. *et al.* (2014) Clinical practice guidelines for delirium management: potential application in palliative care. Journal of Pain and Symptom Management, 48, 2, 249–58.

Clegg, A. and Young, J.B. (2011) Which medications to avoid in people at risk of delirium: a systematic review. Age and Ageing, 40, 23–9.

Cunningham, C. (2011) Systemic inflammation and delirium: important co-factors in the progression of dementia. Biochemical Society Transactions, 39, 4, 945–53.

Cunningham, C., Campion, S., Lunnon, K., Murray, C.L. *et al.* (2009) Systemic inflammation induces acute behavioural and cognitive changes and accelerates neurodegenerative disease. Biological Psychiatry, 65, 4, 304–12.

Dasgupta, M. and Hillier, L.M. (2010) Factors associated with prolonged delirium: a systematic review. International Psychogeriatrics, 22, 3, 373–94.

Davies, P. (1994) Neuronal Abnormalities, Not Amyloid, are the Cause of Dementia in Alzheimer's Disease. In R.D. Terry, R. Katzman and K.I. Bick (eds) Alzheimer Disease. New York, NY: Raven Press.

Davis, D.H., Muniz Terrera, G., Keage, H., Rahkonen, T. *et al.* (2012) Delirium is a strong risk factor for dementia in the oldest-old: a population-based cohort study. Brain, 135, 9, 2809–16.

Department of Health (2009) Living Well with Dementia: a national dementia strategy. Available at www.gov.uk/government/publications/living-well-with-dementia-a-national-dementia-strategy (accessed 6 December 2014).

Department of Health (2013) Improving care for people with dementia. Available at www.gov.uk/government/policies/improving-care-for-people-with-dementia (accessed 6 December 2014).

Doran, T., Kontopantelis, E., Valderas, J.M., Campbell, S. *et al.* (2011) Effect of financial incentives on incentivised and non-incentivised clinical activities: longitudinal analysis of data from the UK Quality and Outcomes Framework. British Medical Journal, 342, d3590.

Fick, D.M., Steis, M.R., Mion, L.C. and Walls, J.L. (2011) Computerized decision support for delirium superimposed on dementia in older adults. Journal of Gerontological Nursing, 37, 4, 39–47.

Fong, T.G., Jones, R.N., Shi, P., Marcantonio, E.R. *et al.* (2009) Delirium accelerates cognitive decline in Alzheimer disease. Neurology, 72, 18, 1570–5.

Gill, D. and Mayou, R. (2012) Delirium. In M.G. Gelder, J.J. Lopóz-Ibor Jr, N.C. Andreasen and J.R. Geddes (eds) New Oxford Textbook of Psychiatry. Oxford: Oxford University Press.

Girard, T.D., Jackson, J.C., Pandharipande, P.P., Pun, B.T. *et al.* (2010) Delirium as a predictor of long-term cognitive impairment in survivors of critical illness. Critical Care Medicine, 38, 1513–20.

Gore, R.L., Vardy, E.R. and O'Brien, J.T. (2014) Delirium and dementia with Lewy bodies: distinct diagnoses or part of the same spectrum? Journal of Neurology, Neurosurgery and Psychiatry, pii, jnnp-2013 306389 [Epub ahead of print].

Heaven, A., Cheater, F., Clegg, A., Collinson, M. *et al.* (2014) Pilot trial of Stop Delirium! (PiTStop): a complex intervention to prevent delirium in care homes for older people: study protocol for a cluster randomised controlled trial. Trials, 15, 47.

Hein, C., Forgues, A., Piau, A., Sommet, A., Vellas, B. and Nourhashémi, F. (2014) Impact of polypharmacy on occurrence of delirium in elderly emergency patients. Journal of the American Medical Directors Association, 15, 11, 850.e11–15.

Henry, W.D. and Mann, A.M. (1965) Diagnosis and treatment of delirium. Canadian Medical Association Journal, 93, 1156–66.

Hölttä, E.H., Laurila, J.V., Laakkonen, M.L., Strandberg, T.E., Tilvis, R.S. and Pitkala, K.H. (2014) Precipitating factors of delirium: stress response to multiple triggers among patients with and without dementia. Experimental Gerontology, 59, 42–46.

Hovens, I.B., Schoemaker, R.G., van der Zee, E.A., Heineman, E., Izaks, G.J. and van Leeuwen, B.L. (2012) Thinking through postoperative cognitive dysfunction: how to bridge the gap between clinical and pre-clinical perspectives. Brain, Behavior, and Immunity, 26, 7, 1169–79.

Inouye, S.K. and Charpentier, P.A. (1996) Precipitating factors for delirium in hospitalized elderly persons: predictive model and interrelationship with baseline vulnerability. Journal of the American Medical Association, 275, 852–7.

Inouye, S.K., Foreman, M.D., Mion, L.C., Katz, K.H. and Cooney, L.M. Jr (2001) Nurses' recognition of delirium and its symptoms: comparison of nurse and researcher ratings. Archives of Internal Medicine, 161, 2467–73.

Inouye, S.K., Westendorp, R.G. and Saczynski, J.S. (2014) Delirium in elderly people. Lancet, 383, 9920, 911–922.

Kalaria, R.N. and Mukaetova-Ladinska, E.B. (2012) Delirium, dementia and senility. Brain, 135, 9, 2582–4.

Kristensen, S.R., McDonald, R. and Sutton, M. (2013) Should pay-for-performance schemes be locally designed? Evidence from the Commissioning for Quality and Innovation (CQUIN) Framework. Journal of Health Service Research and Policy, 18, 2 Suppl., 38–49.

Laurila, J.V., Laakkonen, M.L., Strandberg, T.E. and Tilvis, R.S. (2008) Predisposing and precipitating factors for delirium in a frail geriatric population. Journal of Psychosomatic Research, 65, 249–254.

MacLullich, A.M. and Hall, R.J. (2011) Who understands delirium? Age and Ageing, 40, 4, 412–14.

MacLullich, A.M., Beaglehole, A., Hall, R.J. and Meagher, D.J. (2009) Delirium and long-term cognitive impairment. International Review of Psychiatry, 21, 1, 30–42.

Marcantonio, E.R., Kiely, D.K., Simon, S.E., John Orav, E. *et al.* (2005) Outcomes of older people admitted to postacute facilities with delirium. Journal of the American Geriatrics Society, 53, 6, 963–9.

McDonald, R., Harrison, S., Checkland, K., Campbell, S. and Roland, M. (2007) Impact of financial incentives on clinical autonomy and internal motivation in primary care: ethnographic study. British Medical Journal, 334, 1357–62.

Meagher, D. and Leonard, M. (2008) The active management of delirium: improving detection and treatment. Advances in Psychiatric Treatment, 14, 292–301.

Meagher, D., Leonard, M., Donnelly, S., Conroy, M., Saunders, J. and Trzepacz, P.T. (2010) A comparison of neuropsychiatric and cognitive profiles in delirium, dementia, co-morbid delirium-dementia and cognitively intact controls. Journal of Neurology, Neurosurgery and Psychiatry, 81, 8, 876–81.

Melkas, S., Laurila, J.V., Vataja, R., Oksala, N. *et al.* (2011) Post-stroke delirium in relation to dementia and long-term mortality. International Journal of Geriatric Psychiatry, 27, 401–8.

Mills, J.K., Minhas, J.S. and Robotham, S.L. (2014) An assessment of the dementia CQUIN – an audit of improving compliance. Dementia (London), 13, 5, 697–703.

Morandi, A., Davis, D., Fick, D.M., Turco, R. *et al.* (2014) Delirium superimposed on dementia strongly predicts worse outcomes in older rehabilitation inpatients. Journal of the American Medical Directors Association, Neurology, 72, 18, 1570–5.

Morandi, A., Davis, D., Taylor, J.K., Bellelli, G. *et al.* (2013) Consensus and variations in opinions on delirium care: a survey of European delirium specialists. International Psychogeriatrics, 25, 12, 2067–75.

Morandi, A., McCurley, J., Vasilevskis, E.E., Fick, D.M. *et al.* (2012) Tools to detect delirium superimposed on dementia: a systematic review. Journal of the American Geriatrics Society, 60, 11, 2005–13.

Morgan, D.G., Crossley, M., Kirk, A., D'Arcy, C. *et al.* (2009) Improving access to dementia care: development and evaluation of a rural and remote memory clinic. Aging and Mental Health, 13, 1, 17–30.

National Audit Office (2010) Improving dementia services in England – an Interim Report. London: The Stationery Office. Available at www.nao.org.uk/wp-content/uploads/2010/01/091082.pdf (accessed 10 February 2015).

National Institute for Health and Care Excellence (2010) Delirium: diagnosis, prevention and management. NICE clinical guideline 103. Available at www.nice.org.uk/guidance/cg103/resources/guidance-delirium-pdf (accessed 6 December 2014).

National Institute for Health and Care Excellence (2012) Delirium: Evidence Update April 2012. A summary of selected new evidence relevant to NICE clinical guideline 103 'Delirium: diagnosis, prevention and management' (2010). Available at www.evidence.nhs.uk/search?q=Delirium+evidence+update (accessed 6 December 2014).

NHS England (2011) Innovation, Health and Wealth: Accelerating Adoption and Diffusion in the NHS. Available at http://webarchive.nationalarchives.gov.uk/20130107105354/http://www.dh.gov.uk/prod_consum_dh/groups/dh_digitalassets/documents/digitalasset/dh_134597.pdf (accessed 6 December 2014).

NHS England (2014) Commissioning for Quality and Innovation (CQUIN): 2014/15 guidance. Available at www.england.nhs.uk/wp-content/uploads/2014/02/sc-cquin-guid.pdf (accessed 6 December 2014).

O'Hanlon, S., O'Regan, N., Maclullich, A.M., Cullen, W. *et al.* (2014) Improving delirium care through early intervention: from bench to bedside to boardroom. Journal of Neurology, Neurosurgery and Psychiatry, 85, 2, 207–13.

O'Keeffe, S.T. (1999) Clinical subtypes of delirium in the elderly. Dem Geriatric Cognitive Disorders, 10, 380–5.

O'Keeffe, S.T. and Chonchurhair, N.A. (1994) Postoperative delirium in the elderly. British Journal of Anaesthesia, 73, 5, 709P–724P (182 ref.), 673–87.

O'Malley, G., Leonard, M., Meagher, D. and O'Keeffe, S.T. (2008) The delirium experience: a review. Journal of Psychosomatic Research, 65, 3, 223–8.

Partridge, J.S., Martin, F.C., Harari, D. and Dhesi, J.K. (2013) The delirium experience: what is the effect on patients, relatives and staff and what can be done to modify this? International Journal of Geriatric Psychiatry, 28, 8, 804–12.

Persson, G. and Skoog, I. (1992) Subclinical dementia: relevance of cognitive symptoms and signs. Journal of Geriatric Psychiatry and Neurology, 5, 3, 172–8.

Rockwood, K., Cosway, S., Carver, D., Jarrett, P., Stadnyk, K. and Fisk, J. (1999) The risk of dementia and death after delirium. Age and Ageing, 28, 6, 551–6.

Roland, M. (2004) Linking physician pay to quality of care: a major experiment in the UK. New England Journal of Medicine, 351, 1448–54.

Sakamoto, R., Tsuchiya, K., Yoshida, R., Itoh, Y. *et al.* (2009) Progressive supranuclear palsy combined with Alzheimer's disease: a clinicopathological study of two autopsy cases. Neuropathology, 29, 219–29.

Sampson, E.L., Blanchard, M.R., Jones, L., Tookman, A. and King, M. (2009) Dementia in the acute hospital: prospective cohort study of prevalence and mortality. British Journal of Psychiatry, 195, 1, 61–6.

Saxena, S. and Lawley, D. (2009) Delirium in the elderly: a clinical review. Postgraduate Medicine Journal, 85, 1006, 405–13.

Siddiqi, N., House, A.O. and Holmes, J.D. (2006) Occurrence and outcome of delirium in medical in-patients: a systematic literature review. Age and Ageing, 35, 350–64.

Stern, Y. (2012) Cognitive reserve in ageing and Alzheimer's disease. Lancet Neurology, 11, 11, 1006–12.

Tahir, T.A., Morgan, E. and Eeles, E. (2011) NICE guideline: evidence for pharmacological treatment of delirium. Journal of Psychosomatic Research, 70, 2, 197–8.

Trzepacz, P.T., Meagher, D. and Leonard, M. (2010) Delirium. In J. Levenson (ed.) Textbook of Psychosomatic Medicine. Washington, DC: American Psychiatric Press.

Vardy, E., Holt, R., Gerhard, A., Richardson, A., Snowden, J. and Neary, D. (2014) History of a suspected delirium is more common in dementia with Lewy bodies than Alzheimer's disease: a retrospective study. International Journal of Geriatric Psychiatry, 29, 2, 178–81.

Velilla, N.M., Bouzon, C.A., Contin, K.C., Beroiz, B.I., Herrero, A.C. and Renedo, J.A. (2012) Different functional outcomes in patients with delirium and subsyndromal delirium one month after hospital discharge. Dementia and Geriatric Cognitive Disorders, 34, 5–6, 332–6.

Ward, G., Perera, G. and Stewart, R. (2014) Predictors of mortality for people aged over 65 years receiving mental health care for delirium in a South London Mental Health Trust, UK: a retrospective survival analysis. International Journal of Geriatric Psychiatry, doi: 10.1002/gps.4195 [Epub ahead of print].

Weiner, M.F. (2012) Impact of delirium on the course of Alzheimer disease. Archives of Neurology, 69, 12, 1639–40.

Witlox, J., Eurelings, L.S., de Jonghe, J.F., Kalisvaart, K.J., Eikelenboom, P. and van Gool, W.A. (2010) Delirium in elderly patients and the risk of postdischarge mortality, institutionalization, and dementia: a meta-analysis. Journal of the American Medical Association, 304, 4, 443–51.

Wong, C.L., Holroyd-Leduc, J., Simel, D.L. and Straus, S.E. (2010) Does this patient have delirium? Value of bedside instruments. Journal of the American Medical Association, 304, 7, 779–86.

Young, J., Murthy, L., Westby, M., Akunne, A. and O'Mahony, R. (Guideline Development Group) (2010) Diagnosis, prevention, and management of delirium: summary of NICE guidance. British Medical Journal, 341, c3704.

Young, R.S. and Arseven, A. (2010) Diagnosing delirium. Journal of the American Medical Association, 304, 2125–6.

Chapter 7

CARE AND SUPPORT NETWORKS FOR LIVING BETTER WITH DEMENTIA

'If you find it in your heart to care for somebody else, you will have succeeded.'

Maya Angelou

Introduction

Given the prevalence of dementia and the complexity of dementia care provision, it is undeniable that, historically, dementia service provision and the role of carers has been a relatively neglected issue (Innes, 2002). The reality is that, on receiving a diagnosis of possible dementia, many people find that their community of 'friends' collapses.

Care and support are therefore not synonymous, and careful attention must be put into the relative weights of these for a person living with dementia to avoid power potentially shifting away from a person with dementia in terms of autonomy and dignity. People living with dementia often have multiple co-morbidities, so real attention often has to be put into the accessibility and inclusivity of a physical environment. But in amongst all this discussion it is crucial to get the terminology correct – for example, many spouses of people living with dementia feel extremely uneasy with the term 'carer'.

Caregiving is defined as a chronic stress process that places the carer at risk for negative outcomes. Carers of people living with dementia must manage functional and cognitive impairment and often encounter behavioural problems and personality changes in the people for whom they care (Tooth *et al.*, 2008). Previous research has found that behaviour problems in dementia are more stressful for carers than dealing with the cognitive impairment or the need for assistance with activities of daily living (Kinney and Stephens, 1989).

Because behavioural symptoms shown by persons with dementia in later stages can have such a strong impact on stress and wellbeing, reducing behavioural and psychological symptoms is frequently the aim of interventions for people with dementia and their carers (Hinchliffe *et al.*, 1995). It is noteworthy that these concerns in policy extend to developing countries (Shaji *et al.*, 2009).

Person-centred care and relationship-centred care

There have been, historically, difficulties in defining the word 'carer'.

> The term carer is relatively new in health and social care, though the concept of what a carer is or does is more widely understood. Some people who care are relatives, and prefer to use the word 'relative' to describe themselves. Others have close friendships and are caring for people who are not relatives. Some do not accept that they are carers or even shun the concept. (Carers Trust, RCN, 2013)

At the time of writing this book, the direction of travel by the main political parties in England is a person-centred integrated approach. This is broadly defined thus:

> A person-centred health system is one that supports people to make informed decisions about, and to successfully manage, their own health and care, able to make informed decisions and choose when to invite others to act on their behalf. This requires healthcare services to work in partnership to deliver care responsive to people's individual abilities, preferences, lifestyles and goals. (Health Foundation, 2014, p.2)

A recent literature review and analysis detected four distinct categories of interpretation and usage of the phrase 'patient-centred' (Tanenbaum, 2013). The consumerist interpretation, by eliminating the personhood of the practitioner and reducing him or her to the status of a technical advisor and operator, potentially ignores the relational dimension entirely (Wyer and Silva, 2014). Indeed, Wyer and colleagues (2014) remark that 'coordination and defragmentation of care do not guarantee that the relational dimension of care will be maximized and may not be achievable without it' (p.1366). A systematic review of 43 randomised trials by Lewin and colleagues (2001) assessed the effects of interventions targeting healthcare professionals to promote person-centred care in clinical consultations. The authors concluded that training interventions generally had positive effects on consultation processes such as clarifying patients' concerns and beliefs, communicating about treatment options, levels of empathy, and patients' perception of providers' attentiveness to them and their concerns.

A timely diagnosis of dementia potentially offers carers the opportunity to advance the process of adaptation to the caregiving role. Carers who are better able to adapt to the changes that characterise dementia feel more competent to care and experience fewer psychological problems. However, drawbacks of an early diagnosis may outweigh the benefits if people are left with a diagnosis but little support (de Vugt and Verhey, 2013). Research that supports the persistence of personhood in the later stages of dementia of the Alzheimer type, for example, includes studies that describe periods when people with severe dementia unexpectedly talk or act in a way that reveals an awareness of their situation (Edvardsson, Winblad and Sandman, 2008). The person-centred care approach to dementia (Kitwood, 1990, 1993) also emphasises the personal psychology of an individual, and the social psychology of that individual as a human being in relation to others.

Relationship-centred care (Nolan *et al.*, 2004) considers the importance of connections between all people involved in the care process. For the person with dementia, a supportive and constructive social and interactional context can help to maintain functioning and maximise wellbeing (Kitwood, 1997a; Quinn, Clare and Woods, 2009). Attachment theory has been used as a framework to help understand the social and relational experiences of people with dementia and their carers. Kitwood's understanding of the effect of malignant social psychology upon people with dementia is primarily seen in terms of subjective experience and does not acknowledge the impact of wider social phenomena such as gender, citizenship and marginalisation upon people's experience of dementia (Bartlett, 2000; Bender, 2003).

The term 'person' denotes a holistic humanness and the equal value of individuals (McCormack, 2004), whereas 'patient' has been described as a reductionist, stigmatic term that imputes imperfections or undesired differentness to a person and thereby reduces the humanity of the subject (Goffman, 1968). This sense of 'differentness' is an extremely serious faultline in the policy of dementia-friendly communities, as currently articulated.

The need for a proper analysis of the role of relationships in health and social care was promoted by a major taskforce in the USA that advocated a vision of 'relationship-centred' care as follows:

> The phrase 'relationship-centred' care captures the importance of the interactions among people as the foundation of any therapeutic or teaching activity. Further, relationships are critical to the care provided by nearly all practitioners and a sense of satisfaction and positive outcomes for patients and practitioners. (Ryan *et al.*, 2008, p.78)

Recently, others have argued that, notwithstanding the importance placed upon person-centredness, relationship-centred care provides a more appropriate way of understanding important elements of successful services (Nolan, Davies and Grant, 2001; Nolan *et al.*, 2003, 2004). Others have also called for a more nuanced (inclusive) approach to dementia care but have criticised relationship-centred care and the experience of the senses for being too simplistic and for failing to describe how good relationships develop within dementia care triads (Adams and Gardiner, 2005). In considering how such positive relationships can be created and sustained, Nolan and colleagues have developed the 'Senses Framework' (Nolan *et al.*, 2001, 2003). In essence, this comprises six senses that are seen as prerequisites for good relationships within the context of care and service delivery. The fundamental premise of the vision of relationship-centred care is that good care can only be delivered when all the groups involved experience the senses.

Others have also called for a more inclusive approach to dementia care but have criticised relationship-centred care and the experience of senses for being too simplistic and for failing to describe how good relationships develop within dementia care triads (Adams and Gardiner, 2005). However, it is worth noting that the experience of senses has been developed over several years with the participation of hundreds of older people (some with dementia), family carers, practitioners and student nurses (Ryan *et al.*, 2008). While person-centred care is characterised by the need to value people with dementia, to treat them as individuals, to view the world from their perspective and to create a positive psychosocial environment, relationship-centred care promotes a rather more inclusive vision of dementia care practice and research (Nolan *et al.*, 2002). Inspiration in the English jurisdiction is being drawn from other jurisdictions. In Japan, which globally has the most aged population, there are efforts to create a society where people can lead a decent life even after a diagnosis of dementia; this mainly occurs through the establishment and management of a long-term care insurance system based on the cooperation between central government, local government and care communities (Campbell and Ikegami, 2000). Despite these best efforts, however, the current care system may not be sufficient for patients with dementia (World Health Organization, 2012).

The 'dyadic relationship'

Increasingly, many of the behavioural symptoms experienced by older people with dementia living in residential care are understood as a response to unmet needs (Kovach *et al.*, 2005; Whall and Kolanowski, 2004). These unmet needs often arise as the result of sub-optimal physical and psychosocial environments, in addition to being created by biological factors such as the dementia itself, co-morbid physical, psychiatric illness, or medication issues. The Need-Driven Dementia-Compromised Behaviour model is a holistic model for understanding challenging behavioural symptoms (e.g. passivity, repetitive vocalisations, aggressive behaviours) in persons with dementia in terms of the interaction of background and other factors (Whall and Kolanowski, 2004). This ethos is confirmed in a later paper: 'Our critical constructionist approach facilitates an understanding of the role that education, organisational context and culture and resource issues play in the creation of this psychosocial environment and the attitudes that drive it' (Koehn, Kozak and Drance, 2012, p.734).

Traditionally in the literature, the care recipient has been viewed as a potential stressor and the carer is seen in terms of his or her outcomes (e.g. depression, health). However, the caregiving relationship, by definition, is made up of two people – the iconic 'dyadic relationship'. There is a great deal more to that relationship than just carer outcomes, including the strain both people experience in the relationship and their level of congruence and conflict about the care being provided. Understanding the ways in which the care recipient and carer converge or diverge in their perspectives of situations and each other's needs has implications for how we plan interventions to improve the outcomes of both members of the dyad (Coriell and Cohen, 1995).

Hall and Buckwalter (1987), for example, explained 'dysfunctional' behaviour as the result of a lowered threshold for stress in dementia, where persons with dementia are unable to cope with excessive personal and environmental stress. Dupuis, Wiersma and Loiselle (2012) focus on 'pathologising behaviour' which reflects how behaviours become pathologised and problematised in a long-term care context. For that study, active interviews were conducted with 48 staff members working in a range of positions in long-term care homes in Ontario, Canada. All staff interpreted and placed residents' behaviours in context through a complex process that started with the process of filtering behaviour from a biomedical perspective, and guided how staff then assigned meaning to the behaviours, how they characterised behaviours as 'challenging' and how they ultimately reacted through crisis management.

The Triangle of Care

It is carers who are responsible for care when the professionals are not there and who, as the dementia progresses, are commonly faced with coordinating and managing complex needs.

The main focus has been on 'dyadic' relationships – that is, those between two sets of people: for example, professionals and older people or older people and family carers and, to a lesser extent, family carers and professionals. More recently, there has been increasing recognition of the importance of accounting for the views of all groups – so-called 'triadic' relationships (Brandon and Jack, 1997; McKee, 1999; Qureshi *et al.*, 2000). The Carers Trust (formerly The Princess Royal Trust for Carers) and the National Mental Health Development Unit published a guide entitled *The Triangle of Care – Carers Included: A Guide to Best Practice in Mental Health Care in England* (Carers Trust, RCN, 2013). This emphasises the need for better local strategic involvement of carers and families in the care planning and treatment of people with mental health conditions. The Triangle of Care approach was developed by carers and staff to improve carer engagement in acute inpatient and home treatment services. In this framework, every effort should be made to ensure that the person with dementia is included in decision making. Carers have a crucial role to play in the care of people with dementia, along with people with dementia themselves and 'professionals'. For an illustration of this, please see Figure 7.1.

The upper diagram (a) contrasts with the lower diagram (b):

(a) A disconnected model of involvement like this can lead to carers being excluded at important points. This leads to gaps in practice which can result in the carer being left on the outside and in failure to share information that may be vital to assessment, care planning, and to acting in the best interests of both the person with dementia and the carer.

(b) The Triangle of Care for Dementia builds on the concept of relationship-centred care. The concept of a triangle has been proposed by many carers who wish to be thought of as active partners within the care team. This requires collaboration between the professional, the person with dementia and the carer. An effective Triangle of Care will only be complete if there is a willingness by the professional and carer to engage. Most carers recognise that this three-way partnership between the person with dementia, carer and professional, with all the voices being heard and influencing care, will produce the best outcomes.

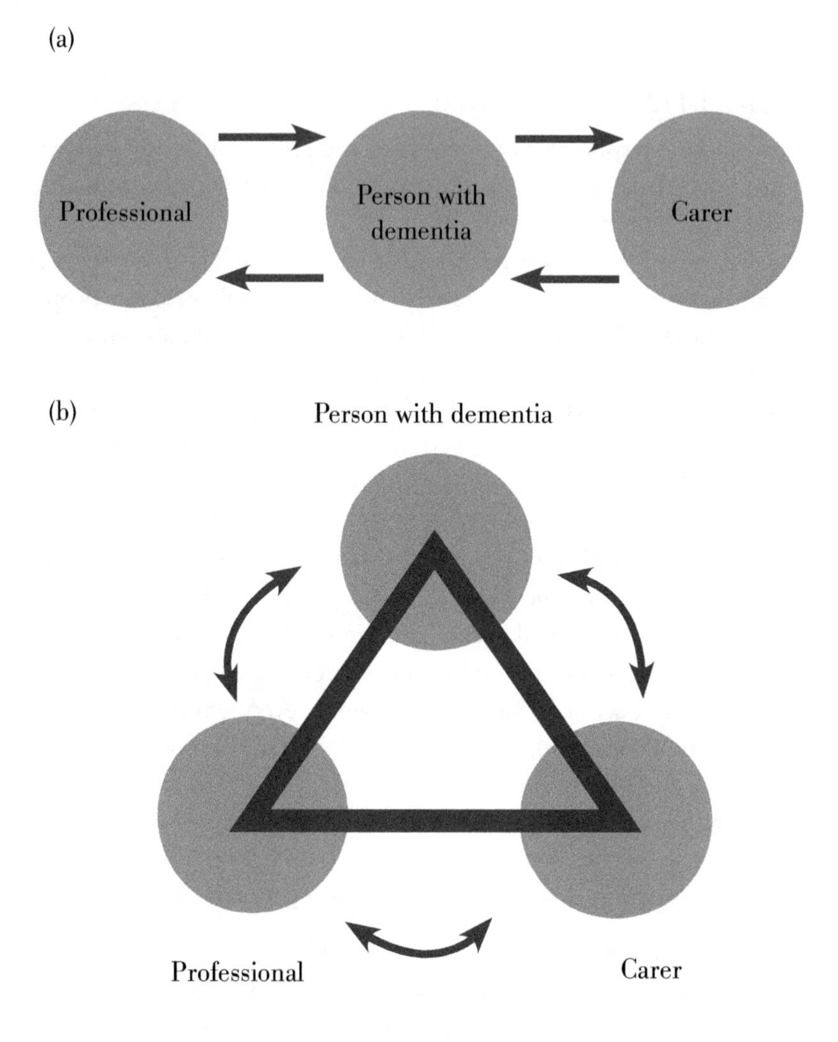

Figure 7.1 The Triangle of Care
SOURCE: CARERS TRUST, RCN, 2013 (REPRODUCED BY KIND PERMISSION OF THE CARERS TRUST)

Research shows that carers of older people with dementia experience greater strain and distress than carers of other older people (Moise, Schwarzinger and Um, 2004). In addition, many carers of people with dementia are older people themselves, with physical frailty and health conditions of their own (The Princess Royal Trust for Carers, 2011).

An interpretation of the Triangle of Care which emphasises effective communication

The Triangle of Care describes a therapeutic relationship between the person with dementia (patient), staff member and carer that promotes safety, supports communication and sustains wellbeing. Carers say their wish to be effective is commonly thwarted by failures in communication. At critical points they can be excluded by staff, and requests for helpful information, support and advice are not heard. Staff who undertake assessment and care planning should have received specific training in how to involve people with dementia and carers. This needs to include training in communication strategies with people with dementia, thus enabling people with dementia to be engaged for as long as possible.

We currently have a relative dearth of research of this triangular relationship – but plenty on the 'dyadic' relationship between professional and carer. Most studies on patient–physician relationships and communication have focused on the dyadic interaction between the parties and the type of exchanges occurring among them. However, up to 60% of medical encounters involving elderly persons involve three parties (Adelman, Greene and Charon, 1987). The features of such relationships differ fundamentally from those of a dyad. The very presence of a third person may affect the basic patient–physician relationship (Keady and Nolan, 2003), either negatively by limiting patients' involvement and assertiveness or actually excluding them from the care discussions (Greene *et al.*, 1994), or positively by enhancing physician–patient communication and consequently superior comprehension and involvement by accompanied rather than unaccompanied patients (e.g. Clayman *et al.*, 2005). A person coming into contact with the health and social care services currently does so from the point of a possible diagnosis.

English dementia policy might learn usefully not only from cancer but also from paediatrics. De Civita and Dobkin (2004) revisited the term 'triadic partnership' in referring to 'the therapeutic triangle in medicine that includes the carer, child, and medical team in facilitating adherence to treatment' (p.157). Optimal health, one may argue, is achieved when patients, carers and healthcare providers collaborate in designing a manageable treatment program (Rapoff, 1999). In time this may impact on the policy for self-care. According to Strachan and colleagues (2014), a better understanding of the individual factors that influence heart failure self-care is necessary for interventions to be more responsive to the needs and preferences of patients. Individual factors known to affect heart failure self-care are thought to include the individual's ability to manage co-morbid conditions, depression or anxiety, sleep disturbances, age/developmental issues, levels of cognitive function and health literacy (Riegel *et al.*, 2009).

Dementia, like cancer, is likely to benefit enormously from the rollout of clinical nursing specialists, especially with the implementation of whole-person care in due course. I will detail how living better with dementia is ideally suited to whole-person care in Chapter 10.

The purpose of the analysis by Dalton (2003) is to describe the construction and initial testing of the theory of collaborative decision making in nursing practice for a triad. The inclusion of a third person (family carer) in the theory required the addition of concepts about the carer, coalition formation and nurse and carer outcomes. And other groups of patients can also helpfully inform on this debate. Patients themselves are increasingly being seen as critical 'partners in care'. Hirsch and colleagues have outlined reasons why partners-in-care approaches are important – for example, in idiopathic Parkinson's disease – including the need to increase social capital, which deals with issues of trust and the value of social networks in linking members of a community (Hirsch *et al.*, 2014).

I feel the answer comes not through dyads or triads, but by considering whole networks of care for the whole person. As observed elsewhere, although each professional group (e.g. nursing, neurology, physiotherapy) makes its own assessment of the needs of the patient, it appears that it is the integration of the assessment and service delivery that is perceived to be the most useful method to address the healthcare needs of these patients (McCabe, Roberts and Firth, 2008). And for me there is no doubt that this involves effective verbal and non-verbal communication all round. Primary care visits of patients with dementia of the Alzheimer type (DAT) often involve communication among patients, family carers and primary care physicians (PCPs). The objective of the study by Schmidt and colleagues was to understand the nature of each individual's verbal participation in these triadic interactions (Schmidt, Lingler and Schulz, 2009). Carers of DAT patients and PCPs maintain active, coordinated verbal participation in primary care visits while patients participate less.

This is why I feel two's company and three's a very good thing for English dementia policy. But I feel that wider networks at large are going to prove to be important for whole-person care, though some agents may possibly be more significant than others.

A network approach to care and support

Kate Swaffer, in a well-received talk entitled 'Prescribed Disengagement, Models of Care and QoL' for the Alzheimer's Disease International Conference in Puerto Rico (2014), discussed her concept of 'prescribed disengagement'. (Swaffer has explained elsewhere her reasons for seeking trademark recognition for this phrase.) Swaffer is currently Chair of Alzheimer's Australia's Dementia Advisory Committee and Co-Founder/Board member of Dementia Alliance International.

The definition she articulates for this notion is:

> People with dementia are told to go home, give up work, give up our pre-diagnosis life, and live for the time they have left.

North America and Europe are presently experiencing a demographic shift towards an elderly population. Currently, 15% of the Canadian population is 65 years or older (Cranswick and Dosman, 2008). The United States and Europe are similar, with those aged 65 or older comprising 12.8% and 17.1% of the population, respectively (Giannakouris, 2011). Köhler and colleagues (2014) cite that in Germany, as in other industrialised countries, most people with dementia are living in their home environment and receiving care from family carers (Alzheimer's Association, 2012). German society and its national health policy emphasise caring for highly dependent older people at home for as long as possible. Also, Awata (2010) describes experience from the Japanese jurisdiction including a need for special medical facilities providing differential diagnosis, emergency and admission services, management of concurrent medical conditions, intervention for patients with difficult social problems, and public enterprises to strengthen the connection between specialists and GPs.

According to Zarit and Edwards (2008), a caregiving relationship emerges when a person becomes dependent on another's assistance to complete tasks. Often carers have a gradual transition into their role, where they increasingly provide help to the care recipient; however, some carers may experience an abrupt entry into their role (Gaugler, Zarit and Pearlin, 2003). It is possible that the various definitions of 'carer burden' lead to vague findings that have been 'difficult to summarise, appraise and apply to clinical and policy settings' (Bastawrous, 2013, p.431). Several studies have been conducted with the aim of identifying factors related to carer burden. Mohamed and colleagues (2010) found that severity of psychiatric symptoms, behavioural disturbances and patient quality of life have a stronger association with carer-experienced burden. It has been argued that carer burden needs to be classified into objective burden and subjective burden because factors contributing to and interventions used to modify those types of burden differ. Objective burden is defined as time spent on care, tasks performed and financial problems faced by the carer, whereas subjective burden refers to the carer's perceived impact of the objective burden on them (Xiao *et al.*, 2014). There has been some concern about the generalisability of research findings from studies that do not provide a rigorous definition of 'carer' (Greenwood *et al.*, 2009). Carers are often responsible for providing physical and emotional support to elderly family members which can limit their ability to participate in regular social activities and decrease their wellbeing (Wade, Legh-Smith and Hewer, 1986). Many variables increasing the risk of carer burden have been identified, and an overview of these risk factors is presented in Table 7.1. This table is based on factors suggested in recent papers, and there is an emerging consensus over these factors.

Table 7.1 Factors that contribute to additional pressure on carers

Possible carer factors	• Advanced age • Carer depression • Educational attainment • Female gender • Hours spent caring • Lack of lifestyle choice • Low income • Poor coping strategies • Poor current relationship with care-recipient • Poor physical health • Social loneliness
Care-recipient factors	• Appetite symptoms • Behavioural symptoms • Cognitive impairment • Medical co-morbidities • Not living with the person with dementia

Source: Adapted from Richardson et al., 2013; Dauphinot et al., 2015; Adelman et al., 2014; Gort et al., 2007

Most studies agree that a minimum criterion for 'family carer' is that the individual must not be paid to provide care. In some literature, the term 'informal carer' is used interchangeably with 'family carer' to reflect this lack of compensation (Hollander, Liu and Chappell, 2009). Other criteria for defining 'family carer' include: (a) the type of assistance they provide (e.g. instrumental or emotional assistance) and (b) the extent of assistance they provide (e.g. hours of care provided, number of times a week care is provided) (Donelan *et al.*, 2002).

Social support is defined as a group or individual who can help and support any person; meanwhile, informal social support is defined as unpaid help or support from any individual (Choo *et al.*, 2003). Historically this has been conceptualised in many different ways. Highlighted features are the structural aspects of social networks (e.g. the size of a person's social circle or the number of resources provided), functional aspects of social support (e.g. emotional support or a sense of acceptance) and enacted support (e.g. provision of specific supportive behaviours, such as reassurance or advice, in times of distress), as well as the subjective perception of support by the recipients (Lakey and Lutz, 1996). Support has been defined in a more interpersonal light as an exchange between providers and recipients. Support interventions are based on the theory that increasing support allows people to cope better, and this enhanced coping will result in fewer psychological or physical symptoms (Cohen and Wills, 1985). Carers of people living with dementia of the Alzheimer type who have reported symptoms of depression have ranged from 28% to 55% (Schulz *et al.*, 1995), with female carers more likely to experience depression than male carers (Stuckey, Neundorfer and Smyth, 1996). Behavioural problems are more significant than cognitive disorders or lack of self-care (van der Lee *et al.*, 2014). It is, however, argued that an intervention that helps carers to utilise their social support networks may help them adapt better to their caregiving responsibilities.

Drentea and colleagues (2006) found that higher levels of emotional support, more visits and having more network members to whom they felt close were all individually predictive of longitudinal changes in social support network satisfaction for those who provide care at home for a spouse with Alzheimer's disease. The findings of Jaglal and colleagues (2007) highlight that family physicians' understanding of dementia and their ability to work with the dyad to become aware of and accept services is an important component in the dyad's satisfaction with the care received, and that this differs by site. This suggests that more attention needs to be paid to increasing the awareness of family physicians concerning their role in dementia care, the availability of services in their communities and how to access these services on behalf of their patients. This would also confirm a previously established observation that family physicians have a role to play in diagnosing dementia, educating families about dementia, providing psychological support for carers and mobilising carer social support networks (Cohen, Pringle and LeDuc, 2001). But there is another reality: the analysis by Peel and Harding (2014) highlights that carers find navigating key issues in dementia care time-consuming, unpredictable and often more difficult than the caring work they undertake. Ultimately, the distress associated with having a partner with dementia in a nursing home versus having such a partner residing at home may indicate that interventions aimed at delaying nursing home admission may be important (Ask *et al.*, 2014).

Family physicians play a key role in dementia care (Cummings *et al.*, 2002; Olafsdóttir, Skoog and Marcusson, 2000). The results from the study by Parmar and colleagues (2014) indicate that there is underuse of diagnostic and functional assessment tools, lack of attention to carer issues, and underuse of community supports (Pimlott *et al.*, 2006). These results, the authors argue, also indicate that quality indicators such as assessment of wandering and driving were inadequately assessed in the primary care setting, which is of concern, as are matters of individual and public safety (Lyketsos *et al.*, 2006). Arguably, the sequelae of a diagnosis of dementia in the medical, mental health and social care context require an interdisciplinary and multi-professional treatment, which needs not just to focus on the person with dementia but also to consider carer relatives together with the individual's social environment. If practitioners were to receive training and the space within which to meet and develop supportive relationships based on trust and recognition, they would be more likely to form solid links with families (Grenier, 2004). There has thus far been relatively little research into the processes that might explain why linkages between families and professional services are so problematic (Brodaty *et al.*, 2005; Lloyd and Stirling, 2011).

The notion of trust is considered fundamental to the creation and maintenance of relationships, as it facilitates decision making, reduces the cost of transactions, encourages cooperation and diminishes uncertainty in complex situations (Weber and Carter, 2002).

As discussed by Carpentier and Grenier (2012), an influential notion has emerged: that of 'social experience', which Dubet (1995) has proposed as a principal parameter for understanding social relations. The idea is that, in circumstances where social roles, socialisation and codes fail to enable individuals to reasonably predict conscious actions, individuals draw on their past experience in their unique social systems as a guide. The relationship between formal and informal networks therefore becomes crucial in this narrative.

Carpentier and Grenier (2012) have helpfully argued recently that the reform of healthcare systems and, in particular, responses to client groups such as persons with dementia require a better grasp of how social relationships that encourage cooperation among various actors in care delivery are formed. Rather than refusing services, it is mooted that carers of people with dementia, who are often under a great deal of perceived strain, find accessing support services challenging and stressful (Peel and Harding, 2014).

Social networks

Social networks depend on both the structural characteristics of the persons with whom one shares social relationships and the perception one has of the quality of the support their network members provide (Amieva *et al.*, 2010). Most evidence suggests that interaction with friends, more than with family, is associated with emotional wellbeing (Bowling, 1994). It is likely that any analysis of social networks has to take place properly in the context of the wider environment or community of the person living with dementia. Housing is one critical factor. Field, Walker and Orrell (2002) reported that 87 residents from three sheltered accommodation schemes for people over 60 years had been interviewed about their physical and mental health, social networks, social support, decision to move in, and how they found living in sheltered housing. Locally integrated social networks were most common (41%). Residents with a private network (16%) were more likely than those with a locally integrated network to have significant activity limitation and to report often being lonely.

Köhler and colleagues (2014) found that the management of dementia patients in an interdisciplinary regional network solely provides measurable advantages with respect to the provision of dementia-specific medication and utilisation of medical treatment – that is, referral rates to specialists. The association between several aspects of social networks and risk of subsequent dementia was examined in this large population-based sample of 2089 elderly participants followed prospectively for up to 15 years (Amieva *et al.*, 2010). Amieva and colleagues found that the only variables associated with subsequent dementia or dementia of the Alzheimer type were those reflecting the quality of relationships. Indeed, in their literature review, Cacioppo and Hawkley (2009) provided data in favour of the importance of perceived social connectedness on cognitive and mood outcomes. And, in fairness, there might be a plausible neuroscientific substrate for this. Martin Webber and colleagues (2015) reported recently the findings of a qualitative study which used ethnographic field methods in six sites in England to investigate how workers helped people recovering from psychosis to enhance their social networks. Intriguingly, they found that the extent to which the agency engaged with its local community appeared to influence its ability to develop service users' personal networks.

Participation in social networks – arguably an informal form of brain-activating rehabilitation – may serve to enhance patients' motivation and maximise the use of their remaining function, recruiting a compensatory functional distributed neuronal network and preventing the disuse of residual brain function as considered by Yamaguchi and colleagues in their review (2010). The authors argue that the primary expected effect would be that patients recover a desire for life, as well as their self-respect. In this construct, according to the authors, enhanced motivation could lead to improvements in cognitive function, and melioration of the behavioural and psychological symptoms of dementia and improvements in activities of daily living can also be expected due to the renewed positive attitude towards life. Social capital is increasingly being recognised as important for health and mental wellbeing (Van Der Gaag and Webber, 2007). It is also increasingly being articulated as a useful concept for social work (Hawkins and Maurer, 2012; Webber, 2005), particularly as it could assist in the development of new social interventions, which may support an individual's recovery from a mental health problem.

Family carers

The issue of who does the caregiving is a very relevant one. Family carers provide the majority of hands-on care to older adults with dementia, and most of this care is provided in community settings.

Schulz and Martire (2004) helpfully reviewed the literature on this as it was at the time; older adults no longer with spouses often receive beneficial assistance from adult children, particularly adult daughters and daughters-in-law. The consequences of carer stress have been shown to be moderated by resources such as social support (Wilks and Croom, 2008), race and ethnicity (Hilgeman *et al.*, 2009) and the combination of relationship quality (mutuality) and perceived carer preparedness for caregiving tasks (Schumacher, Stewart and Archbold, 2007). Several variables have been found to be protective resources for family carers of patients with dementia. For example, social support moderated the effects of these carers' perceived stress and resilience (Wilks and Croom, 2008) and decreased the likelihood of their depression (Huang *et al.*, 2013). In addition to personal and social resources, dyadic relational variables such as relationship quality have been identified as protective resources; indeed, the quality of the carer/care-receiver relationship before the onset of illness was found to decrease carers' depressive symptoms (Williamson and Schulz, 1995).

Informal carers provide care to those who need help out of love or a sense of moral duty. This is often not a conscious choice but a gradual adaptation to changes in their family member (de Vugt and Verhey, 2013). Family members most often notice the first symptoms of dementia, as patients can be unaware of their memory impairment (Lopez *et al.*, 1994). Recognition of the problem by family members is triggered by behavioural changes rather than by cognitive or functional impairment (Eustace *et al.*, 2007). Another important factor was a high level of predictability, which tended to decrease role strain. Finally, the association between care-receiver cognitive functioning and carer role strain was influenced by the level of mutuality between carer and care receiver. More specifically, high levels of mutuality diminished role strain in carers of patients with mild dementia (Yang, Liu and Shyu, 2014).

The caregiving relationship includes two members: a primary carer (CG) and a care recipient (CR) (Lyons *et al.*, 2002). The changes that occur as dementia progresses may influence both individual factors and factors shared between the CGs and CRs such as their relationship, reciprocal interaction and level of interdependence (Moon and Adams, 2013). Some spousal carers manage to maintain wellbeing and health in the face of a progressing illness. Heru and colleagues (2004) examined spousal dementia carers of moderately disabled partners and found that some carers perceived more reward than burden. Additionally, both negative and positive changes experienced by caregiving spouses may co-exist (Narayan *et al.*, 2001). In fact, spouses may report perceiving caring as fulfilling, satisfying and affirming, while concurrently experiencing negative responses, such as relational deprivation with their partner (de Vugt *et al.*, 2003). Older couples are also likely to share a history of joint problem solving and coping, and of adapting their interactions appropriately around events such as childbirth or retirement (Martin and Wight, 2008). Braun and colleagues (2009) have deduced that the majority of studies neglect the individual with dementia by exclusively assessing carer variables or only indirectly including patients' characteristics.

Family carers amongst others provide care for individuals with dementia in the home (Callahan *et al.*, 2012). Healthcare providers in service provision are likely to have to recognise that family carers often present as secondary patients; given the importance of these carers to patients with dementia of the Alzheimer type and other dementias, arguably it is vital to understand the risk factors that impact carer health and wellbeing (Richardson *et al.*, 2013). Indeed, the evidence suggests that some carers are at increased risk for serious illness (Kiecolt-Glaser *et al.*, 1996). Advances made in accurately diagnosing the early symptoms of dementia offer additional opportunities for interventions before the onset of significant stressors. Thus, an intervention that includes both members of the care dyad may represent an optimal approach in early-stage dementia (Whitlatch *et al.*, 2006). Carers of people with dementia incur significant strain and have substantial need for a variety of services; nevertheless, many carers were not using support services, mainly because of perceived lack of need or lack of awareness (Brodaty *et al.*, 2005).

It is likely that there is a strong cultural component to the ability of carers to cope; culture might influence family carers' burdens and play an important part in the development of a holistic model for family-centred care; it is reported that, in many Asian countries, the family is the primary long-term carer and an important resource for persons with dementia (Chan, 2010).

An introduction to clinical nursing specialists including Admiral Nurses

At the time of writing, there are just over 130 Admiral Nurses (Rachel Thompson, personal communication), compared to 3942 Macmillan Nurses (Macmillan, 2015). It is estimated that one in three people will care for a person with dementia in their lifetime (Carers Trust, RCN, 2013). The potential contribution of clinical nursing specialists in proactive case management in whole-person care could be enormous.

The Admiral Nurse Service aims to improve the quality of life of people with dementia and their carers by providing a specialist nursing service for the carers of people with dementia and by raising awareness and providing education and training for carers, professionals and the public. The literature cites various methods and approaches to nurse-led interventions, and prior research lends support to the argument that nurses can effectively manage chronic medical conditions. In one review, nurses identified three factors important to the success of their clinics: (1) management of symptoms, (2) prevention of complications, and (3) client satisfaction (Wong and Chung, 2006). Burton and Hope (2005) have nonetheless described that 'the desire to fulfil a case-management role while attempting to provide a service that is of a specialist nature and of limited capacity generated tensions' (p.359). Dewing and Traynor (2005) have developed a competency framework which will enable Admiral Nurses to demonstrate their level of specialist practice, as individuals and collectively as a service. The authors also propose that this framework promotes the principles of nurses as life-long learners. Admiral Nurses are UK-based qualified mental health nurses who have specialised in dementia care. Admiral Nurses can also work with the carer/care-recipient dyad to identify dementia care services appropriate to their needs. Adelman and colleagues (1987) suggested that the presence of the third person can significantly change the dynamic of the doctor–patient relationship. The third person may facilitate or inhibit a trusting doctor–patient relationship, and the doctor's and patient's perceptions of this third person may differ. A study by Quinn and colleagues illuminated the triadic relationship between the carer, person with dementia and Admiral Nurse (Quinn *et al.*, 2013). This study proposed that the triadic relationship between carer, care-recipient and Admiral

Nurse can be encompassed under an overarching process entitled 'negotiating the balance'.

A support network for carers

That carers should have support needs addressed is a top policy priority around the world. A network, active in a national (not fragmented) way, appears to be an appropriate vehicle to harness mutual peer support, foster learning and discuss coping strategies. The Dementia Action Alliance is an organic movement with the simple aim of bringing about a society-wide response to dementia. It encourages and supports communities and organisations across England to take practical actions to enable people to live well with dementia and to reduce the risk of costly crisis intervention.

Carers save the economy a substantial amount of money. It is mooted that properly identifying and supporting carers will prevent escalation and demand on statutory services (Newbronner *et al.*, 2013). The new legal changes in care arguably provide new opportunities to engage and for commissioners to fund and deliver better early intervention and support.

Launched by the Dementia Action Alliance, the 'Call to Action' had five key aims for carers of people with dementia – that carers:

» have recognition of their unique experience – 'given the character of the illness, people with dementia deserve and need special consideration in designing packages of care and support that meet their and their carers needs' (Alzheimer's Disease International/Bupa, 2013, p.28)

» are recognised as essential partners in care – valuing their knowledge and the support they provide to enable the person with dementia to live well

» have access to expertise in dementia care for personalised information, advice, support and coordination of care for the person with dementia

» have assessments and support to identify the ongoing and changing needs to maintain their own health and wellbeing

» have confidence that they are able to access good-quality care, support and respite services that are flexible, culturally appropriate, timely and provided by skilled staff for both the carer and the person for whom they care.

It was hoped that this initiative would bring about some change, ensuring that the diverse needs of carers were both acknowledged and respected as essential partners in care, and were supported with easy access to the information and the advice they needed to assist them in carrying out their role. Indeed, it is widely felt that this policy aim was achieved. While the Dementia Action Alliance ended, as planned, late March 2015, there are plans for a new national network to empower carers of people living with dementia at a national level.

The real heart of the Call to Action remains, however, the production of the action and the communication of this action to others. This is the 'Dementia Declaration'.

Box 7.1 The National Dementia Declaration – Action Plan

The National Dementia Declaration lists seven outcomes that the DAA are seeking to achieve for people with dementia and their carers. How would you describe your organisation's role in delivering better outcomes for people with dementia and their carers?

The Department of Health's work centres around three strategic objectives – better health and wellbeing for all, better care for all and better value for all. In relation to dementia, this means ensuring that public funds are used efficiently and effectively to provide health and social care services which meet the needs of people with dementia and their carers.

The Department published its revised, outcomes-focused implementation plan for Living Well with Dementia – A National Dementia Strategy on 28 September 2010. The implementation plan sets out the Department's priority objectives for securing improvements in dementia care, which are:

* good-quality early diagnosis and intervention for all;
* improved quality of care in general hospitals;
* living well with dementia in care homes; and
* reduced use of anti-psychotic medication.

The implementation plan also sets out for health and social care localities and their delivery partners:

* the Department of Health's role and priorities during 2010/11 for supporting local delivery of and local accountability for the implementation of the National Dementia Strategy;
* the Strategy's fit with the new vision for the future of health and social care set out in the White Paper Equity and Excellence: Liberating the NHS; and
* the fit with the consultation document Liberating the NHS: Transparency in Outcomes – a framework for the NHS.

The Department, in conjunction with the National End of Life Care Programme, is working with and supporting key partners such as the National Council for Palliative Care and national dementia charities to help improve end of life care for all adults, including those with dementia.

The Department also has a key role in influencing the public, communities and organisations in both the private and voluntary sectors to be more supportive of people with dementia and their carers.

SOURCE: DEMENTIA ACTION ALLIANCE, 2015 (REPRODUCED BY KIND PERMISSION OF THE DEMENTIA ACTION ALLIANCE)

These aims are supported by a 20-point checklist of what good support for the needs and rights of family carers should look like. Box 7.2 summarises these points.

Box 7.2 Top 20 Checklist for Commissioners – examples of services supporting family carers of people living with dementia

1. Pre-diagnosis support from the point of GP referral to Memory Clinic.
2. Post diagnosis education for the family and person with dementia.
3. A dementia adviser/support worker/Admiral Nurse to provide on-going and timely access to local, face to face, personalised, dementia expertise and practical advice as well as psychological and emotional support.
4. On-going and timely access to dementia specific local information, resources and support in a variety of accessible formats.
5. Support for family carers that provides a clear, collaborative pathway of action and plan of care once GPs have identified a family carer.
6. Carer Peer Support Groups specifically for family members/carers/friends of people living with dementia, which meets the cultural needs of the local population and age range of those affected.
7. Health and social care staff (including third sector services) who have knowledge & expertise in dementia to complete personalised assessments of a person who has dementia and their family carers.
8. An expert clinician in dementia to support and supervise Care Co-ordinators/ Social Care Staff/Health Care Practitioners with their role in assessing, treating

and managing the impact of co-morbidities of the person with dementia and thus supporting the family carer.

9. Support to remain active and integrated in the local community, thus reducing impact of loneliness and social isolation of both the person with dementia and their carer, e.g. dementia friendly communities, health prescriptions, community transport, age appropriate activities.

10. Access to appropriate and timely respite opportunities by the hour, day or week in a range of settings.

11. Age appropriate support for the impact of young onset dementia, e.g. supporting younger family members, loss of income and roles.

12. Culturally appropriate, accessible information and support for people with dementia and their family carers from Black and ethnic minority communities.

13. Culturally appropriate, accessible information and support for people with dementia and their family carers from Lesbian, Gay, Bisexual and Transgender communities.

14. Dementia advocacy services – e.g. to capture the wishes, values and beliefs of a family carer and strategies to ensure people living with dementia have a person-centred assessment, support for completing legal and financial issues.

15. Community Health & care services that are delivered by those who have training and expertise in dementia (not just dementia awareness), e.g. dentist, nutrition, opticians, podiatry, hairdressers who specialise in dementia and offer domiciliary visits.

16. Training in dementia care for Health & Social Care professionals.

17. Glossary/overview/jargon buster concerning what professions/services mean and what they can do for you.

18. Dementia awareness promotion within local communities and businesses including 'Dementia Friends', dementia friendly communities and environments, Local Dementia Action Alliance initiatives.

19. Support for employers to enable carers to continue working.

20. Support, and training as necessary, for family carers and people living with dementia to have a voice to influence and support change locally. This requires a 'meaningful community engagement' so that commissioning services is based on the evidence of need of the local population.

Source: Dementia Action Alliance, 2014 (reproduced by kind permission of the Dementia Action Alliance)

Care homes and community visitors

Moving individuals from their homes to an institution, whether living with dementia or not, always poses a significant challenge, since this often involves a drastic change in lifestyle resulting from a loss of autonomy; many perceive institutionalisation as a process leading to loss of liberty, abandonment by relatives and proximity to death (Medeiros de A Nunes *et al.*, 2014). In England, commercial companies and not-for-profit organisations are the main formal providers of long-term care (in care homes, with and without on-site nursing) for older people. Approximately 17% of people aged over 85 live in a care home and the number of residents is projected to rise (Laing and Buisson, 2009).

In 2012, the Dementia and Neurodegenerative Diseases research network (DeNDRoN) set up an online resource for researchers working in care homes, care home staff, residents and family members, and began to build a network of 'research-ready' care homes. The overall project title chosen was ENRICH – Enabling Research in Care Homes (Davies *et al.*, 2014). Care homes are increasingly being viewed as 'communities of care' and have the potential to be active partners in research (Goodman *et al.*, 2011). Reports of poor-quality care for people with dementia in many care home settings remains a serious concern (Marshall, 2001). In the UK, steps towards a more regulatory approach including inspections (e.g. Department of Health, 2006) has led to concerns that a checklist-based exercise will not promote person-centred care. Fossey and colleagues (2006) reported that agitated and challenging behaviours could be managed without drug use if staff were trained in individualised approaches to patient care. Staff often felt they did not have time for this approach, although it is perhaps worth noting that Zimmerman and colleagues (2005) have found that person-centred attitudes were related to greater job satisfaction among those working in long-term care settings.

The design of buildings, if regarded as a therapeutic resource, can promote wellbeing and functioning of people with dementia (Day, Carreon and Stump, 2000). A dementia-friendly environment is argued to compensate for disability and should consider both the importance for the person with dementia of his/her experiences within the environment and also the social, physical and organisational environments which impact on these experiences (Davis *et al.*, 2009). Davis and colleagues (2009) argue that shifting thinking from 'condition' to 'experience' has the potential to facilitate the culture change needed to create environments that allow for active participation in everyday life. The role that care homes play in providing care and support to people with dementia at the end of their lives is an area of increasing policy and research interest (National Council for Palliative Care and the NHS End of Life Care Programme, 2006).

A useful report entitled '"Put yourself in my place": designing and managing care homes for people with dementia' by Caroline Cantley and Robert Wilson (2012) reviewed the needs of care home providers. It was a contemporary synthesis based on the experiences of seven specialist homes to advise on how to create and maintain a good place for people with dementia to live. This report, notably, had some overlap with another report produced by the Joseph Rowntree Foundation (2012) at roughly the same time, entitled 'My home life: promoting quality of life in care homes'.

Cantley and Wilson (2012) note, however, that 'although good dementia care homes must share the same broad set of values and principles there may be differences in emphasis' (p.4). In July 2014 the government announced legislation which introduced fundamental standards for health and social care providers. Subject to parliamentary approval, these were due to become law in April 2015. The new measures were being introduced as part of the government's response to the Francis Inquiry's recommendations, and were intended to help improve the quality of care and transparency of providers by ensuring that those responsible for poor care can be held to account.

Design of care homes plugs into the potent issue of the social determinants of health, which can impact on the wellbeing of a person living with dementia. I carry out an analysis of how housing is about more than the raw structure of buildings, however, in Chapter 11.

Intermediate care

The National Service Framework for Older People (Department of Health, 2001) set out the requirements for the NHS and local authorities to provide enhanced intermediate care services at home or in designated care settings. These services aim to prevent unnecessary admission to hospital and long-term residential care, and to provide effective rehabilitation to facilitate early discharge from hospital. One study of hospitals in the UK in 2006–07 found that 1.6% of all 50 million bed-days were caused by delayed discharges (Godden, McCoy and Pollock, 2009). During the delay, seven out of the 58 people developed new medical problems including hospital-acquired chest and *Clostridium difficile* infections, and three deaths occurred as a result of pulmonary embolism, bronchopneumonia and *C. difficile* infection. Although the study did not state how many patients had dementia, delayed discharge was more likely in older patients and those with confusion at the time of admission (Jasinarachchi *et al.*, 2009). The Health Foundation (2011) proposes that intermediate care services should be multi-disciplinary, involve short-term interventions lasting one to six weeks, and be designed to maximise independence and facilitate the elderly person being able to live safely at home.

Moving into a care home

The World Alzheimer Report (Alzheimer's Disease International/Bupa, 2013) states a preference for the term 'transition into a care home' rather than the term 'institutionalisation', generally a marker of particularly high needs for care, although other factors can be involved. Predictors of transition into a care home in the USA have been studied in a review including 77 reports across 12 data sources that used longitudinal designs and community-based samples. Cognitive impairment was the health condition that most strongly predicted transition, with a 2.5-fold increased risk. Other major chronic conditions also conferred an increased risk – separately, hypertension, cancer and diabetes – but these were modest compared with the risk associated with cognitive impairment.

In a study conducted in Sweden, dementia was the main predictor of transition into a care home, with a population attributable figure of 61% (Aguero-Torres *et al.*, 2001). Family members also bring knowledge of ways to preserve personhood when a person with dementia is admitted to long-term care. New residents face an unfamiliar institutional environment and disrupted routines. Family carers can serve as the link between the resident with dementia and the long-term care staff. Photos, personalised items, stories and observations from family members can foster understanding of the resident's past, relationships, needs and preferences. Palmer (2013) argues that application of the carers' knowledge of the care of the person with dementia can help to guide the practice of nurses in the promotion of personhood in long-term care and other settings.

Although a developing field of research (McKeown, Clarke and Repper, 2006), the use of life story and family biographical approaches in aged care has advanced the aim of how best to deliver sensitive and effective support that empowers staff to relate confidently to family and residents and engage in flexible, inclusive care practices informed by life story (Clarke, Hanson and Ross, 2003; Keady and Williams, 2007). From the findings of the systematic review by Beerens and colleagues (2013), it can be concluded that mood – and especially depressive symptoms – is a consistent factor which is negatively related to self-rated quality of life of people with dementia living in long-term care facilities, indicating that more depressive symptoms are related to lower quality of life. The complex needs of people with dementia can be difficult to meet, leading to need-driven dementia-compromised behaviours – also called behavioural and psychological symptoms of dementia or unmet need behaviours (Kitwood, 1997b). Use of person-centred care, which can be learned by use of education and staff support, is becoming more common in residential care, because it can reduce need-driven dementia-compromised behaviours and help maintain personhood (Edvardsson *et al.*, 2008).

Incontinence can be a reason why persons living with dementia might find themselves moving into a care home. This relates to a general sphere of work on the 'unmet needs' of people living with dementia. I discuss incontinence in the context of a person with dementia's aspiration to live better with dementia in Chapter 9.

Acute hospital care

> 'Dementia is a challenge for hospitals. Surveys show that around a quarter of hospital beds are occupied by somebody with dementia; a figure which increases in older people and individuals with a superimposed delirium.'
>
> Royal College of Nursing (RCN), 2013

Wellbeing in dementia 'is influenced by a number of factors including neurological impairment, physical health, individual biography, personality and physical and social environment' (RCN, 2013, p.7). An acute hospital admission can be a significant event for older people and their relatives, and can threaten older people's sense of identity and involvement (Bridges, Flatley and Meyer, 2010). A number of reports across jurisdictions have been important in establishing the direction of travel for acute hospital care: for example, 'Dementia care in the acute hospital setting: issues and strategies: a report for Alzheimer's Australia' (Alzheimer's Australia, 2014); 'Spotlight on dementia care: a Health Foundation Improvement Report' (Health Foundation, 2011); and 'Dementia: commitment to the care of people with dementia in hospital settings' (RCN, 2013).

To improve outcomes for people with dementia in the acute hospital setting, there are a number of different issues which could be addressed constructively. These include:

» better identification of cognitive impairment in our hospitals

» increased training for all staff, including how to communicate with a person with dementia and how to respond to behavioural and psychological symptoms

» more extensive and systematic involvement of all carers, including paid carers and informal carers, as partners in the health care of people with dementia

» creation of appropriate physical hospital environments to reduce the confusion and distress of people with dementia.

This leads to a range of strategies to improve the outcomes for people with dementia.

RCN Principle 1: Supporting staff need to be informed, skilled and have enough time to care

The workforce of the health and social care sectors in England themselves have often claimed to be better trained in dementia than they actually are, as the traditional time devoted to these studies currently is minimal.

A number of themes emerged from the systematic review and synthesis of qualitative studies describing older patients' and/or their relatives' experiences of care in acute hospital settings by Bridges and colleagues (2010).

RCN Principle 2: Family carers and friends are seen as partners in care

The involvement of carers, friends and family is a welcome move in policy. It is certainly true that effective care acknowledges the needs of friends, families and carers who have been supporting the person with dementia in the home, usually for some time and with limited support. It is important to learn from all carers, including paid carers and informal family carers, about the person with dementia and how people living with dementia function best in everyday life. A 'care for the carer approach' has also contributed to the development of psychosocial interventions towards informal carers to people with dementia (Pusey, 2003).

Involving carers or care coordinators in developing care pathways with specialist nurses could also help deliver quality care, and care packages tailored to the person with dementia and the informal carer could help identify what care is available (Hunter *et al.*, 1997). Also important is support for informal carers so they can continue to care without the need for residential care, and can recognise health problems early so they can be sorted before a crisis point is reached (Health Foundation, 2011).

RCN Principle 3: A dementia assessment will be offered to all those at risk, to support early identification and appropriate care

An accurate assessment of a person living with dementia by experienced and skilled practitioners is essential here. Care of long-term conditions, which involves health promotion, prevention, self-management, disease control, treatment and disease palliation (Martin and Sturmberg, 2009) as applied to patients with dementia, requires interdisciplinary teams formed by professionals who provide distinct health and social services and ensure continuity of care with patient and family commitment (Innes, 2002). The ideal is to identify and manage dementia at hospital admission and plan for discharge from the outset. A specialist multi-disciplinary team input should be available, ideally, to assess and coordinate appropriate in-patient care when a person is admitted to hospital, so that all health needs can be addressed (Health Foundation, 2011). The inability of persons with dementia to live on their own was cited as a 'stressor' leading to crisis situations such as unplanned institutionalisation or emergency hospital admission (Villars *et al.*, 2010). An approach of prevention, detection and treatment by the general practitioner of acute medical conditions (e.g. syncope and collapse, pneumonia, urinary tract infections, hip fractures and dehydration) and malnutrition is considered useful to reduce emergency hospital admissions (Rafferty *et al.*, 1989). Nourhashemi and colleagues (2001) recommended improved information for carers with structured follow-up after emergency admission and early management and treatment for persons with dementia, although it is unclear what this entails.

RCN Principle 4: Care plans will be person-centred, responsive to individual needs and support nutrition, dignity, comfort, continence, rehabilitation, activity and palliative care

A principal aim of policy will now be to reduce 'avoidable hospital admissions'. Hospitals are not always the best place for people with dementia to receive care. In some situations, it is best for people with dementia to receive care within the home or within specialised residential aged care facilities. Hospitalisations of aged care facility residents could also be reduced. Strategies such as specialised care units can provide more intensive medical care for periods of time for people with dementia. Research has found that these units can significantly reduce rates of hospitalisation from residential care (Nobili *et al.*, 2008). Timely access to medical services, including general practitioners, specialists, nurse practitioners and physiotherapists, as well as appropriate palliative care services, has also been shown to reduce the need for hospitalisation for people in residential care (Australian Institute of Health and Welfare, 2013).

RCN Principle 5: Environments will be dementia-friendly and support independence and wellbeing

In my previous book *Living Well with Dementia: The Importance of the Person and the Environment for Wellbeing*, I outlined the importance of the design of home and ward environments (Rahman, 2014).

Conclusion

There are particular activities which load heavily into the experience of quality of life. One of them is eating. Care and support for a person living with dementia means paying particular attention to the mealtime environment as well as the actual food itself.

Chapter 8 is concerned with eating well while living better with dementia.

References

Adams, T. and Gardiner, P. (2005) Developing a theory for relationship-centred care. Dementia, 4, 2, 185–205.

Adelman, R.D., Greene, M.G. and Charon, R. (1987) The physician–elderly patient–companion triad in the medical encounter: the development of a conceptual framework and research agenda. Gerontologist, 27, 6, 729–34.

Adelman, R.D., Tmanova, L.L., Delgado, D., Dion, S. and Lachs, M.S. (2014) Caregiver burden: a clinical review. Journal of the American Medical Association, 311, 10, 1052–1060.

Aguero-Torres, H., von Strauss, E., Viitanen, M., Winblad, B. and Fratiglioni, L. (2001) Institutionalization in the elderly: the role of chronic diseases and dementia. Cross-sectional and longitudinal data from a population-based study. Journal of Clinical Epidemiology, 54, 8, 795–801.

Alzheimer's Association (2012) Alzheimer's disease facts and figures. Alzheimer's and Dementia, 8, 2, 131–68.

Alzheimer's Australia (2014) Dementia care in the acute hospital setting: issues and strategies: a report for Alzheimer's Australia. Available at https://fightdementia.org.au/sites/default/files/Alzheimers_Australia_Numbered_Publication_40.PDF (accessed 6 December 2014).

Alzheimer's Disease International/Bupa (2013) World Alzheimer Report 2013. Journey of caring: an analysis of long-term care for dementia. Available at www.alz.co.uk/research/WorldAlzheimerReport2013.pdf (accessed 6 December 2014).

Amieva, H., Stoykova, R., Matharan, F., Helmer, C., Antonucci, T.C. and Dartigues, J.F. (2010) What aspects of social network are protective for dementia? Not the quantity but the quality of social interactions is protective up to 15 years later. Psychosomatic Medicine, 72, 9, 905–11.

Ask, H., Langballe, E.M., Holmen, J., Selbæk, G., Saltvedt, I. and Tambs, K. (2014) Mental health and wellbeing in spouses of persons with dementia: the Nord-Trøndelag Health Study. BMC Public Health, 14, 413.

Australian Institute of Health and Welfare (2013) Dementia Care in Hospitals: Costs and Strategies. Available at www.aihw.gov.au/WorkArea/DownloadAsset.aspx?id=60129542819 (accessed 11 February 2015).

Awata, S. (2010) New national health program against dementia in Japan: the medical center for dementia. Psychogeriatrics, 10, 2, 102–6.

Bartlett, R. (2000) Dementia as a disability: can we learn from disability studies and theory? Journal of Dementia Care, 8, 5, 33–6.

Bastawrous, M. (2013) Caregiver burden: a critical discussion. International Journal of Nursing Studies, 50, 3, 431–41.

Beerens, H.C., Zwakhalen, S.M., Verbeek, H., Ruwaard, D. and Hamers, J.P. (2013) Factors associated with quality of life of people with dementia in long-term care facilities: a systematic review. International Journal of Nursing Studies, 50, 9, 1259–70.

Bender, M. (2003) Explorations in Dementia. London: Jessica Kingsley Publishers.

Bowling, A. (1994) Social networks and social support among older people and implications for emotional wellbeing and psychiatric morbidity. International Review of Psychiatry, 6, 1, 41–58.

Brandon, D. and Jack, R. (1997) Struggling for Services. In I.J. Norman and S. Redfern (eds) Mental Health Care for Elderly People. Edinburgh: Churchill Livingstone.

Braun, M., Scholz, U., Bailey, B., Perren, S., Hornung, R. and Martin, M. (2009) Dementia caregiving in spousal relationships: a dyadic perspective. Aging and Mental Health, 13, 3, 426–36.

Bridges, J., Flatley, M. and Meyer, J. (2010) Older people's and relatives' experiences in acute care settings: systematic review and synthesis of qualitative studies. International Journal of Nursing Studies, 47, 1, 89–107.

Brodaty, H., Thomson, C., Thompson, C. and Fine, M. (2005) Why caregivers of people with dementia and memory loss don't use services. International Journal of Geriatric Psychiatry, 20, 6, 537–46.

Burton, J. and Hope, K.W. (2005) An exploration of the decision-making processes at the point of referral to an Admiral Nurse team. Journal of Psychiatric and Mental Health Nursing, 12, 3, 359–64.

Cacioppo, J.T. and Hawkley, L.C. (2009) Perceived social isolation and cognition. Trends in Cognitive Sciences, 13, 447–54.

Callahan, C.M., Arling, G., Tu, W., Rosenman, M.B. *et al.* (2012) Transitions in care for older adults with and without dementia. Journal of the American Geriatrics Society, 60, 5, 813–20.

Campbell, J.C. and Ikegami, N. (2000) Long-term care insurance comes to Japan. Health Affairs, 19, 26–39.

Cantley, C. and Wilson, R.C. (2012) 'Put yourself in my place': designing and managing care homes for people with dementia (a Joseph Rowntree Foundation Paper). Available at www.jrf.org.uk/sites/files/jrf/1861348118.pdf (accessed 6 December 2014).

Carers Trust, Royal College of Nursing (RCN) (2013) The Triangle of Care – Carers Included: A Guide to Best Practice for Dementia Care. Available at www.rcn.org.uk/__data/assets/pdf_file/0009/549063/Triangle_of_Care_-_Carers_Included_Sept_2013.pdf (accessed 14 May 2015).

Carpentier, N. and Grenier, A. (2012) Successful linkage between formal and informal care systems: the mobilization of outside help by caregivers of persons with Alzheimer's disease. Qualitative Health Research, 22, 10, 1330–44.

Chan, S.W. (2010) Family caregiving in dementia: the Asian perspective of a global problem. Dementia and Geriatric Cognitive Disorders, 30, 6, 469–78.

Choo, W.Y., Karina, R., Poi, P.J.H., Ebenezer, E. and Prince, M.J. (2003) Social support and burden among caregivers of patients with dementia in Malaysia. Asia-Pacific Journal of Public Health, 15, 1, 23–9.

Clarke, A., Hanson, E.J. and Ross, H. (2003) Seeing the person behind the patient: enhancing the care of older people using a biographical approach. Journal of Clinical Nursing, 12, 697–706.

Clayman, M.L., Roter, D., Wissow, L.S. and Bandeen-Roche, K. (2005) Autonomy-related behaviors of patient companions and their effect on decision-making activity in geriatric primary care visits. Social Science and Medicine, 60, 1583–91.

Cohen, C.A., Pringle, D. and LeDuc, L. (2001) Dementia caregiving: the role of the primary care physician. Canadian Journal of Neurological Sciences, 28, Suppl. 1, S72–6.

Cohen, S. and Wills, T.A. (1985) Stress, social support, and the buffering hypothesis. Psychological Bulletin, 98, 310–57.

Coriell, M. and Cohen, S. (1995) Concordance in the face of a stressful event: when do members of a dyad agree that one person supported the other? Journal of Personality and Social Psychology, 69, 289–99.

Cranswick, K. and Dosman, D. (2008) Eldercare: what we know today. Canadian Social Trends, 86, 48–56.

Cummings, J.L., Frank, J.C., Cherry, D., Kohatsu, N.D. *et al.* (2002) Guidelines for managing Alzheimer's disease. Part II: Treatment. American Family Physician, 65, 12, 2525–34.

Dalton, J.M. (2003) Development and testing of the theory of collaborative decision making in nursing practice for triads. Journal of Advanced Nursing, 41, 1, 22–33.

Dauphinot, V., Delphin-Combe, F., Mouchoux, C., Dorey, A., et al. (2015) Risk factors of caregiver burden among patients with Alzheimer's disease or related disorders: a cross-sectional study. Journal of Alzheimer's Disease, 44, 3, 907–916.

Davies, S.L., Goodman, C., Manthorpe, J., Smith, A., Carrick, N. and Iliffe, S. (2014) Enabling research in care homes: an evaluation of a national network of research ready care homes. BMC Medical Research Methodology, 14, 47.

Davis, S., Byers, S., Nay, R. and Koch, S. (2009) Guiding design of dementia friendly environments in residential care settings: considering the living experiences. Dementia, 8, 185–203.

Day, K., Carreon, D. and Stump, C. (2000) The therapeutic design of environments for people with dementia: a review of the empirical research. Gerontologist, 40, 397–416.

De Civita, M. and Dobkin, P.L. (2004) Pediatric adherence as a multidimensional and dynamic construct, involving a triadic partnership. Journal of Pediatric Psychology, 29, 3, 157–69.

Dementia Action Alliance (2014) Top 20 Checklist for Commissioners – Examples of Services Supporting Family Carers of People Living with Dementia. Available at www.dementiaaction.org.uk/carers/examples_of_services_and_support (accessed 19 February 2015).

Dementia Action Alliance (2015) Action Plan, National Dementia Declaration. Available at www.dementiaaction.org.uk/members_and_action_plans/69-department_of_health (accessed 19 February 2015).

Department of Health (2001) National Service Framework for Older People (DH publication number 23633). London: Department of Health.

Department of Health (2006) Care Homes for Older People, National Minimum Standards, Care Home Regulations 2001 (3rd edition 2003, third impression 2006). London: The Stationery Office.

de Vugt, M.E. and Verhey, F.R. (2013) The impact of early dementia diagnosis and intervention on informal caregivers. Progress in Neurobiology, 110, 54–62.

de Vugt, M.E., Stevens, F., Aalten, P., Lousberg, R. *et al.* (2003) Behavioural disturbances in dementia patients and quality of the marital relationship. International Journal of Geriatric Psychiatry, 18, 149–54.

Dewing, J. and Traynor, V. (2005) Admiral nursing competency project: practice development and action research. Journal of Clinical Nursing, 14, 6, 695–703.

Donelan, K., Hill, C.A., Hoffman, C., Scoles, K. *et al.* (2002) Challenged to care: informal caregivers in a changing health system. Health Affairs, 21, 222–31.

Drentea, P., Clay, O.J., Roth, D.L. and Mittelman, M.S. (2006) Predictors of improvement in social support: five year effects of a structured intervention for caregivers of spouses with Alzheimer's disease. Social Science and Medicine, 63, 4, 957–67.

Dubet, F. (1995) Sociologie de l'experience [Experiences and Sociology]. Paris, France: Seuil. Cited in N. Carpentier and A. Grenier (2012) Successful linkage between formal and informal care systems: the mobilization of outside help by caregivers of persons with Alzheimer's disease. Qualitative Health Research, 22, 10, 1330–44.

Dupuis, S.L., Wiersma, E. and Loiselle, L. (2012) Pathologizing behavior: meanings of behaviors in dementia care. Journal of Aging Studies, 26, 162–73.

Edvardsson, D., Winblad, B. and Sandman, P.O. (2008) Person-centred care of people with severe Alzheimer's disease: current status and ways forward. Lancet Neurology, 7, 4, 362–7.

Eustace, A., Bruce, I., Coen, R., Cunningham, C. *et al.* (2007) Behavioural disturbance triggers recognition of dementia by family informants. International Journal of Geriatric Psychiatry, 22, 6, 574–9.

Field, E.M., Walker, M.H. and Orrell, M.W. (2002) Social networks and health of older people living in sheltered housing. Aging and Mental Health, 6, 4, 372–86.

Fossey, J., Ballard, C., Juszczak, E., James, I. *et al.* (2006) Effect of enhanced psychosocial care on antipsychotic use in nursing home residents with severe dementia: cluster randomised trial. British Medical Journal, 332, 756–61.

Gaugler, J.E., Zarit, S.H. and Pearlin, L.I. (2003) The onset of dementia and its longitudinal implications. Psychology and Aging, 18, 2, 171–80.

Giannakouris, K. (2011) Ageing characterises the demographic perspectives of the European societies. Eurostat: Statistics in Focus. Available at http://polennu.dk/sites/default/files/Eurostat%20befolkningsprognose%202008-2060.pdf (accessed 6 December 2014).

Godden, S., McCoy, D. and Pollock, A. (2009) Policy on the rebound: trends and causes of delayed discharges in the NHS. Journal of the Royal Society of Medicine, 102, 22–8.

Goffman, E. (1968) Stigma: Notes on the Management of Spoiled Identity. Harmondsworth: Penguin.

Goodman, C., Baron, N.L., Machen, I., Stevenson, E. *et al.* (2011) Culture, consent, costs and care homes: enabling older people with dementia to participate in research. Aging and Mental Health, 15, 4, 475–81.

Gort, A.M., Mingot, M., Gomez, X., Soler, T., et al. (2007) Use of the Zarit scale for assessing caregiver burden and collapse in caregiving at home in dementias. International Journal of Geriatric Psychiatry, 22, 10, 957–962.

Greene, M.G., Majerovitz, S.D., Adelman, R.D. and Rizzo, C. (1994) The effects of the presence of a third person on the physician–older patient medical interview. Journal of the American Geriatrics Society, 42, 413–19.

Greenwood, N., Mackenzie, A., Cloud, G.C. and Wilson, N. (2009) Informal primary carers of stroke survivors living at home – challenges, satisfactions and coping: a systematic review of qualitative studies. Disability and Rehabilitation, 31, 5, 337–51.

Grenier, A. (2004) Older Women Negotiating Uncertainty in Everyday Life: Contesting Risk Management Systems. In L. Davies and P. Leonard (eds) Critical Social Work in a Corporate Era: Practices of Power and Resistance. Aldershot: Ashgate.

Hall, G. and Buckwalter, K. (1987) Progressively lowered stress threshold: a conceptual model for care of adults with Alzheimer's disease. Archives of Psychiatric Nursing, 1, 399–406.

Hawkins, R.L. and Maurer, K. (2012) Unravelling Social Capital: Disentangling a Concept for Social Work British Journal of Social Work, 42, 353–70.

Health Foundation (2011) Spotlight on dementia care: a Health Foundation Improvement Report. Available at www.health.org.uk/public/cms/75/76/4181/2703/Spotlight_Dementia%20Care.pdf?realName=1pWJno.pdf (accessed 6 December 2014).

Health Foundation (2014) Helping measure person-centred care: a review of evidence about commonly used approaches and tools used to help measure person-centred care. Available at www.health.org.uk/public/cms/75/76/313/4697/Helping%20measure%20person-centred%20care.pdf?realName=lnet6X.pdf (accessed 6 December 2014).

Heru, A.M., Ryan, C.E. and Iqbal, A. (2004) Family functioning in the caregivers of patients with dementia. International Journal of Geriatric Psychiatry, 19, 536–7.

Hilgeman, M.M., Durkin, D.W., Sun, F., DeCoster, J. *et al.* (2009) Testing a theoretical model of the stress process in Alzheimer's caregivers with race as a moderator. Gerontologist, 49, 2, 248–61.

Hinchliffe, A.C., Hyman, I.L., Blizard, B. and Livingston, G. (1995) Behavioural complications of dementia: can they be treated? International Journal of Geriatric Psychiatry, 10, 10, 839–47.

Hirsch, M.A., Sanjak, M., Englert, D., Iyer, S. and Quinlan, M.M. (2014) Parkinson patients as partners in care. Parkinsonism and Related Disorders, 20, Suppl. 1, S174–9.

Hollander, M.J., Liu, G. and Chappell, N.L. (2009) Who cares and how much? The imputed economic contribution to the Canadian Healthcare System of middle-aged and older unpaid caregivers providing care to the elderly. Healthcare Quarterly, 12, 42–9.

Huang, H.L., Kuo, L.M., Chen, Y.S., Liang, J. *et al.* (2013) A home-based training program improves caregivers' skills and dementia patients' aggressive behaviors: a randomized controlled trial. American Journal of Geriatric Psychiatry, 21, 11, 1060–70.

Hunter, R., McGill, L., Bosanquet, N. and Johnson, N. (1997) Alzheimer's disease in the United Kingdom: developing patient and carer support strategies to encourage care in the community. Quality in Health Care, 6, 3, 146–52.

Innes, A. (2002) The social and political context of formal dementia care provision. Ageing and Society, 22, 483–99.

Jaglal, S., Cockerill, R., Lemieux-Charles, L., Chambers, L.W., Brazil, K. and Cohen, C. (2007) Perceptions of the process of care among caregivers and care recipients in dementia care networks. American Journal of Alzheimer's Disease and Other Dementias, 22, 2, 103–11.

Jasinarachchi, K., Ibrahim, I., Keegan, B., Mathialagan, R. *et al.* (2009) Delayed transfer of care from NHS secondary care to primary care in England: its determinants, effect of hospital bed days, prevalence of acute medical conditions and deaths during delay, in older adults aged 65 years and over. BMC Geriatrics, 9, 4.

Joseph Rowntree Foundation (October 2012) My home life: promoting quality of life in care homes. Available at www.jrf.org.uk/sites/files/jrf/care-home-quality-of-life-summary.pdf (accessed 6 December 2014).

Keady, J. and Nolan, M. (2003) The Dynamics of Dementia: Working Together, Working Separately, or Working Alone? In M.R. Nolan, U. Lundh, G. Grant and J. Keady (eds) Partnerships in Family Care: Understanding the Care-Giving Career. Buckingham: Open University Press.

Keady, J. and Williams, S. (2007) Co-constructed inquiry: a new approach to generating, disseminating and discovering knowledge in qualitative research. Quality in Ageing, 8, 27–36.

Kiecolt-Glaser, J.K., Glaser, R., Gravenstein, S., Malarkey, W.B. and Sheridan, J. (1996) Chronic stress alters the immune response to influenza virus vaccine in older adults. Proceedings of the National Academy of Sciences of the USA, 93, 3043–7.

Kinney, J.M. and Stephens, M.A.P. (1989) Caregiving hassles scale: assessing the daily hassles of caring for a family member with dementia. Gerontologist, 29, 3, 328–32.

Kitwood, T. (1990) The dialectics of dementia: with particular reference to Alzheimer's disease. Ageing and Society, 10, 177–96.

Kitwood, T. (1993) Towards a theory of dementia care: the interpersonal process. Ageing and Society, 13, 51–67.

Kitwood, T. (1997a) Dementia Reconsidered: The Person Comes First. Buckingham: Open University Press.

Kitwood, T. (1997b) The experience of dementia. Aging and Mental Health, 1, 13–22.

Koehn, S.D., Kozak, J.-F. and Drance, E. (2012) 'The problem with Leonard': a critical constructionist view of need-driven dementia-compromised behaviours. Dementia, 11, 725–41.

Köhler, L., Meinke-Franze, C., Hein, J., Fendrich, K. *et al.* (2014) Does an interdisciplinary network improve dementia care? Results from the IDemUck-study. Current Alzheimer Research, 11, 6, 538–48.

Kovach, C.R., Noonan, P.E., Schlidt, A.M. and Wells, T. (2005) A model of consequences of need-driven, dementia-compromised behavior. Journal of Nursing Scholarship, 37, 2, 134–40.

Laing, W. and Buisson, E. (2009) Care of Elderly People: UK Market Survey. London: Laing and Buisson.

Lakey, B. and Lutz, C.J. (1996) Social Support and Preventive and Therapeutic Interventions. In G.R. Pierce, B.R. Sarason and I.G. Sarason (eds) Handbook of Social Support and the Family. New York, NY: Plenum.

Lewin, S.A., Skea, Z.C., Entwistle, V., Zwarenstein, M. and Dick, J. (2001) Interventions for providers to promote a patient-centred approach in clinical consultations. Cochrane Database of Systematic Reviews, 4.

Lloyd, B.T. and Stirling, C. (2011) Ambiguous gain: uncertain benefits of service use for dementia carers. Sociology of Health and Illness, 33, 4, 1–15.

Lopez, O.L., Becker, J.T., Somsak, D., Dew, M.A. and DeKosky, S.T. (1994) Awareness of cognitive deficits and anosognosia in probable Alzheimer's disease. European Neurology, 34, 277–82.

Lyketsos, C.G., Colenda, C.C., Beck, C., Blank, K. *et al.* Task Force of American Association for Geriatric Psychiatry (2006) Position statement of the American Association for Geriatric Psychiatry regarding principles of care for patients with dementia resulting from Alzheimer disease. American Journal of Geriatric Psychiatry, 14, 7, 561–72.

Lyons, K., Zarit, S., Sayer, A. and Whitlatch, C.J. (2002) Caregiving as a dyadic process: perspectives from caregiver and receiver. Journals of Gerontology, Series B: Psychological Sciences and Social Sciences, 57, 195–204.

Macmillan (2015) Macmillan Nurses. Available at www.macmillan.org.uk/information-and-support/coping/getting-support/macmillan-nurses (accessed 27 May 2015).

Marshall, M. (2001) The challenge of looking after people with dementia. British Medical Journal, 323, 410–11.

Martin, C. and Sturmberg, J. (2009) Complex adaptive chronic care. Journal of Evaluation in Clinical Practice, 15, 571–7.

Martin, M. and Wight, M. (2008) Dyadic Cognition in Old Age: Paradigms, Findings, and Directions. In S.M. Hofer and D.F. Alwin (eds) Handbook of Cognitive Ageing: Interdisciplinary Perspectives. Thousand Oaks, CA: Sage Publications.

McCabe, M.P., Roberts, C. and Firth, L. (2008) Satisfaction with services among people with progressive neurological illnesses and their carers in Australia. Nursing and Health Sciences, 10, 3, 209–15.

McCormack, B. (2004) Person-centredness in gerontological nursing: an overview of the literature. International Journal of Older People Nursing, 13, 31–8.

McKee, K. (1999) This is Your Life: Research Paradigm in Dementia Care. In T. Adams and C.I. Clarke (eds) Dementia Care: Developing Partnerships in Practice. London: Baillière Tindall.

McKeown, J., Clarke, A. and Repper, J. (2006) Life story work in health and social care: systematic literature review. Journal of Advanced Nursing, 55, 237–47.

Medeiros de A Nunes, V., Alchieri, J.C., Azevedo, L.M., Varela de Oliveira, K.M. and Pereira, D.A. (2014) Cognitive assessment in elderly residents of long-stay institutions. Dementia and Geriatric Cognitive Disorders, 37, 1–2, 27–33.

Mohamed, S., Rosenheck, R., Lyketsos, C.G. and Schneider, L.S. (2010) Caregiver burden in Alzheimer disease: cross-sectional and longitudinal patient correlates. American Journal of Geriatric Psychiatry, 18, 917–27.

Moise, P., Schwarzinger, M. and Um, M.Y. (2004) Dementia Care in 9 OECD Countries: A Comparative Analysis. OECD Health Working Paper No. 13 (OECD). Available at www.oecd.org/health/health-systems/33661491.pdf (accessed 11 February 2015).

Moon, H. and Adams, K.B. (2013) The effectiveness of dyadic interventions for people with dementia and their caregivers. Dementia (London), 12, 6, 821–39.

Narayan, S., Lewis, M., Tornatore, J., Hepburn, K. and Corcoran-Perry, S. (2001) Subjective responses to caregiving for a spouse with dementia. Journal of Gerontological Nursing, 27, 3, 19–28.

National Council for Palliative Care and the NHS End of Life Care Programme (2006) Introductory Guide to End of Life Care in Care Homes. London: Department of Health.

Newbronner, L., Chamberlain, R., Borthwick, R., Baxter, M. and Glendinning, C./Carers Trust (2013) A Road Less Rocky – Supporting Carers of People with Dementia. London: Carers Trust. Available at www.carers.org/sites/default/files/dementia_report_road_less_rocky_final_low.pdf (accessed 11 February 2015).

Nobili, A., Piana, I., Pasina, L., Matucci, M., Tarantola, M. and Trevisan, S. (2008) Alzheimer special care units compared with traditional nursing home for dementia care: are there differences at admissions and in clinical outcomes? Alzheimer Disease and Associated Disorders, 22, 4, 352–61.

Nolan, M.R., Davies, S., Brown, J., Keady, J. and Nolan, J. (2004) Beyond 'person-centred' care: a new vision for gerontological nursing. Journal of Clinical Nursing, 13, 45–53.

Nolan, M.R., Davies, S. and Grant, G. (eds) (2001) Working with Older People and Their Families: Key Issues in Policy and Practice. Buckingham: Open University Press.

Nolan, M.R., Lundh, U., Grant, G. and Keady, J. (eds) (2003) Partnerships in Family Care: Understanding the Caregiving Career. Maidenhead: Open University Press.

Nolan, M.R., Ryan, T., Enderby, P. and Reid, D. (2002) Towards a more inclusive vision of dementia care practice and research. Dementia: The International Journal of Social Research and Practice, 1, 2, 193–211.

Nourhashemi, F., Andrieu, S., Sastres, N., Ducasse, J.L. *et al.* (2001) Descriptive analysis of emergency hospital admissions of patients with Alzheimer disease. Alzheimer Disease and Associated Disorders, 15, 1, 21–5.

Olafsdóttir, M., Skoog, I. and Marcusson, J. (2000) Detection of dementia in primary care: the Linköping study. Dementia and Geriatric Cognitive Disorders, 11, 4, 223–9.

Palmer, J.L. (2013) Preserving personhood of individuals with advanced dementia: lessons from family caregivers. Geriatric Nursing, 34, 3, 224–9.

Parmar, J., Dobbs, B., McKay, R., Kirwan, C. *et al.* (2014) Diagnosis and management of dementia in primary care: exploratory study. Canadian Family Physician, 60, 5, 457–65.

Peel, E. and Harding, R. (2014) 'It's a huge maze, the system, it's a terrible maze': dementia carers' constructions of navigating health and social care services. Dementia (London), 13, 5, 642–61.

Pimlott, N.J.G., Siegel, K., Persaud, M., Slaughter, S. *et al.* (2006) Management of dementia by family physicians in academic settings. Canadian Family Physician, 52, 1108–9.

Pusey, H. (2003) Psychosocial Interventions with Carers of People with Dementia. In J. Keady, C.L. Clarke and T. Adams (eds) Community Mental Health Nursing and Dementia Care: Practice Perspective. Maidenhead: Open University Press.

Quinn, C., Clare, L., McGuinness, T. and Woods, R.T. (2013) Negotiating the balance: the triadic relationship between spousal caregivers, people with dementia and Admiral Nurses. Dementia (London), 12, 5, 588–605.

Quinn, C., Clare, L. and Woods, R.T. (2009) The impact of the quality of relationship on the experiences and wellbeing of caregivers of people with dementia: a systematic review. Aging and Mental Health, 13, 143–54.

Qureshi, H., Bamford, C., Nicholas, E., Patmore, C. and Harris, J.C. (2000) Outcomes in Social Care Practice: Developing an Outcome Focus in Care Management and Use Surveys, Social Policy Research Unit, University of York.

Rafferty, J., Smith, R.G., Lewis, S.J. and Levack, H. (1989) The functional status of elderly people admitted to a local authority residential home. Health Bulletin (Edinburgh), 47, 3, 141–9.

Rahman, S. (2014) Living Well with Dementia: The Importance of the Person and the Environment for Wellbeing. Oxford: Radcliffe Health.

Rapoff, M.A. (1999) Adherence to Pediatric Medical Regimens. New York: Kluwer Academic/Plenum.

Richardson, T.J., Lee, S.J., Berg-Weger, M. and Grossberg, G.T. (2013) Caregiver health: health of caregivers of Alzheimer's and other dementia patients. Current Psychiatry Reports, 15, 7, 367.

Riegel, B., Moser, D.K., Anker, S.D., Appel, L.J. *et al.* (2009) State of science: promoting self care in persons with heart failure: a scientific statement from the American Heart Association. Circulation, 120, 1141e63.

Royal College of Nursing (RCN) (2013) Dementia: commitment to the care of people with dementia in hospital settings. Available at www.rcn.org.uk/__data/assets/pdf_file/0011/480269/004235.pdf (accessed 6 December 2014).

Ryan, T., Nolan, M., Reid, D. and Enderby, P. (2008) Using the Senses Framework to achieve relationship-centred dementia care services: a case example. Dementia, 7, 1, 71–93.

Schmidt, K.L., Lingler, J.H. and Schulz, R. (2009) Verbal communication among Alzheimer's disease patients, their caregivers, and primary care physicians during primary care office visits. Patient Education and Counseling, 77, 2, 197–201.

Schulz, R. and Martire, L.M. (2004) Family caregiving of persons with dementia: prevalence, health effects, and support strategies. American Journal of Geriatric Psychiatry, 12, 3, 240–9.

Schulz, R., O'Brien, A.T., Bookwala, J. and Fleissner, K. (1995) Psychiatric and physical morbidity effects of dementia caregiving: prevalence, correlates, and causes. Gerontologist, 35, 771–91.

Schumacher, K.L., Stewart, B.J. and Archbold, P.G. (2007) Mutuality and preparedness moderate the effects of caregiving demand on cancer family caregiver outcomes. Nursing Research, 56, 6, 425–33.

Shaji, K.S., George, R.K., Prince, M.J. and Jacob, K.S. (2009) Behavioural symptoms and caregiver burden in dementia. Indian Journal of Psychiatry, 51, 1, 45–9.

Strachan, P.H., Currie, K., Harkness, K., Spaling, M. and Clark, A.M. (2014) Context matters in heart failure self-care: a qualitative systematic review. Journal of Cardiac Failure, 20, 6, 448–55.

Stuckey, J.C., Neundorfer, M.M. and Smyth, K.A. (1996) Burden and wellbeing: the same coin or related currency? Gerontologist, 36, 68–93.

Swaffer, K. (2014) Prescribed Disengagement, Models of Care and QoL. A presentation at the Alzheimer's Disease International Conference, Puerto Rico, 2014. Available at www.alz.co.uk/sites/default/files/conf2014/OC091.pdf (accessed 6 December 2014).

Tanenbaum, S.J. (2013) What is patient-centered care? A typology of models and missions. Health Care Analysis, June 2013 [Epub ahead of print].

The Princess Royal Trust for Carers (2011) Always on Call; Always Concerned. A Survey of the Experiences of Older Carers (The Princess Royal Trust for Carers). Available at www.carers.org/sites/default/files/always_on_call_always_concerned.pdf (accessed 6 December 2014).

Tooth, L., Russell, A., Lucke, J., Byrne, G. *et al.* (2008) Impact of cognitive and physical impairment on carer burden and quality of life. Quality of Life Research, 17, 267–73.

Van Der Gaag, M. and Webber, M. (2007) Measurement of Individual Social Capital: Questions, Instruments and Measures. In I. Kawachi, S.V. Subramanian and D. Kim (eds) Social Capital and Health. New York: Springer.

van der Lee, J., Bakker, T.J., Duivenvoorden, H.J. and Dröes, R.M. (2014) Multivariate models of subjective caregiver burden in dementia: a systematic review. Ageing Research Reviews, 15, 76–93.

Villars, H., Oustric, S., Andrieu, S., Baeyens, J.P. *et al.* (2010) The primary care physician and Alzheimer's disease: an international position paper. Journal of Nutrition, Health and Aging, 14, 2, 110–20.

Wade, D.T., Legh-Smith, J. and Hewer, R.L. (1986) Effects of living with and looking after survivors of a stroke. British Medical Journal Clinical Research, 293, 418–20.

Webber, M. (2005) Social capital and mental health. In J. Tew (ed.) Social Perspectives in Mental Health: Developing Social Models to Understand and Work with Mental Distress. London: Jessica Kingsley Publishers.

Webber, M., Reidy, H., Ansari, D., Stevens, M. and Morris, D. (2015) Enhancing social networks: a qualitative study of health and social care practice in UK mental health services. Health and Social Care in the Community, 23, 2, 180–9.

Weber, L.R. and Carter, A.I. (2002) The Social Construction of Trust. New York, NY: Springer.

Whall, A.L. and Kolanowski, A.M. (2004) The need-driven dementia-compromised behavior model – a framework for understanding the behavioural symptoms of dementia. Aging and Mental Health, 8, 2, 106–8.

Whitlatch, C.J., Judge, K., Zarit, S.H. and Femia, E. (2006) Dyadic intervention for family caregivers and care receivers in early-stage dementia. Gerontologist, 46, 5, 688–94.

Wilks, S.E. and Croom, B. (2008) Perceived stress and resilience in Alzheimer's disease caregivers: testing moderation and mediation models of social support. Aging and Mental Health, 12, 3, 357–65.

Williamson, G.M. and Schulz, R. (1995) Caring for a family member with cancer: past communal behavior and affective reactions. Journal of Applied Social Psychology, 25, 2, 93–116.

Wong, F.K. and Chung, L.C. (2006) Establishing a definition for a nurse-led clinic: structure, process, and outcome. Journal of Advanced Nursing, 53, 3, 358–69.

World Health Organization (2012) Dementia: a public health priority. World Health Organization and Alzheimer's Disease International. Geneva: WHO. Available at http://whqlibdoc.who.int/publications/2012/9789241564458_eng.pdf (accessed 6 December 2014).

Wyer, P.C. and Silva, S.A. (2014) Through a glass, darkly: the challenge of integration of the science and the art of medicine: analysis of the discussion paper: 'The care of the patient and the soul of the clinic: person-centered medicine as an emergent model of modern clinical practice' by Andrew Miles and Juan E. Mezzich, IJPCM 2011, 1, 2, 207–22. European Journal of Person Centered Healthcare, 2, 1, 46–53.

Wyer, P.C., Alves Silva, S., Post, S.G. and Quinlan, P. (2014) Relationship-centred care: antidote, guidepost or blind alley? The epistemology of 21st century health care. Journal of Evaluation in Clinical Practice, 20, 6, 881–9.

Xiao, L.D., Wang, J., He, G.P., De Bellis, A., Verbeeck, J. and Kyriazopoulos, H. (2014) Family caregiver challenges in dementia care in Australia and China: a critical perspective. BMC Geriatrics, 14, 6.

Yamaguchi, H., Maki, Y. and Yamagami, T. (2010) Overview of non-pharmacological intervention for dementia and principles of brain-activating rehabilitation. Psychogeriatrics, 10, 4, 206–13.

Yang, C.T., Liu, H.Y. and Shyu, Y.I. (2014) Dyadic relational resources and role strain in family caregivers of persons living with dementia at home: a cross-sectional survey. International Journal of Nursing Studies, 51, 4, 593–602.

Zarit, S.H. and Edwards, A.B. (2008) Family Caregiving: Research and Clinical Intervention. In R.T. Woods and L. Clare (eds) Handbook of the Clinical Psychology of Ageing, 2nd edition. Chichester: Wiley.

Zimmerman, S., Williams, C., Reed, P., Boustani, M., Preisser, J., Heck, E. and Sloane, P.D. (2005) Attitudes, stress, and satisfaction of staff who care for residents with dementia. Gerontologist, 45, 96–105.

Chapter 8

EATING AND LIVING BETTER WITH DEMENTIA

'One cannot think well, love well, sleep well, if one has not dined well.'

Virginia Woolf, *A Room of One's Own* (1929)

Introduction

'Eating well' can literally mean that someone has the amount of energy (calories) and nutrients (protein, fats, carbohydrates, fibre, vitamins and minerals) that they need every day to maintain their body processes and to protect their body from ill health (Crawley and Hocking, 2011).

But this is sometimes not what happens in care environments. This chapter will look at how, for the person living with dementia, *what* he or she eats matters, and so does *how* he or she eats.

Edgar Schein (1984, p.3) defined 'organisational culture' as follows:

> ...the pattern of basic assumptions that a given group has invented, discovered or developed in learning to cope with its problem of external adaptation and internal integration, and that have worked well enough to be considered valid, and, therefore, to be taught, to new members as the correct way to perceive, think, and feel in relation to these problems.

Ray and colleagues (2014) have recently discussed how one in four adults are estimated to be at medium to high risk of malnutrition when screened using the 'Malnutrition Universal Screening Tool' upon admission to hospital in the United Kingdom. The Need for Nutrition Education/Innovation Programme (NNEdPro) was developed to address this issue, and the Nutrition Education and Leadership for Improved Clinical Outcomes (NELICO) was an innovative method to promote nutrition awareness in tomorrow's doctors. These doctors were shown the enthusiasm and drive to be nutrition champions.

Organisational change is difficult. The problem is that studies tracking various types of organisational changes indicate that 70% or more of significant organisational changes either fail to achieve the desired results, fail altogether or make things worse (Senge, 1999). The characteristics of 'change champions', defined by Warrick (2009, p.15) as 'a person at any level of the organization who is skilled at initiating, facilitating, and implementing change'. Warrick (2009) furthermore emphasises the need to build strategic alliances and commitment from stakeholders and the need for feedback mechanisms to identify any progress.

Bikhchandani, Hirshleifer and Welch, in 'A theory of fads, fashion, custom, and cultural change as informational cascades' (1992), offer a useful and coherent explanation of the phenomenon known as 'information cascading', best known in the marketing and knowledge transfer disciplines. Information cascades in terms of 'herd behaviour' – what happens when somebody follows the person ahead of them, irrespective of their own knowledge base. Endurance suggests that the change has staying power over a length of time. The ability of an organisation to change, in terms of its 'inertia', might be related to its fundamental architecture (Hannah, Polos and Carroll, 2003). It is also interesting to observe how bandwagons develop: adoption by certain organisations can promote future adoption because these organisations increase the social or economic value of adoption (Tolbert and Zucker, 1983). Another explanation is that adoption by certain organisations sets off bandwagons because these adopters better reveal information about the value of adoption (Rao, Greve and Davis, 2001).

Making sure older people have nutritious food and drinks is fundamental to good care. The report by the Care Commission entitled 'Promoting nutrition in care homes for older people' (2009) evaluated a programme aimed at improving nutrition in Scotland's care homes for older people. This initiative urged a role for nutrition champions in care homes. They concluded that, overall, the programme was highly valued by the participants.

The 'nutrition champions' felt the programme gave them, for example (Care Commission, 2009, pp.2–3):

- an excellent grounding in nutrition, which allowed them to make a change in their care home
- essential support from other nutrition champions, including the chance to share their experiences and resolve problems together
- knowledge and new skills and confidence in all aspects of practice, including managing change, involving people, gathering and using evidence, providing support and feedback, and project planning the chance to challenge and change current care practice in their care homes, including staff attitudes, and raising staff awareness of ways of improving nutrition.

Nutrition standards and care homes

In England, meanwhile, the Care Quality Commission (CQC) carried out unannounced inspections at 100 acute NHS hospitals in England between March and June 2011, using teams made up of CQC inspectors, a practising and experienced nurse, and an 'expert by experience' – someone with experience of caring or receiving care, trained and supported by Age UK. This was reported on, promptly, in October 2011.

Malnutrition

According to National Institute for Health and Care Excellence (NICE, 2006) guidance on nutrition support in adults (NICE clinical guidance CG32), malnutrition is defined as:

- a body mass index (BMI) of less than 18.5 kg/m^2
- unintentional weight loss greater than 10% within the last three to six months
- a BMI of less than 20 kg/m^2 and unintentional weight loss greater than 5% within the last three to six months.

Malnutrition is both a cause and consequence of disease and illness, and there can be many contributing factors. The Malnutrition Task Force (2013) proposed that prevention and treatment of malnutrition should be at the heart of everything society does to ensure older people can live more independent, fulfilling lives. The Task Force outlined five main principles and offered guidance on implementing changes using the wealth of existing guides and tools readily available.

Eating behaviours in dementia and the use of volumetric neuroimaging

Food is a relatively undeveloped research subject in health and social welfare, particularly with respect to older people (Mennell, Murcott and van Otterloo, 1992), but some inroads have been made into understanding the specific neural substrates underlying abnormal eating behaviours for persons living with dementia. It is probably fair to say that the dementia syndromes in which eating behaviours have been investigated the most include dementia of the Alzheimer type (at first signposted by problems in attention and new learning and memory; DAT), behavioural variant frontotemporal dementia (at first signposted by problems in personality and behaviour; bvFTD) and temporal variant frontotemporal dementia (including problems in semantic knowledge; semantic dementia or SD).

First of all, it is important to appreciate that eating abnormalities are more likely in certain types of dementia than others. For example, the frequencies of symptoms in all five domains, except swallowing problems, might be higher in bvFTD than in DAT (Ikeda *et al.*, 2002); conversely, changes in food preference and eating habits were greater in SD than in DAT. In bvFTD, the first symptom reported was altered eating habits or appetite increase. Indeed, eating abnormalities form one of the major criteria for the diagnosis of bvFTD (Rascovsky *et al.*, 2011). Patients typically develop changes in appetite, binge-eating behaviour and increased carbohydrate and sugar intake (Ikeda *et al.*, 2002). In DAT, the pattern was not clear, although swallowing problems developed in relatively early stages.

Understanding which parts of the brain go wrong in producing these symptoms has proved to be productive. Turning to the neuroanatomical implications of their findings, Ikeda and colleagues (2002) have proposed that the changes in eating behaviours reflect the involvement of a common network in both variants of frontotemporal dementia – namely, the ventral (orbitobasal) frontal lobe, the temporal pole and the amygdala (e.g. Cummings and Duchen, 1981). The ventromedial frontal lobe is affected from an early stage in patients with bvFTD and SD, either by direct pathological involvement or indirectly through damage to the temporal pole and amygdala, which are heavily interconnected with the ventromedial frontal lobe (Mummery *et al.*, 2000). Klüver–Bucy syndrome has been known about by neurologists for some time for its distinct cluster of symptoms. Bilateral degeneration of the amygdaloid nuclear complex in monkeys and surgical removal of the temporal lobes in humans result in Klüver–Bucy syndrome which is characterised by hyperorality, overeating and the eating of quasi-food items (Bucy and Klüver, 1955, cited in Ikeda *et al.*, 2002).

A study by Howard Rosen and colleagues (2005) examined neuroanatomical correlates of behavioural abnormalities, as measured by the famous rating scale known as the 'Neuropsychiatric Inventory', in 148 patients with dementia using a brain-imaging technique called voxel-based morphometry (VBM). The methodology of VBM has revolutionised our understanding of eating abnormalities in dementia. The aim of VBM is to identify differences in the local composition of brain tissue, while discounting large-scale differences in gross anatomy and position.

Flavour identification performance in the combined FTD cohort was significantly associated with changes in distinct regions of the brain: grey-matter volume in the left entorhinal cortex, hippocampus, parahippocampal gyrus and temporal pole. This profile, in fact, comprises brain substrates in the anteromedial temporal lobe which have been previously implicated in the associative processing of chemosensory stimuli (e.g. Gorno-Tempini *et al.*, 2004). Some people living with dementia may eat too much and gain excess weight. This can be due to changes in food preferences, memory loss or boredom. In an interesting VBM study by Whitwell and colleagues (2007), the authors found distinct neuroanatomical signatures of different abnormalities of eating behaviour (pathological sweet tooth and increased food consumption or hyperphagia) in individuals with FTD. The development of pathological sweet tooth has been associated with grey-matter loss in a distributed brain network including bilateral posterolateral orbitofrontal cortex (Brodmann areas 12/47) and right anterior insula. Hyperphagia was associated with more focal grey-matter loss in anterolateral orbitofrontal cortex bilaterally (Brodmann area 11).

Carers' reports of changes in eating behaviour show that various forms of increased eating are commonly found at some stage in the course of dementia (Morris, Hope and Fairburn, 1989). According to Keene and Hope (1998), studies showed that hyperphagia is a stable condition, generally occurring as a single episode. Duration of hyperphagia varied, ranging from four months to more than three years in a few subjects. This is likely to be an underestimate as the end of the hyperphagia was often masked by the preventive measures taken by the carer. Hyperphagia and associated eating changes occur frequently in DAT and lead to considerable morbidity. However, the neurochemical basis for these neuropsychiatric behaviours is at present unclear. Medications known as selective serotonin reuptake inhibitors (SSRIs) have shown efficacy in the treatment of bulimia nervosa and binge-eating disorders (Milano *et al.*, 2005), as well as suppressing rebound hyperphagia in rats (Inoue *et al.*, 1997). Tsang and colleagues (2010) measured serotonin transporters and receptors 5-HT1A, 5-HT2A and 5-HT4 using radioligand binding assays in the post-mortem temporal cortex of a cohort of controls and patients with dementia of the Alzheimer type longitudinally assessed for hyperphagia.

The 'human sweet tooth' and living well with dementia

Older people with dementia may choose sweet foods over savoury ones, and it has been shown that a craving for sweet foods is part of the clinical syndrome for dementia at some stages (Crawley and Hocking, 2011). If people eat only sweet foods – for example, if they just eat desserts – they will not get all the nutrients they need. An important consideration is, of course, the potential for weight gain: if excess weight gain is a problem, it might be worth trying an artificial sweetener instead. Marked disturbances in eating behaviour, such as overeating and preference for sweet foods, are also commonly reported in bvFTD. It has been thought for some time that this might have something to do with a small area of the brainstem known as the hypothalamus. The hypothalamus plays a critical role in feeding regulation, yet the relation between pathology in this region and eating behaviour in bvFTD is unknown.

A pictorial representation of the 'human sweet tooth' is given in Figure 8.1.

The study by Piquet and colleagues (2011) identified significant atrophy of the hypothalamus in persons with bvFTD. Indeed, persons with prominent eating disturbance exhibited significant atrophy of the posterior hypothalamus. Features of eating disturbance, such as increased appetite, preference for sweet foods and an increased tendency to eat the same foods, were found in that study to be present in the bvFTD group, but were not observed in the healthy controls.

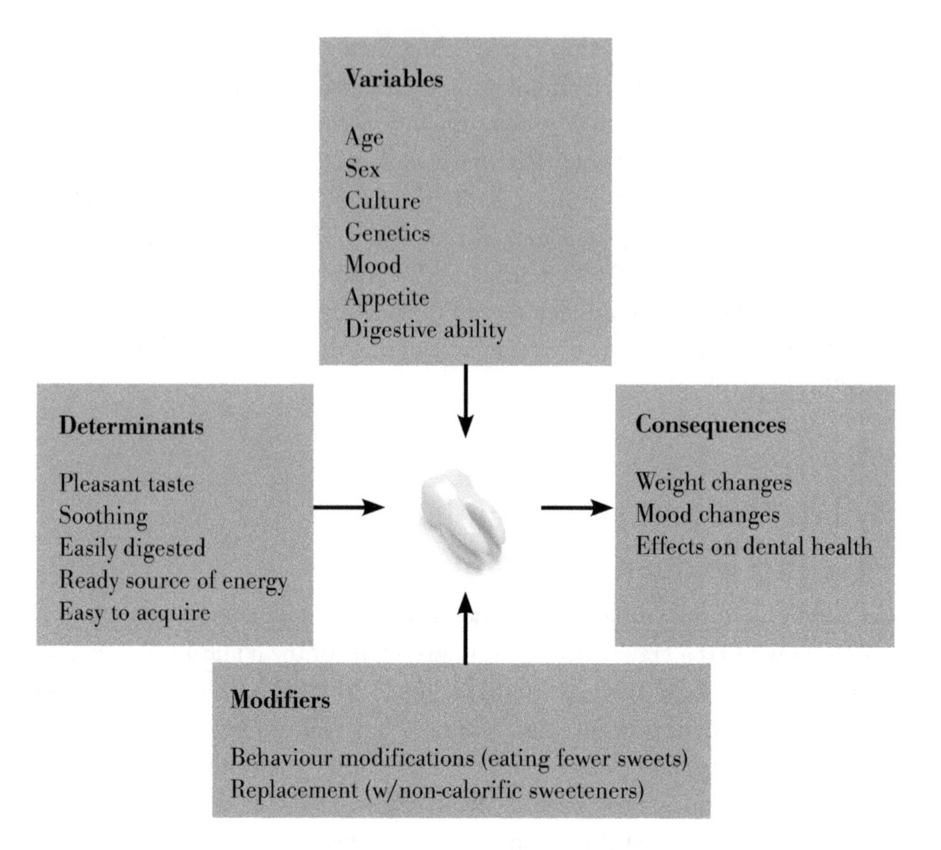

Figure 8.1 The 'human sweet tooth'
Source: Reed and McDaniel, 2006 (reproduced under the Open Government Licence v3.0)

Metabolism and dementia

It has been found that patients with bvFTD and those with SD have increased triglyceride and insulin levels and lower HDL cholesterol levels compared with controls, suggesting a state of peripheral insulin resistance. These factors have been found to affect prognosis in motor neurone disease favourably, although insulin resistance has been proposed as a mechanism promoting neurodegeneration. Insulin inhibits the phosphorylation of tau, and thus a low brain insulin concentration could lead to the hyperphosphorylation of tau and the formation of neurofibrillary tangles (Craft and Watson, 2004).

Nutrition and diet

The Mediterranean Diet (MeDi) has received much attention for its role in the prevention of dementia of the Alzheimer type. The MeDi is characterised by a high intake of vegetables, legumes, fruits, cereals, fish and unsaturated fatty acids (mostly in the form of olive oil), low intake of saturated fatty acids, meat and poultry, low-to-moderate intake of dairy products (mostly cheese and yoghurt) and a regular but moderate amount of alcohol (mostly wine and generally with meals). Epidemiological studies suggest that fish consumption can reduce the risk of dementia, including dementia of the Alzheimer type, especially among APOE ε4 non-carriers, and frequent consumption of fruits and vegetables might decrease the risk of dementia of the Alzheimer type (Barberger-Gateau *et al.*, 2007). A medium or great proportion of fruits and vegetables in the diet, compared with a small proportion or none, was associated with a decreased risk of dementia including dementia of the Alzheimer type (Hughes *et al.*, 2010).

This diet includes many dietary components reported to be beneficial in reducing risk of dementia of the Alzheimer type (Scarmeas *et al.*, 2006). For example, many vegetables, fruits, legumes and cereals contain antioxidants, which combat oxidative stress. Previous studies have found that higher adherence to the MeDi was associated with lower risk of dementia of the Alzheimer type (e.g. Féart *et al.*, 2009). A study in France found that the MeDi may reduce the rate of cognitive decline in older adults (Tangney *et al.*, 2011). Higher adherence to a MeDi has been implicated with lower risk for dyslipidemia, hypertension, abnormal glucose metabolism and coronary heart disease (reviewed in Gardener *et al.*, 2012) – all thought to increase DAT risk.

Contributory factors to the development of dementia of the Alzheimer type

There is a huge range of factors which are thought to affect the likelihood of developing dementia of the Alzheimer type. Elucidating these factors in the future will be good for helping with prevention of this dementia; however, at worst, it might mean people will feel 'to blame' if they develop a dementia.

Genetic architecture

The genetic architecture of dementia of the Alzheimer type is complex, as it includes multiple susceptibility genes and likely non-genetic factors. As summarised by Ringman and Coppola (2013), rare but highly penetrant autosomal dominant mutations explain a small minority of the cases but have allowed tremendous advances in understanding disease pathogenesis. The identification of susceptibility genes has opened new avenues for exploration of the underlying disease mechanisms. In addition to detecting novel risk factors in large samples, next-generation sequencing approaches can deliver novel insights with even small numbers of patients (Bettens, Sleegers and Van Broeckhoven, 2013).

The identification of a strong genetic risk factor, apolipoprotein E (APOE), reshaped the field and introduced the notion of genetic risk for dementia of the Alzheimer type. Furthermore, such studies have renewed a focus on the interaction between genetic risk and the environment. For example, Huang and colleagues (2005) reported on associations of lean fish vs fatty fish (tuna or other fish) intake with dementia of the Alzheimer type and vascular dementia, and in relation to APOE ε4 allele status, in the Cardiovascular Health Cognition Study (CHCS). In the CHCS, consumption of fatty fish was associated with a reduced risk of dementia and Alzheimer's disease for those without the APOE ε4 allele.

Antioxidants

Inflammatory reactions invariably mean increased production of oxidants, and hence an increased need for antioxidants such as vitamin A, beta-carotene and vitamins C and E, all of which have been shown to be low in those with dementia of the Alzheimer type (Holford, 2004). Vitamin E is a lipid-soluble antioxidant that has been found to confer neuroprotection by inhibiting oxidative stress (Guan *et al.*, 2011). However, at present, there is not a reliable consensus of opinion on the efficacy of vitamin E in the prevention or treatment of people with Alzheimer's disease, and more research is therefore needed (see, for example, Mgekn, Quinn and Tabet, 2008).

Omega-3 fatty acids

Current evidence suggests that elevated intake of polyunsaturated fatty acids might be beneficial for dementia of the Alzheimer type (Boudrault, Bazinet and Ma, 2009). Dietary supplementation of omega-3 polyunsaturated fatty acids was reported to affect expression of genes that might influence the inflammatory process (Vedin *et al.*, 2012).

Nutritional supplements

Alzheimer's Disease International (ADI) (2014) argues that there is no current evidence that nutritional supplementation, whether with micronutrients or macronutrients, can modify the course of dementia (cognitive and functional decline). ADI also argued that there is currently insufficient evidence to recommend the use of any medical food; however, data are emerging that may indicate some potential for therapeutic benefit, and trials are ongoing. Vitamin E shows some promise, but at doses that may lead to harmful side effects. Lauque and colleagues (2004) and Young and colleagues (2004) reported on the effect of giving nutritional supplements to older people with dementia. Lauque and colleagues (2004) found an increase in body weight of 70% in the intervention group after three months of giving nutritional supplements. This increase was sustained for three months after the trial. On the other hand, Young and colleagues (2004) found that nutritional supplements were of less benefit to participants with a low BMI than participants with a high BMI, because those with a low BMI tended to eat less food for lunch after being given a supplement in the morning. As a result, participants with a higher BMI gained weight whereas those with a lower BMI did not.

Mealtime environments

According to a recent report (Alzheimer's Disease International, 2014), attention to staff training and mealtime environment in care homes can lead to significant enhancement in calorie intake among residents. Eating is a social activity, and more thought should be given to how this can be optimised, normalised and made a core aspect of person-centred care. The ADI report argued that sensitive and inclusive design of dining rooms, kitchens, furniture and tableware could all make important contributions. Traditionally, the focus of research efforts has been somewhat misdirected. For example, Manthorpe and Watson (2003) identify that studies into dementia and eating have a tendency to focus on problems with providing food rather than issues with the experience of those receiving food.

Mealtimes provide an opportunity for social activity and emotional connection (Keller *et al.*, 2010). The environment in which a person with dementia eats can have a huge impact on the mealtime experience – it can affect a person's enjoyment of food and how much food they eat. Poor recognition of food and drink can be an issue for a person with dementia; this may be due to food being placed outside their immediate field of attention (Williams and Weatherhead, 2013). Visual changes may make it hard for the patient physically to see food on a patterned plate; simple single-coloured crockery can help, preferably white, though the clinician should make sure the table or tray background is of a different colour so plates can easily be identified. A good resource here is 'The eating environment' from the Social Care Institute for Excellence in their Dementia Gateway (2013).

Other useful recommendations include acknowledging that a person with dementia may not be comfortable eating with other people or in an unfamiliar environment. They may have difficulty eating food, and this can only make feelings of embarrassment worse if they are sitting with others. As a result, they may leave food uneaten. While some family care partners are innovative and develop strategies to overcome these issues (Keller, Edward and Cook, 2006), mealtimes continue to be a source of tension, frustration and disappointment for others (Kellaher, 2000). Furthermore, it is important to be aware that some people with dementia may experience visual impairments that make it difficult to see the food in front of them. Therefore, mealtime difficulty encompasses eating and feeding behaviours occurring in advanced dementia, and must be considered within the environment and include complex social interactions surrounding a meal (Keller *et al.*, 2006).

Carers have identified several specific strategies that they employed to promote pleasurable mealtimes for themselves and the persons for whom they cared. These specific strategies have ranged from assisting with making food choices when eating out to having family members involved in total feeding assistance, according to Keller and colleagues (2006). A recent comprehensive review examined the effectiveness of mealtime interventions aimed at improving behavioural symptoms in elderly people living with dementia in residential care. A total of 6118 articles were identified in that published study (Whear *et al.*, 2014). The authors concluded that there is some evidence to suggest that mealtime interventions improve behavioural symptoms in elderly people with dementia living in residential care, although weak study designs limited the generalisability of the findings.

Chewing and swallowing

Dysphagia, or swallowing impairment, is a growing concern in dementia and can lead to malnutrition, dehydration, weight loss, functional decline and fear of eating and drinking, as well as a decrease in quality of life or wellbeing. Prevalence of swallowing difficulties in patients with dementia ranged from 13% to 57%. Dysphagia developed during the late stages of frontotemporal dementia, but it was seen during the early stage of dementia of the Alzheimer type (Alagiakrishnan, Bhanji and Kurian, 2013). Problems with chewing and swallowing are commonly encountered, with managing food in the mouth or aspiration when swallowing being key difficulties (Candy, Sampson and Jones, 2009).

Weight loss

A key finding of the report by Alzheimer's Disease International (2014) is that while weight loss is a common problem for people with dementia, undernutrition can and should be avoided. Proof of concept comes from a new review of the use of oral nutritional supplements, indicating that it is possible to stabilise or even increase the weight of people with dementia over relatively long periods. The nutritional benefit of education and training for carers was less apparent, although such interventions were popular and there are likely to be other benefits. Weight loss is common among older people with dementia, so it is particularly important to look for signs of unintended weight loss. Weight loss is caused by insufficient energy (calorie) intake, so it may be necessary to offer extra drinks and nutritious snacks during the day, or to fortify meals with extra calories (Crawley and Hocking, 2011). Possible causes of low food intake in older adults with dementia was the most popular area of study (Berkhout, Cools and Houwelingen, 1998; Lin, Watson and Wu, 2010). Decline in cognition impacting on the person's ability to cook or handle cutlery properly, cerebral degeneration causing changes and disturbances in smell and taste, behavioural symptoms, affective disorders and possible co-morbidity can all cause weight loss (Williams and Weatherhead, 2013).

Reduced concentration

Reduced concentration may mean that the person with dementia can no longer continue to focus on eating until a meal is finished; care must be taken by care providers not to assume that the person has finished. Easy-to-manage 'finger foods' should be considered as an alternative if attention span is short (Williams and Weatherhead, 2013).

Conclusion

Eating is an inevitability of life. Going to the toilet is also an inevitability. Chapter 9 looks at a topic that many people prefer not to discuss openly; it is a good example of a subject that many find embarrassing and stigmatising, for all sorts of reasons, including control and dependence. The next chapter is on incontinence and living better with dementia.

References

Alagiakrishnan, K., Bhanji, R.A. and Kurian, M. (2013) Evaluation and management of oropharyngeal dysphagia in different types of dementia: a systematic review. Archives of Gerontology and Geriatrics, 56, 1, 1–9.

Alzheimer's Disease International (2014) Nutrition and dementia: a review of available research. Available at www.alz.co.uk/sites/default/files/pdfs/nutrition-and-dementia.pdf (accessed 20 April 2015).

Barberger-Gateau, P., Raffaitin, C., Letenneur, L., Berr, C. *et al.* (2007) Dietary patterns and risk of dementia: the Three-City cohort study. Neurology, 69, 20, 1921–30.

Berkhout, A.M., Cools, H.J. and Houwelingen, H.C. (1998) The relationship between difficulties in feeding oneself and loss of weight in nursing-home patients with dementia. Age and Ageing, 27, 5, 637–41.

Bettens, K., Sleegers, K. and Van Broeckhoven, C. (2013) Genetic insights in Alzheimer's disease. Lancet Neurology, 12, 1, 92–104.

Bikhchandani, S., Hirshleifer, D. and Welch, I. (1992) A theory of fads, fashion, custom, and cultural change as informational cascades. Journal of Political Economy, 10, 5, 992–1026.

Boudrault, C., Bazinet, R.P. and Ma, D.W.L. (2009) Experimental models and mechanisms underlying the protective effects of n-3 polyunsaturated fatty acids in Alzheimer's disease. Journal of Nutritional Biochemistry, 20, 1, 1–10.

Candy, B., Sampson, E.L. and Jones, L. (2009) Enteral tube feeding in older people with advanced dementia: findings from a Cochrane systematic review. International Journal of Palliative Nursing, 1, 8, 396–404.

Care Commission (2009) Promoting nutrition in care homes for older people. Available at www.dignityincare.org.uk/_library/Resources/Dignity/CSIPComment/promotingnutritionincare_homes1.pdf (accessed 6 December 2014).

Care Quality Commission (2011) Dignity and nutrition inspection programme: national overview. Available at www.cpa.org.uk/cpa/docs/CQC_Dignity_and_nutrition_inspection_report_October2011.pdf (accessed 6 December 2014).

Craft, S. and Watson, G.S. (2004) Insulin and neurodegenerative disease: shared and specific mechanisms. Lancet Neurology, 3, 3, 169–78.

Crawley, H. and Hocking, E. (on behalf of the Caroline Walker Trust) (2011) Eating well: supporting older people and older people with dementia. Practical guide. Available at www.gov.im/lib/docs/socialcare/RI/eatingwellsupportingolderpeople.pdf (accessed 6 December 2014).

Cummings, J.L. and Duchen, L.W. (1981) Klüver–Bucy syndrome in Pick disease: clinical and pathologic correlations. Neurology, 31, 1415–22.

Féart, C., Samieri, C., Rondeau, V., Amieva, H. *et al.* (2009) Adherence to a Mediterranean diet, cognitive decline, and risk of dementia. Journal of the American Medical Association, 302, 6, 638–48.

Gardener, S., Gu, Y., Rainey-Smith, S.R., Keogh, J.B. et al. (AIBL Research Group) (2012) Adherence to a Mediterranean diet and Alzheimer's disease risk in an Australian population. Translational Psychiatry, 2, e164.

Gorno-Tempini, M.L., Rankin, K.P., Woolley, J.D., Rosen, H.J., Phengrasamy, L. and Miller, B.L. (2004) Cognitive and behavioural profile in a case of right anterior temporal lobe neurodegeneration. Cortex, 40, 4–5, 631–44.

Guan, J.-Z., Guan, W.-P., Maeda, T. and Makino, N. (2011) Effect of vitamin E administration on the elevated oxygen stress and the telomeric and subtelomeric status in Alzheimer's disease. Gerontology, 58, 1, 62–9.

Hannah, M.T., Polos, L. and Carroll, G.R. (2003) Cascading organisational change. Organisational Science, 14, 5, 463–82.

Holford, P. (2004) Alzheimer's and dementia: the nutrition connection. Primary Care Mental Health, 2, 1, 5–12.

Huang, T.L., Zandi, P.P., Tucker, K.L., Fitzpatrick, A.L. *et al.* (2005) Benefits of fatty fish on dementia risk are stronger for those without APOE epsilon4. Neurology, 65, 9, 1409–14.

Hughes, T.F., Andel, R., Small, B.J., Borenstein, A.R. *et al.* (2010) Midlife fruit and vegetable consumption and risk of dementia in later life in Swedish twins. American Journal of Geriatric Psychiatry, 18, 5, 413–20.

Ikeda, M., Brown, J., Holland, A.J., Fukuhara, R. and Hodges, J.R. (2002) Changes in appetite, food preference, and eating habits in frontotemporal dementia and Alzheimer's disease. Journal of Neurology, Neurosurgery and Psychiatry, 73, 4, 371–6.

Inoue, K., Kiriike, N., Fujisaki, Y., Kurioka, M. and Yamagami, S. (1997) Effects of fluvoxamine on food intake during rebound hyperphagia in rats. Physiology and Behavior, 61, 603–8.

Keene, J. and Hope, T. (1998) Natural history of hyperphagia and other eating changes in dementia. International Journal of Geriatric Psychiatry, 13, 10, 700–6.

Kellaher, L. (2000) A Choice Well Made: 'Mutuality' as a Governing Principle in Residential Care. London: Centre for Policy on Ageing.

Keller, H.H., Edward, H.G. and Cook, C. (2006) Mealtime experiences of families with dementia. American Journal of Alzheimer's Disease and Other Dementias, 21, 6, 431–8.

Keller, L.J., Martin, L.S., Dupuis, S., Genoe, R., Edward, H.G. and Cassolato, C. (2010) Mealtimes and being connected in the community-based dementia context. Dementia, 9, 2, 191–213.

Lauque, S., Arnaud-Battandier, F., Gillette, S., Plaze, J.M. *et al.* (2004) Improvement of weight and fat-free mass with oral nutritional supplementation in patients with Alzheimer's disease at risk of malnutrition: a prospective randomized study. Journal of the American Geriatrics Society, 52, 10, 1702–7.

Lin, L.C., Watson, R. and Wu, S.C. (2010) What is associated with low food intake in older people with dementia? Journal of Clinical Nursing, 19, 1–2, 53–9.

Malnutrition Task Force (2013) Malnutrition in Later Life: Prevention and Early Intervention Best Practice Principles and Implementation Guide: Care Homes. Available at www.malnutritiontaskforce.org.uk/wp-content/uploads/2014/07/Prevention_Early_Intervention_Of_Malnutrition_in_Later_Life_Care_Home.pdf (accessed 6 December 2014).

Manthorpe, J. and Watson, R. (2003) Poorly served? Eating and dementia. Journal of Advanced Nursing, 41, 2, 162–9.

Mennell, S., Murcott, A. and van Otterloo, A. (1992) The Sociology of Food: Eating, Diet and Culture. London: Sage.

Mgekn, I., Quinn, R. and Tabet, N. (2008) Vitamin E for Alzheimer's disease and mild cognitive impairment. Cochrane Database of Systematic Reviews, CD002854.

Milano, W., Siano, C., Putrella, C. and Capasso, A. (2005) Treatment of bulimia nervosa with fluvoxamine: a randomized controlled trial. Advances in Therapy, 22, 278–83.

Morris, C.H., Hope, R.A. and Fairburn, C.G. (1989) Eating habits in dementia: a descriptive study. British Journal of Psychiatry, 154, 801–6.

Mummery, C.J., Patterson, K., Price, C.J., Ashburner, J., Frackowiak, R.S. and Hodges, J.R. (2000) A voxel-based morphometry study of semantic dementia: relationship between temporal lobe atrophy and semantic memory. Annals of Neurology, 47, 1, 36–45.

National Institute for Health and Care Excellence (NICE) (2006) Nutrition support in adults: oral nutrition support, enteral tube feeding and parenteral nutrition (NICE clinical guideline 32). Available at www.nice.org.uk/guidance/cg32/resources/guidance-nutrition-support-in-adults-pdf (accessed 6 December 2014).

Piquet, O., Petersén, A., Yin Ka Lam, B., Gabery, S. *et al.* (2011) Eating and hypothalamus changes in behavioural-variant frontotemporal dementia. Annals of Neurology, 69, 2, 312–19.

Rao, H., Greve, H.R. and Davis, G.F. (2001) Fool's gold: social proof in the initiation and abandonment of coverage by Wall Street analysts. Administrative Science Quarterly, 46, 3, 502–26.

Rascovsky, K., Hodges, J.R., Knopman, D., Mendez, M.F. *et al.* (2011) Sensitivity of revised diagnostic criteria for the behavioural variant of frontotemporal dementia. Brain, 134, 2456–77.

Ray, S., Laur, C., Douglas, P., Rajput-Ray, M. *et al.* (2014) Nutrition education and leadership for improved clinical outcomes: training and supporting junior doctors to run 'Nutrition Awareness Weeks' in three NHS hospitals across England. BMC Medical Education, 14, 109.

Reed, D.R. and McDaniel, A.H. (2006) The human sweet tooth. BioMed Central Oral Health, 15, 6, Suppl 1, S17.

Ringman, J.M. and Coppola, G. (2013) New genes and new insights from old genes: update on Alzheimer disease. Continuum (Minneapolis, Minn.), 19 (2 Dementia), 358–71.

Rosen, H.J., Allison, S.C., Schauer, G.F., Gorno-Tempini, M.L., Weiner, M.W. and Miller, B.L. (2005) Neuroanatomical correlates of behavioural disorders in dementia. Brain, 128, 11, 2612–25.

Scarmeas, N., Stern, Y., Tang, M.X., Mayeux, R. and Luchsinger, J.A. (2006) Mediterranean diet and risk for Alzheimer disease. Annals of Neurology, 59, 6, 912–21.

Schein, E.H. (1984) Coming to a new awareness of organizational culture. Sloan Management Review, 25, 2, 3–16.

Senge, P. (1999) The Dance of Change. New York, NY: Currency Doubleday.

Social Care Institute for Excellence (SCIE) (2013) Eating well for people with dementia: 4. The eating environment. Dementia Gateway. Available at www.scie.org.uk/publications/dementia/living-with-dementia/eating-well/files/the-eating-environment.pdf (accessed 6 December 2014).

Tangney, C.C., Kwasny, M.J., Li, H., Wilson, R.S., Evans, D.A. and Morris, M.C. (2011) Adherence to a Mediterranean type dietary pattern and cognitive decline in a community population. American Journal of Clinical Nutrition, 93, 601–7.

Tolbert, P.S. and Zucker, L.G. (1983) Institutional sources of change in the formal structure of organisations: the diffusion of civil service reform. Administrative Science Quarterly, 28, 1, 22–39.

Tsang, S.W., Keene, J., Hope, T., Spence, I. *et al.* (2010) A serotoninergic basis for hyperphagic eating changes in Alzheimer's disease. Journal of the Neurological Sciences, 288, 1–2, 151–5.

Vedin, I., Cederholm, T., Freund-Levi, Y., Basun, H. *et al.* (2012) Effects of DHA-rich n-3 fatty acid supplementation on gene expression in blood mononuclear leukocytes: the omegAD study. PLoS ONE, 7, 4, e35425.

Warrick, D.D. (2009) Developing organisation change champions a high payoff investment! OD Practitioner, 41, 1, 14–19.

Whear, R., Abbott, R., Thompson-Coon, J., Bethel, A. *et al.* (2014) Effectiveness of mealtime interventions on behavior symptoms of people with dementia living in care homes: a systematic review. Journal of the American Medical Directors Association, 15, 3, 185–93.

Whitwell, J.L., Sampson, E.L., Loy, C.T., Warren, J.E. *et al.* (2007) VBM signatures of abnormal eating behaviours in frontotemporal lobar degeneration. Neuroimage, 35, 1, 207–13.

Williams, K. and Weatherhead, I. (2013) Improving nutrition and care for people with dementia. British Journal of Community Nursing, May, Suppl., S20–5.

Young, K.W., Greenwood, C.E., van Reekum, R.V. and Binns, M.A. (2004) Providing nutrition supplements to institutionalised seniors with probable Alzheimer's disease is least beneficial to those with low body weight status. Journal of the American Geriatrics Society, 52, 8, 1305–12.

Chapter 9

INCONTINENCE AND LIVING BETTER WITH DEMENTIA

> 'Community equipment helps older people to remain independent. But the provision of community equipment is often delayed with unacceptable variation in access and availability across the country. Incontinence is distressing for the individual, and for their carers, and is the second most common reason for admission to residential care. Continence services have not been readily available to all those who need them.'
>
> Department of Health, *National Service Framework for Older People* (2001)

Introduction

Incontinence, like dementia, does not just affect 'old people'. That incontinence is somehow closely linked to dementia is no surprise, but it is indeed noteworthy that 'the prevalence of somatic diseases was not greater than among continent patients' (Ekelund and Rundgren, 1987). Some people living with dementia experience persistent problems with toileting and incontinence which are difficult to manage. This difficulty can contribute to depression in the person with dementia and is stressful for family carers. It is a significant factor in decisions to move the person with dementia to a care home.

A national policy in England, the 'Single Assessment Process', was introduced across agencies from April 2004, aimed at improving assessments by the use of shared procedures and assessment tools. According to Clarkson and colleagues (2012), recognition for those with dementia, grooming, toileting and incontinence difficulties was significantly improved after the policy. The International Continence Society defines urinary incontinence as the 'involuntary loss of urine that is objectively demonstrable and presents a social or hygiene problem' (Hägglund, Olsson and Leppert, 1999, p.506).

Urinary incontinence rates are noted to be higher in those with dementia (53%), compared with those without dementia (13%) (Campbell, Reinken and McCosh, 1985). Neurogenic incontinence is common in multiple cerebral infarction and dementia with Lewy bodies (DLB), and in both diseases walking difficulty and falls are common. In a retrospective examination of DLB patients, urinary incontinence and constipation were the most commonly documented autonomic symptoms, occurring in 97% and 83%, respectively, whereas syncope occurred in 28% (Horimoto *et al.*, 2003). In particular, the negative effect of autonomic symptoms is reported to be considerable in non-Alzheimer's dementias. The identification of such symptoms is important because of the detrimental effect of these symptoms upon physical activity, depression, activities of daily living and quality of life (Allan *et al.*, 2006).

According to Professor Murna Downs (2013) at the University of Bradford, a further illustration of the issue of body and control for those living with dementia is the apparent inevitability of dementia meaning loss of bodily control. The meaning of dementia for the lay public and professionals, including people with dementia, is intimately connected to loss of control of the body, most notably continence. The consequences of incontinence are both physical and sociopsychological. For example, the person living with incontinence can experience skin irritation and pressure ulcers, falls and fractures, and is more predisposed to urinary tract infections. Incontinence in a person with dementia increases their level of dependency and places a heavier care burden on carers, resulting in earlier transfer into residential settings (Rabins, Mace and Lucas, 1982). Numerous risk factors of falls, including urinary incontinence and behavioural symptoms, have been identified among elderly people in long-term care settings. Urinary incontinence has been identified as a risk factor for recurrent falls but not for injurious falls; in contrast, behavioural symptoms were an independent risk factor for injurious but not for recurrent falls (Hasegawa, Kuzuya and Iguchi, 2010). And there is an important consideration of intimacy in care settings. Carers have long reported the range of problems caused by incontinence and their impact on persons living with dementia (Drennan, Cole and Iliffe, 2011). Male carers have reported feeling distressed and uncomfortable taking on intimate tasks which they were not accustomed to, such as their wife's personal hygiene (Toot *et al.*, 2013).

As the number of elderly persons living with dementia who choose to die at home continues to rise, it is important to ascertain how cognitive impairment is associated with symptom experience and end-of-life care received at home. Data were obtained from the Dying Elderly at Home (DEATH) project, a multi-centre observational study conducted in Japan. The following information was collected: decedent characteristics, observed symptoms and end-of-life care provided during the last 48 hours of life (Hirasawa *et al.*, 2006). It was found that people living with dementia had incontinence during the last days of their lives. Covinsky and colleagues (2003) similarly suggested that elderly patients with cognitive impairment have a particularly high rate of incontinence compared with elderly patients without cognitive impairment.

Cognition and incontinence

Yap and Tan (2006), in a wide-ranging review, helpfully include a description of the cognitive deficits in patients with dementia such as loss of gnostic and visuospatial abilities, apraxia, procedural memory loss and frontal lobe dysfunction (causing socially inappropriate and disinhibited behaviour) that can interfere with the ability to:

- recognise the need to go to the toilet
- hold on until it is appropriate to go
- find the toilet
- recognise the toilet
- disrobe and use the toilet properly.

Apathy and depression occur commonly in dementia and could also account for poor volition to maintain continence. Specifically, recent evidence points towards mixed incontinence to be associated with executive control deficits in community-dwelling older women (Lussier *et al.*, 2013). It could be argued that the association between urinary incontinence and executive function is, in fact, caused by a shared variable: frailty. Indeed, frailty, a clinical syndrome, is associated with early cognitive decline, incident falls, worsening mobility or disability in activities of daily living, hospitalisation and death (Fried *et al.*, 2001).

Predictors of incontinence in dementia

Damage to various different levels of the neurosystem can result in urinary incontinence. Jirovec and Wells (1990) have summarised these factors to be the presence of an adequate stimulus to initiate the micturition reflex, neuromuscular and structural integrity of the genitourinary system, the cognitive ability to interpret and respond to the sensation of a full bladder, and the motivation to want to inhibit the passage of urine. The individual must also be mobile enough to be able to react to a full bladder before the urge to urinate overwhelms inhibiting ability. It therefore makes intuitive sense that two important predictors of incontinence in dementia are the severity of cognitive impairment and the degree of immobility (Berrios, 1986; Teri *et al.*, 1989).

Immobility increases the likelihood of incontinence among nursing home residents by preventing them from getting to the toilet; dementia reduces their motivation to do so. There is also ample evidence of dysfunction in the lower urinary tract among nursing home residents (Resnick and Yalla, 1987; Schnelle, 1990). Any intervention in the nursing home setting, however, must consider immobility and dementia as first-stage treatment priorities. Treating the bladder abnormalities alone will not alleviate urinary incontinence, especially if the resident lacks consistent access to and motivation to use a toilet. Mobility problems and the inability to transfer have been shown to be greater predictors of incontinence than severity of actual dementia (Resnick and Yalla, 1987).

Certain types of dementia can be especially associated with incontinence:

» normal pressure hydrocephalus

» vascular dementia

» frontotemporal dementia if there is damage to the cortical inhibitory centre for micturition.

Detrusor hyperactivity, or detrusor overactivity (DOA), was traditionally thought to be the principal cause of incontinence in dementia (Brocklehurst and Dillane, 1966). The problem here is what to do about it pharmacologically. Central cholinergic stimulation is a major pharmacological management strategy for some symptoms of some dementias. In contrast, to date, the use of anticholinergic medications for DOA in the elderly is still under wide consideration (Sakakibara *et al.*, 2008). DOA is defined as phasic contractions of the detrusor during bladder filling. The vesical pressure rises, but the abdominal pressure remains steady. DOA is often associated with urgency and an overactive bladder, but can sometimes be seen in normal individuals with no symptoms (Rai and Parkinson, 2014). Furthermore, as Ryuji Sakakibara and colleagues explain, the use of medications with anticholinergic side effects in older persons is a concern, particularly when there is a risk of exacerbating cognitive impairment. After they are ingested and absorbed from the intestine, anticholinergic drugs are systemically circulated. If they cross the blood–brain barrier, they reach the central nervous system and might block cholinergic receptors in the cerebral or in the basal ganglia.

Strategies on how to prevent incontinence in persons with dementia have therefore considered the overall level of physical activity of persons trying to live better with dementia. For example, a controlled trial by Sung and colleagues (2006) of older adults with dementia in a nursing home found the forms of movement and music preferred by patients were beneficial in managing agitation and recommended that these be incorporated into care routines.

Evaluation of incontinence

Potentially reversible causes of incontinence should be identified (Resnick, 1984, cited in Yap and Tan, 2006). A thorough history, physical examination and review of medications is imperative.

Per rectal examination is a high-yield yet simple procedure that should not be forgotten in clinical evaluation. It may reveal an enlarged prostate or faecal impaction, both of which can result in increased residual urine or urinary retention. Measurement of post-void residual urine should also be done. Urinary retention can result in overflow incontinence. Volumes greater than 200ml indicate inadequate emptying. Possible reasons include constipation, drugs (e.g. anti-cholinergics), bladder outlet obstruction or a hypocontractile bladder.

Yap and Tan (2006, p.239) provide a useful approach for evaluating urinary incontinence, including the identification of the incontinence issue as 'active' or 'passive', a description of the problem, exclusion of any reversible causes, analysis of the contributions of cognitive deficits, behavioural or mobility/motor problems, and evaluation of established causes where appropriate.

Categorising incontinence as passive or active can be helpful in elucidating the aetiology of the problem. Although stress testing is usually done in a routine assessment, it is understandably difficult to perform in persons with cognitive impairment (Ouslander *et al.*, 1989).

Aspects of management

Whatever the management strategy, it is essential that this strategy is articulated to all involved, including the person living with dementia and carers. (This chapter is predominantly to do with non-medical aspects, and does not include surgery at all.)

Conservative management of incontinence has been defined as 'any therapy that does not involve pharmacological or surgical intervention' (Wilson *et al.*, 2005, p.857) – for example, behavioural therapies. Behavioural therapies such as prompted voiding have been described as the mainstay of urinary incontinence in groups such as the frail elderly (DuBeau *et al.*, 2010), although there is little differentiation between the setting of care home and individual residence. The setting is, however, important in considering the feasibility and effectiveness of conservative interventions for the prevention of incontinence and management of incontinence.

The reader is strongly advised to refer to the article 'Conservative management for urinary incontinence' by Kate Moore (2000) for an excellent description of current conservative management strategies. There are two broad strategies: general measures, designed to lessen factors that raise intra-abdominal pressure, and specific measures, designed to improve the contractile strength of the levator ani muscles. Transient or occasional urinary incontinence can be resolved in older people – for example, by treatment of symptomatic urinary tract infections, respiratory tract infections with cough, confusion conditions, temporary and difficult constipation and changes in the environment (Hägglund, 2010).

The mechanism of pelvic muscle training is described elsewhere (Delancey, 1988). The minimum duration required to achieve benefit is thought to be between 15 and 20 weeks, for muscular fitness in general (Bo, 1995).

Although electrostimulation therapy has been used for detrusor instability, results have been highly variable (for a review, see Wheeler, Walter and Cai, 1993). However, the use of a 10Hz current is generally thought to inhibit detrusor contractility (as opposed to a 50Hz current which is believed to stimulate the skeletal muscles of the pelvic floor to contract). Webb and Powell (1992) have reported considerable benefit when they applied a current across the skin of the S3 dermatome using TENS stimulation.

Garments

It is not always clear whether incontinence is caused mainly by the progress of the dementia syndrome or whether it is associated with social issues, such as not getting enough assistance and support for visiting the toilet, a lack of rehabilitation or having medication with side effects that increase the risk of incontinence (Schnelle and Leung, 2004). However, it is possible that continence could be supported by the material (Namazi and DiNatale Johnson, 1991) and psychosocial care environment. Garments may have the potential to support the continence of people with dementia, but there is a lack of such products and no studies that assess their value.

Image and appearance have become vital considerations in recent strands of research in dementia care (Ward and Campbell, 2013). In their work on clothing and dementia, Iltanen-Tähkävuori, Wikberg and Topo (2012) considered garments specifically designed for wear in 'institutionalised settings'. They investigated the possible use of a 'patient overall' to prevent undressing in socially inappropriate situations and/or to stop the user from removing an incontinence pad. This article was based on interviews of designers of medical textiles and patients and family carers in Finland.

Communication

Effective communication is often key to alleviating caregiving problems in dementia. Being stubborn and uncooperative during activities such as toileting and bathing is often seen as difficult behaviour on the part of the person living with dementia. Remembering that toileting is a very private issue to everyone can help to further understanding of the resistance sometimes encountered during caregiving.

I devoted a whole chapter to communication in my book *Living Well with Dementia* (Rahman, 2014).

Crises

Crises are common in people with dementia and can lead to care home and hospital admissions (Banerjee *et al.*, 2003). A recent systematic review on crisis intervention teams for older people with mental health problems concluded that they were likely to reduce the number of acute admissions (Toot, Devine and Orrell, 2011). Drennan and colleagues (2011) have described the results of interviews about toileting strategies according to 32 family carers of people with dementia living in their own homes, recruited through primary care, specialist community mental health services and voluntary organisations. These authors concluded that primary care professionals could be more proactive in enquiry, repeated over time, about toileting and incontinence problems and in giving advice and information to reduce crises and problems.

Day care

Day care, as a type of care in between residential care and home help, has been available for several years in many jurisdictions, and is often referred to as an adequate alternative form of care for people with dementia. The goal of day care is generally to create a meaningful day for participants, offer family carers respite and provide care for persons with dementia.

The aim of a Swedish study by Måvall and Malmberg (2007) was to describe day-care clients with dementia problems over a 12-month period, and to discuss what distinguished those who discontinued day care from those who stayed with it. There were very few persons entering day care who lived alone and also needed help with toileting. The personal home of an individual living with dementia is a very different environment to a care home. People with dementia or cognitive impairment and incontinence problems, living at home, are likely to require tailored, evidence-based interventions and advice from their primary care and specialist health professionals (Drennan *et al.*, 2012). In their study, Drennan and colleagues (2012) found that clinical guidance on continence assessment and management for community nurses in many parts of England does not address the specific needs of people with dementia living at home or their carers.

Incontinence in different clinical diagnoses of dementia

Urge incontinence occurs in 50–90% of patients with diffuse Lewy body disease (DLBD) (Ransmayr *et al.*, 2008), presenting in some cases before the onset of manifestations of Parkinsonism. Lower urinary tract dysfunction is a common feature in DLBD, due not only to dementia and immobility but also to central and peripheral types of somato-autonomic dysfunction (Sakakibara *et al.*, 2005). In the early stages of dementia of the Alzheimer type, the prevalence of urge incontinence is lower than in DLBD (Ransmayr *et al.*, 2008).

In the context of bladder dysfunction in dementia, it is also relevant to consider a possible idiopathic normal pressure hydrocephalus (INPH). This condition is a clinical symptom complex that includes cognitive decline, gait disturbance and urinary and fecal incontinence. Urodynamic studies have shown that the majority of INPH patients present urinary urgency and increased urinary frequency, due to detrusor overactivity (Poggesi *et al.*, 2008).

Prompted voiding

The best predictor of responsiveness to prompted voiding has been a resident's ability to toilet appropriately during the first two to three days of the intervention. Residents who were appropriately toileted (defined as the number of continent voids divided by continent plus incontinent voids) 65% of the time or more during a three-day trial period tended to maintain continence with a toileting programme over longer time periods (Ouslander *et al.*, 1995; Schnelle, 1990). It can be envisaged that residents can be stratified into two groups; it becomes more feasible for staff to maintain consistent toileting assistance for the group consisting of residents who are most responsive to prompted voiding (Leung and Schnelle, 2008).

Incontinence aids

When all attempts at keeping the person continent fail, the use of continence aids is a last recourse. In this circumstance, the goals are to maintain hygiene and cleanliness, prevent skin irritation and breakdown, reduce the risk of infections, decrease falls and ease the caregiving task. Indwelling and external catheters are discouraged as they can predispose to urinary tract infections (Hirsh, Fainstein and Musher, 1979).

Beth Britton, in an excellent blogpost (2013), has described an experience of unacceptable rationing of pads in care homes. The EVIDEM-C is a study at University College London concerned with promoting continence and managing incontinence with people with dementia living at home. There is little clinical guidance for primary care professionals tailored to this population living at home.

Co-morbidity

Co-morbidity is an extremely important consideration in considering the needs of persons wishing to live better with dementia. I will return to this issue in my conclusion (Chapter 18). The International Continence Society Committee for the Frail Elderly argued that the management of urinary incontinence in the frail elderly must be multi-component, address co-morbidities and take into account other impairments and preferences (DuBeau *et al.*, 2010). Indeed, a recent UK retrospective cohort study reported on the effect of comprehensive geriatric assessment combined with such a multi-component management approach to incontinence in 112 frail, community-dwelling patients, of whom 30% had dementia (Harari and Igbedioh, 2009). Further research is needed in this area.

Moving into a care home

It is well accepted that urinary incontinence predicts both death and long-term transfer into residential settings in the general aged population. However, this observation is mainly explained by the close association of urinary incontinence itself with dementia (Tilvis *et al.*, 1995). People living with dementia often move into care homes as their needs become too complex or expensive for them to remain in their own homes. Little is known about how well their needs are met within care homes. O'Donnell and colleagues (1992) studied the factors predicting the early transfer into residential settings of patients living with dementia using a sample of 143 outpatients, of which 51 patients became institutionalised. They found that increased global severity of dementia, the presence of 'difficult behaviours' and incontinence increased the likelihood of institutionalisation. An unmet need may be described as a situation in which an individual has significant problems for which there is an appropriate intervention that could potentially meet the need (Orrell and Hancock, 2004; Stevens and Gabbay, 1991). In the UK, the National Service Framework for Older People (Department of Health, 2001) emphasises the importance of addressing older people's needs on an individual basis, taking into account the abilities and preferences of each person.

In order to achieve individualised, good-quality and effective care to meet the needs of people with dementia living in residential care, a person-centred approach is arguably required. In a relatively recent study, 238 people with dementia were recruited from residential care homes nationally to identify the unmet needs of people with dementia in care and the characteristics associated with high levels of needs, using the Camberwell Assessment of Needs for the Elderly (CANE) (Hancock *et al.*, 2006). Incontinence needs were often found to be unmet.

Conclusion

Incontinence is just one example of a health and social care issue which can only sensibly be managed through coordinated action from professionals and non-professionals known to the person with dementia. Incontinence is an extremely sensitive and delicate issue. It is inconceivable to envisage that incontinence for a person aspiring to live better following a diagnosis of dementia should come under the 'silo' of a single generalist or specialist, whether a physical health doctor, mental health doctor or social care practitioner. A medical doctor, for example, cannot fail to be interested in the psychological impact of physical disease. Chapter 10 introduces the rationale for whole-person care for the English jurisdiction.

References

Allan, L., McKeith, I., Ballard, C. and Kenny, R.A. (2006) The prevalence of autonomic symptoms in dementia and their association with physical activity, activities of daily living and quality of life. Dementia and Geriatric Cognitive Disorders, 22, 3, 230–7.

Banerjee, S., Murray, J., Foley, B., Arkins, L., Schneider, J. and Mann, A. (2003) Predictors of institutionalisation in people with dementia. Journal of Neurology, Neurosurgery and Psychiatry, 74, 1315–[AQ]16.

Berrios, G. (1986) Urinary incontinence and the psychopathology of the elderly with cognitive failure. Gerontology, 32, 2, 119–24.

Bo, K. (1995) Pelvic floor muscle exercise for the treatment of stress urinary incontinence: an exercise physiology perspective. International Urogynecology Journal, 6, 282–91.

Britton, B. (2013) An urgent need to understand. D4Dementia blog, Wednesday 5 June. Available at http://d4dementia.blogspot.co.uk/2013/06/an-urgent-need-to-understand.html (accessed 11 February 2015).

Brocklehurst, J. and Dillane, J. (1966) Studies of the female bladder in old age. II: cystometrograms in 100 incontinent women. Gerontologia Clinica, 8, 306–19.

Campbell, A., Reinken, J. and McCosh, L. (1985) Incontinence in the elderly: prevalence and prognosis. Age and Ageing, 14, 65–70.

Clarkson, P., Abendstern, M., Sutcliffe, C., Hughes, J. and Challis, D. (2012) The identification and detection of dementia and its correlates in a social services setting: impact of a national policy in England. Dementia, 11, 5, 617–32.

Covinsky, K.E., Eng, C., Lui, L.Y., Sands, L.P. and Yaffe, K. (2003) The last two years of life: functional trajectories of frail older people. Journal of the American Geriatrics Society, 51, 492–8.

Delancey, J.O.L. (1988) Anatomy and mechanics of structures around the vesical neck: how vesical neck position might affect its closure. Neurourology and Urodynamics, 7, 161–2.

Department of Health (2001) National Service Framework for Older People. London: Department of Health. Available at www.gov.uk/government/uploads/system/uploads/attachment_data/file/198033/National_Service_Framework_for_Older_People.pdf (accessed 6 December 2014).

Downs, M. (2013) Embodiment: the implications for living well with dementia. Dementia (London), 12, 3, 368–74.

Drennan, V.M., Cole, L. and Iliffe, S. (2011) A taboo within a stigma? A qualitative study of managing incontinence with people with dementia living at home. BMC Geriatrics, 11, 75.

Drennan, V.M., Greenwood, N., Cole, L., Fader, M. *et al.* (2012) Conservative interventions for incontinence in people with dementia or cognitive impairment, living at home: a systematic review. BMC Geriatrics, 12, 77.

DuBeau, C.E., Kuchel, G.A., Johnson, T. II, Palmer, M.H. and Wagg, A. (2010) Incontinence in the frail elderly: report from the 4th International Consultation on Incontinence. Neurourology and Urodynamics, 29, 165–78.

Ekelund, P. and Rundgren, A. (1987) Urinary incontinence in the elderly with implications for hospital care consumption and social disability. Archives of Gerontology and Geriatrics, 6, 1, 11–18.

Fried, L.P., Tangen, C.M., Walston, J., Newman, A.B. *et al.* (2001) Frailty in older adults: evidence for a phenotype. Journals of Gerontology: Series A, Biological Sciences and Medical Sciences, 56, M146–56.

Hägglund, D. (2010) A systematic literature review of incontinence care for persons with dementia: the research evidence. Journal of Clinical Nursing, 19, 3–4, 303–12.

Hägglund, D., Olsson, H. and Leppert, J. (1999) Urinary incontinence: an unexpected large problem among young females. Results from a population-based study. Family Practice, 16, 5, 506–9.

Hancock, G.A., Woods, B., Challis, D. and Orrell, M. (2006) The needs of older people with dementia in residential care. International Journal of Geriatric Psychiatry, 21, 1, 43–9.

Harari, D. and Igbedioh, C. (2009) Restoring continence in frail older people living in the community: what factors influence successful treatment outcomes? Age and Ageing, 38, 228–33.

Hasegawa, J., Kuzuya, M. and Iguchi, A. (2010) Urinary incontinence and behavioural symptoms are independent risk factors for recurrent and injurious falls, respectively, among residents in long term care facilities. Archives of Gerontology and Geriatrics, 50, 1, 77–81.

Hirasawa, Y., Masuda, Y., Kuzuya, M., Kimata, T., Iguchi, A. and Uemura, K. (2006) End-of-life experience of demented elderly patients at home: findings from DEATH project. Psychogeriatrics, 6, 2, 60–7.

Hirsh, D., Fainstein, C. and Musher, D. (1979) Do condom catheter collecting systems cause urinary tract infection? Journal of the American Medical Association, 242, 340.

Horimoto, Y., Matsumoto, M., Akatsu, H., Ikari, H. *et al.* (2003) Autonomic dysfunctions in dementia with Lewy bodies. Journal of Neurology, 250, 530–3.

Iltanen-Tähkävuori, S., Wikberg, M. and Topo, P. (2012) Design and dementia: a case of garments designed to prevent undressing. Dementia, 11, 1, 49–59.

Jirovec, M.M. and Wells, T.J. (1990) Urinary incontinence in nursing home residents with dementia: the mobility-cognition paradigm. Applied Nursing Research, 3, 112–17.

Leung, F.W. and Schnelle, J.F. (2008) Urinary and fecal incontinence in nursing home residents. Gastroenterology Clinics of North America, 37, 3, 697–707.

Lussier, M., Renaud, M., Chiva-Razavi, S., Bherer, L. and Dumoulin, C. (2013) Are stress and mixed urinary incontinence associated with impaired executive control in community-dwelling older women? Journal of Clinical and Experimental Neuropsychology, 35, 5, 445–54.

Måvall, L. and Malmberg, B. (2007) Day care for persons with dementia: an alternative for whom? Dementia, 6, 1, 27–43.

Moore, K.H. (2000) Conservative management for urinary incontinence. Best Practice and Research: Clinical Obstetrics and Gynaecology, 14, 2, 251–89.

Namazi, K.H. and DiNatale Johnson, B. (1991) Environmental effects on incontinence problems in Alzheimer's disease patients. American Journal of Alzheimer's Disease and Other Dementias, 6, 6, 16–21.

O'Donnell, B.F., Drachman, D.A., Barnes, H.J., Peterson, K.E., Swearer, J.M. and Lew, R.A. (1992) Incontinence and troublesome behaviors predict institutionalization in dementia. Journal of Geriatric Psychiatry and Neurology, 5, 1, 45–52.

Orrell, M. and Hancock, G. (2004) Camberwell Assessment of Need for the Elderly, CANE. London: Gaskell.

Ouslander, J., Leach, G., Staskin, D., Abelson, S. *et al.* (1989) Prospective evaluation of an assessment strategy for geriatric urinary incontinence. Journal of the American Geriatrics Society, 37, 8, 715–24.

Ouslander, J., Schnelle, J.F., Uman, G., Fingold, S. *et al.* (1995) Predictors of successful prompted voiding among incontinent nursing home residents. Journal of the American Medical Association, 273, 17, 1366–70.

Poggesi, A., Pracucci, G., Chabriat, H., Erkinjuntti, T. *et al.* (2008) Urinary complaints in nondisabled elderly people with age-related white matter changes: the Leukoaraiosis And DISability (LADIS) Study. Journal of the American Geriatrics Society, 56, 9, 1638–43.

Rabins, P., Mace, N. and Lucas, M. (1982) The impact of dementia on the family. Journal of the American Medical Association, 248, 333–5.

Rahman, S. (2014) Living Well with Dementia: The Importance of the Person and the Environment for Wellbeing. Oxford: Radcliffe Health.

Rai, J. and Parkinson, R. (2014) Urinary incontinence in adults. Surgery – Oxford International Edition, 32, 6, 286–91.

Ransmayr, G.N., Holliger, S., Schletterer, K., Heidler, H. *et al.* (2008) Lower urinary tract symptoms in dementia with Lewy bodies, Parkinson disease, and Alzheimer disease. Neurology, 70, 4, 299–303.

Resnick, N.M. (1984) Urinary incontinence in the elderly. Medical Grand Rounds, 3, 281–90.

Resnick, N.M. and Yalla, S.V. (1987) Detrusor hyperactivity with impaired contractile function: an unrecognized but common cause of incontinence in elderly patients. Journal of the American Medical Association, 257, 3076–81.

Sakakibara, R., Ito, T., Uchiyama, T., Asahina, M. *et al.* (2005) Lower urinary tract function in dementia of Lewy body type. Journal of Neurology, Neurosurgery and Psychiatry, 76, 5, 729–32.

Sakakibara, R., Uchiyama, T., Yamanishi, T. and Kishi, M. (2008) Dementia and lower urinary dysfunction: with a reference to anticholinergic use in elderly population. International Journal of Urology, 15, 9, 778–88.

Schnelle, J.F. (1990) Treatment of urinary incontinence in nursing home patients by prompted voiding. Journal of the American Geriatrics Society, 38, 356–60.

Schnelle, J.F. and Leung, F.W. (2004) Urinary and fecal incontinence in nursing homes. Gastroenterology, 126, Suppl. 1, S41–7.

Stevens, A. and Gabbay, J. (1991) Needs assessment, needs assessment. Health Trends, 23, 20–3.

Sung, H.C., Chang, S.M., Lee, W.L. and Lee, M.S. (2006) The effects of group music with movement intervention on agitated behaviors of institutionalized elders with dementia in Taiwan. Complementary Therapies in Medicine, 14, 113–19.

Teri, L., Borson, S., Kiyak, H.A. and Yamagishi, M. (1989) Behavioural disturbance, cognitive dysfunction, and functional skill: prevalence and relationship in Alzheimer's disease. Journal of the American Geriatrics Society, 37, 2, 109–16.

Tilvis, R.S., Hakala, S.M., Valvanne, J. and Erkinjuntti, T. (1995) Urinary incontinence as a predictor of death and institutionalization in a general aged population. Archives of Gerontology and Geriatrics, 21, 3, 307–15.

Toot, S., Devine, M. and Orrell, M. (2011) The effectiveness of crisis resolution/home treatment teams for older people with mental health problems: a systematic review and scoping exercise. International Journal of Geriatric Psychiatry, 26, 1221–30.

Toot, S., Hoe, J., Ledgerd, R., Burnell, K., Devine, M. and Orrell, M. (2013) Causes of crises and appropriate interventions: the views of people with dementia, carers and healthcare professionals. Aging and Mental Health, 17, 3, 328–35.

Ward, R. and Campbell, S. (2013) Mixing methods to explore appearance in dementia care. Dementia (London), 12, 3, 337–47.

Webb, R.J. and Powell, P.H. (1992) Transcutaneous electrical nerve stimulation in patients with idiopathic detrusor instability. Neurourology and Urodynamics, 11, 327–8.

Wheeler, J.S., Walter, J.S. and Cai, W. (1993) Electrical stimulation for urinary incontinence. Critical Reviews in Physical and Rehabilitation Medicine, 5, 31–56.

Wilson, P.D., Berghmans, B., Hagen, S., Hay-Smith, J. *et al.* (2005) Adult conservative management. In Incontinence, 3rd International Consultation on Incontinence (Vol. 2). Health Publication Ltd.

Yap, P. and Tan, D. (2006) Urinary incontinence in dementia – a practical approach. Australian Family Physician, 35, 4, 237–41.

Chapter 10

HOW IS 'WHOLE-PERSON CARE' RELEVANT TO A PERSON LIVING BETTER WITH DEMENTIA?

'Wherever people are in this disjointed system, some or all of one person's needs will be left unmet.'

Andy Burnham MP, Shadow Secretary of State for Health (2011–)

Introduction

'Integrated care' means different things to different people, though it is worth noting that some healthcare providers sell products under the brand name of 'integrated care'. At best, it engages a philosophy of joining up the features important for someone's health and wellbeing, including social care, and tackling the wider 'social determinants of health' or inequalities (such as housing and transport). This happens to be what makes 'dementia communities' 'friendly'.

What is driving the cost of the NHS budget in England is technology, not the ageing population; half of England's current NHS budget goes to people below the age of 65 (Iliffe and Manthorpe, 2014). Certainly, electronic patient records shared between entities would help. But there is a temptation, and indeed danger, that 'whole-person care' becomes a wish list for multinational corporations – 'big is best' – and implementation of massive information technology (IT) projects. Focusing on a person's beliefs, concerns and expectations, however, has been done successfully by many family doctors, who have been subject to the same principles of regulation over confidentiality and disclosure as those that are relevant to IT systems.

In May 2015 the UK Government received a mandate to implement integrated care, which, like whole-person care, aims to bring health and care together. There are features of 'whole-person care' worth noting though. Precise details about devolution of policy remain uncertain at the time of writing. The 'whole-person care' approach – treating the person as a whole, not as a list of separate problems – has a delicate balance to run between recognising specialist clinical care in dementia – for example, through Admiral Nurses, in England – and avoiding the creation of new 'silos' – for example, whole-person care nurses in dementia. Creation of new silos, apart from all else, encourages insurance-based funding mechanisms for single diseases rather than mechanisms that encourage fair treatment of the whole person in an equitable way. The strength of the 'whole-person care' construct is that persons have their physical health, social care and mental health needs considered in the round, with an understanding that co-morbidities can act both ways: physical illness can cause mental illness, and vice versa.

Background

The course of dementia varies from person to person, and levels of awareness are variable even in the early stages of the disease (Aalten *et al.*, 2005). There are, notwithstanding, a huge number of different causes of dementia. It remains a sad fact that, despite considerable work spanning decades, 'whole-person care', which promotes a more tightly coordinated, comprehensive system (e.g. Butler *et al.*, 2008; Collins *et al.*, 2010), has been slow to gain policy momentum. Whole-person perspective focuses on improving a person's health and wellbeing by addressing the person's physical health (body), mental/psychological health (mind) and the mind–body connection.

Dementia is a very good example of how a physical disease, such as dementia of the Alzheimer type, can produce symptoms of the mind – for instance, problems in cognition or mood disorders. Illnesses such as coronary heart disease and cancer may be helped with adjunctive management strategies that promote changes in patients' behaviours (e.g. improvements in eating, sleeping and exercise habits) and psychological states. Psychological problems can indeed help to bring about or exacerbate physical disease, such as anxiety/stress and stomach ulcers, which is only to be expected when one considers how the brain can initiate a cascade of neuroendocrine activity through hormones present in the body. What ends up being provided in healthcare systems, however, tends to support the needs of the provider rather than the need of the person using these services.

The concept of care for a whole person is, of course, by no means new. The modern concept of person-centred care is derived from an approach developed by Carl Rogers in the late 1940s. This model was based on the assumption that 'no one can make decisions for another, act for them or solve their problems because these are matters of personal responsibility and choice' (Graham, 1989, cited in Lane, 2000, p.311).

I have previously described in great length the importance of personhood and the interaction of the person living well with dementia with his or her own environment (Rahman, 2014). The economic strength of whole-person care is that overall it discourages utilisation of technology-intensive disease-focused interventions, and it can possibly lead to care more focused on personhood, encouraging a person to be able to contribute fully to society, including 'productivity' for employers (this is discussed fully in Herman, 2013). Managing physical disease does not abolish the reactions to disease. Furthermore, whole-person care is necessarily involved in supporting a person continuously over time, rather than only supporting a patient for discrete episodes or events when ill. This approach will only induce a change in the behaviour of a person in a sustainable way if the system is not simply 'reactive' (Dixon-Fyle *et al.*, 2012).

There is now a convincing case for change. In an influential report by the Institute for Public Policy Research entitled 'Towards whole person care', Sarah Bickerstaffe writes in the executive summary:

> There is clear local enthusiasm for delivering more integrated health and social care services. Moves towards whole person care should build on this momentum rather than unpick it, making this the core aim of service improvement over the next decade, with the same political focus that waiting times have had in the past. (Bickerstaffe, 2014, p.3)

Wellbeing is essentially how comfortable a person feels with himself or herself and his or her local environment. A particular strength of policy has been to acknowledge the potent social determinants of health. A person's health will be determined by the social milieu, including factors such as housing, employment, access to law, access to health and nutrition.

Whatever the jurisdiction, it is clearly distressing for a person to navigate through numerous uncoordinated systems. A lack of coordination among health and social care services is a major cause of frustration, along with provision that does not meet people's needs, such as 15-minute time slots for social care visits (see, for example, Unison, 2013).

In a document prepared by John Snow, Inc., a 'triple aim' is proposed:

> [W]e posit that expanding the notion of integration beyond the health sector to include coordination of a broad range of health, behavioural health, and social services holds the most promise for achieving the Triple Aim…of improved health outcomes, improved patient experience, and reduced per-capita costs while also reducing health disparities and optimizing use of public resources. We focus on the notion of whole-person care because of its broad application to a range of contexts. (Maxwell *et al.*, 2014, p.4)

This 'triple aim' is shown in Figure 10.1.

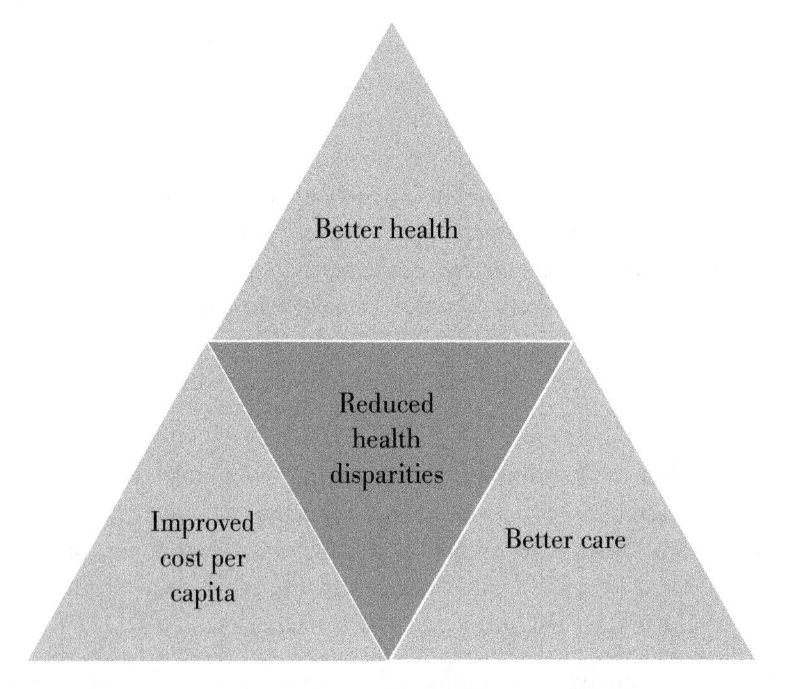

Figure 10.1 Achieving the 'triple aim'

SOURCE: MAXWELL ET AL., 2014 (P.5), ADAPTED FROM THE INSTITUTE FOR HEALTHCARE IMPROVEMENT (WWW.IHI.ORG) (REPRODUCED BY KIND PERMISSION OF JOHN SNOW, INC.)

A holistic viewpoint

Curing is an action carried out by the healthcare practitioner to eradicate disease or correct a problem, while healing is a process leading to a greater sense of integrity and wholeness in response to an injury or disease that occurs within the patient, which can be facilitated by the healthcare practitioner (Mount and Kearney, 2003). Great strides have been made in the study of whole-person health care. The integration of body, mind and spirit has become a key dimension of health education and disease prevention and treatment (Schultz and Valentina, 2013).

Seeing yourself and your patients as social, emotional, physical and spiritual beings can allow for effective and meaningful communication that promotes healing and therapeutic relationships. These ideas are generating considerable momentum. Ennis and Kazer (2013) argue that attention to spirituality is beneficial not only to the patient but to carers and nurses/healthcare providers as well. Research indicates that the memory needed to explore one's spirituality may be spared the effects of dementia. The concept of spirituality in health care has gained increasing attention over the last decade, as evidenced by the increasing number of conceptual and empirical articles published (Buck, 2006). There is widespread agreement among nursing scholars that spiritual care is a valued and integral component of quality holistic nursing care (McEwen, 2005). However, there is no overall consensus with regard to a definition of spirituality (Ennis and Kazer, 2013).

Person- vs patient-centredness

The concepts of person-centredness and patient-centredness are also frequently used synonymously in the academic journals; however, these two concepts are slightly but importantly different.

The term 'person' denotes a holistic humanness and the equal value of individuals (McCormack, 2004), whereas 'patient' has been described as a reductionist, stigmatic term that imputes imperfections or undesired 'otherness' to a person and thereby reduces the humanity of the subject (Goffman, 1968). Indeed, stigma was frequently mentioned in the study by Martin and colleagues (2013) as a barrier to 'self-care', representing a challenge to and object of self-management. Stigmatising attitudes by healthcare professionals and service providers lead to a lack of support for self-management. Education is needed for the public and professionals as to what living with dementia is like (Koch and Iliffe, 2010). One approach to deliver person-centred care incorporates biographical knowledge of the person with dementia into their clinical care (Clarke, 2000). As such, the biographical information helps staff to shift the focus from the disease and its symptoms towards recognition of the person as an individual.

There have been various thoughts on the delivery of 'a person-centred approach' to dementia care (such as Edvardsson, Winblad and Sandbam, 2008). Box 10.1 lists possible strategies for promoting person-centred dementia care.

Box 10.1 Possible strategies for promoting person-centred dementia care

* A focus on the wellbeing of the person with dementia.
* Drive to preserve 'self', e.g. identification of key biographical knowledge of the person with dementia (life story).
* Adequate staffing.
* Effective verbal and non-verbal communication, including minimisation of interruptions.
* Excellent staff-resident relationship.
* Carers who are properly supported.
* A motivated and well-trained workforce.
* Responding to concerns of the immediate network such as friends and family.
* Personalised care plans.
* Personalisation of the environment.
* A determined effort to identify 'unmet needs' and individual preferences.
* Opportunities for social interaction.
* Reminiscence.
* Avoidance of routines.
* Avoidance of arguments.
* A positive learning culture for all staff.

When a person becomes a patient is an important time, and one might have imagined that the literature on 'patient-centred care' might have helped overwhelmingly here. However, the optimum method of measuring the process and outcomes of patient-centred care has historically proved to be confused (Mead and Bower, 2000). Unfortunately, definitions of patient-centredness have been somewhat elusive. Edith Balint (1969, p.269) describes patient-centred medicine as 'understanding the patient as a unique human being', while for Byrne and Long (1976) it represents a style of consulting where the doctor uses the patient's knowledge and experience to guide the interaction. According to Mead and Bower (2000), five conceptual dimensions have emerged: the biopsychosocial perspective; 'patient-as-person'; sharing power and responsibility; therapeutic alliance; and 'doctor-as-person'.

Broadening the explanatory perspective on illness to include social and psychological factors has expanded the remit of medicine into the realm of 'healthy' bodies. Again, this has been particularly evident in general practice. For Stott and Davis (1979), the 'exceptional potential' of the primary care consultation is not confined to managing acute and chronic (physical and psychosocial) disorders, but also includes possibilities for health promotion and the modification of help-seeking behaviour. The promotion of wellbeing must surely be seen as integral to that. Wellbeing in general measures 'individuals' subjective perceptions that life as a whole is good' (George, 2010, pp.331–2), and therefore there is a strong link to the fulfilment of needs (Kaufmann and Engel, 2014). A care and support plan should truly reflect the full range of individuals' needs and goals, bringing together the knowledge and expertise of both the professional and the person, and it should give equal importance to mental and physical health needs (Department of Health, 2014).

Patient-centred medicine promotes the ideal of an egalitarian doctor–patient relationship, differing fundamentally from the conventional 'paternalistic' relationship envisaged by Parsons (1951). Parsons considers that patient deference to medical authority is an important part of the social function of medicine, serving the interests of both parties. The asymmetrical relationship between doctor and patient (whereby authority and control lie with the former) is seen as an inevitable consequence of the information asymmetry between medical expert and lay patient. However, Parsons' model of social relations has been much criticised for its assumptions of mutuality and reciprocity between the two parties. For example, Friedson (1970) argues that conflict between medical authority and patient autonomy is fundamental to the doctor–patient relationship. In reality, people living with dementia are somewhat resentful of the perceived stranglehold that the medical profession seems to exert in all aspects of care. Besides, although 'patient-centred' consulting skills are increasingly seen as crucial for the delivery of effective primary care, there is significant lack of clarity over the precise definition of the term, optimal methods of measurement, and the relationship between patient-centred care and patient outcomes (Mead and Bower, 2002).

Stechl and colleagues (2006), cited in Kaufmann and Engel (2014), identify in their self-report research the need for autonomy, continuity of lifestyle, security and social acceptance/respect, stressing that they vary between individuals and are closely interrelated. Despite the limitations conceded by the authors themselves, the findings from the Kaufmann and Engel study arguably also strengthen the case that individuals with dementia are potentially important informants of their subjective wellbeing. The deference to medical authority may not be justified by the sheer power of knowledge that patients have about themselves. Cassel (1982) describes the different facets of a person as having a past, having a cultural background, roles and relationships with 'others', being political and doing things, including action and creation. Cassel further stresses that no person exists without 'others', and it is through relationship with 'others' that experience of a full sense of being a person evolves.

The relationship between the person with dementia and the rest of his or her family may not be assumed to be harmonious. Peisah, Brodaty and Quadrio (2006) reported on family conflict in cases of dementia referred to the Guardianship Tribunal of New South Wales, Australia. They found that family conflict was most commonly seen in mild to moderate dementia. The person with dementia was usually involved in the conflict or in alliance with one or other of the family members in conflict, especially when paranoid ideation had been somehow fuelled by family members. Common themes included accusations of neglect, exploitation, lack of communication or sequestration of the person with dementia. They concluded that 'dementia may be a great family divider, particularly when there are cracks in family solidarity' (p.485).

On a happier note, a supportive family can aid 'self-care', discussed in some detail later in this chapter. Woods (1999), in a now famous article entitled 'Promoting wellbeing and independence for people with dementia', cites a single-case study in a family context as reported by Pinkston and Linsk (1984). In this example, family members were taught to use differential attention to modify the self-care of a 70-year-old lady with dementia. She was praised for brushing her teeth, combing her hair or having a bath, and ignored when behaving inappropriately. Near maximum levels of self-care function were rapidly attained.

Policies to promote shared decision making are becoming prominent in the UK (Department of Health, 2010), partly because of a recognition of the ethical imperative to properly involve patients in decisions about their care (Mulley, 2009).

The dynamics in shared decision making are incredibly interesting (for an elegant paper on this, see de Haes, 2006). Sharing decisions constitutes a separate field in the literature regarding doctor–patient communication (Charles, Gafni and Whelan, 1997). At the same time, this is one of the elements commonly considered important in patient-centred care. After a paternalistic era, sharing decisions has also become the ideal model for doctor–patient decision making. It is supported, again, by relevant governmental bodies.

To take things even further, especially in life-threatening situations, physicians may have to hold patients back from taking some decisions rather than sharing them. As is well known from clinical experience, patients may revert to unproven therapy. Empirical evidence supports the existence of such 'anomalies'. Jansen and colleagues (2001) asked patients with breast cancer whether or not they would like to undergo chemotherapy given a certain level of benefit. Interestingly, it turned out that as many as 40% of them would choose to undergo chemotherapy, even if zero benefit was expected. Similarly, Locadia and colleagues (2006) found that about 30% of respondents would prefer to start anti-retroviral therapy (HAART) rather than wait without any evidence for the effectiveness of early treatment for HIV. In other words, when patients make irrational choices, physicians should dissuade them rather than share decisions.

The basic dimensions of whole-person care are shown in Box 10.2.

Box 10.2 Policy considerations for 'whole-person care'

* Person- vs patient-centredness
* The multi-disciplinary team
* Data sharing
* Collaborative leadership
* Physical health conditions associated with dementia
* Parity of esteem for mental health
* Care coordinators
* Primary care
* Social care
* Self-management and self-care
* Assistance technology and ambient assisted living

The multi-disciplinary team and whole-person care

Ideally, there would be seamless handovers between different teams of different disciplines (Strategy&, 2013). It is anticipated that the GP practice will have close contact with staff working principally in the community, such as district nurses, pharmacists and social workers (Department of Health, 2014). Participants in this 'extended ecosystem' might include practitioners in physical health (physicians, dieticians, occupational therapy, physiotherapy, pharmacy, primary care, hospital doctors), mental health (clinical psychologists, cognitive neuropsychologists, psychiatrists, psychotherapists, community psychiatric nurses) and social care (e.g. long-term care providers). Clearly the number of people comprising any multi-disciplinary team should not be intimidating to the person with dementia or any carers involved.

In north-west London, multi-disciplinary teams in an integrated care pilot have found weekly case review meetings extremely valuable (e.g. Harris *et al.*, 2012). However, Kelly and Coons (2012), from the US jurisdiction, have published a very helpful article emphasising that integrated care might involve multi-disciplinary teams, but the two are not the same. It is common for people to discuss the care plan of a person living with dementia from the separate perspectives of neurology, medicine, psychology, psychiatry, nutrition/diet, occupational therapy, physiotherapy and so on. What sets integrated care apart, however, is collaboration and communication across all aspects of care (Kelly and Coons, 2012).

Data sharing

Goodwin and colleagues (2012, p.7) noted that:

> the absence of a robust shared electronic patient record that is accessible to and used by all those involved in providing care to people with complex conditions is a major drawback to supporting a more appropriate and integrated response to people's needs.

The recent furore in the English jurisdiction over 'care.data' (NHS England, 2015) is an illustration of the concern of many members of the general public that data sharing about patients might be too easy, with perceived blurred lines between presumed consent and valid consent.

Patients clearly have a right to privacy and confidentiality, but these can act as barriers to information sharing. There remain political, financial, social and technical barriers to sharing data (Poline *et al.*, 2012), but the current Government and NHS England remain strongly committed to improving information sharing between health and care providers (Department of Health, 2014). There are many situations where it can be mutually beneficial for two or more entities to share data because the usefulness or value of the combined data exceeds that of the data held individually (Morris *et al.*, 2014).

A PwC report from 2011 asks, 'Who knows what about me?' (PwC, 2011, p.9). It is yet to be seen whether traditional approaches to professional consent will be able to match up to the regulation of free sharing of person data. The sharing of data brings with it concerns of privacy and security, and in the UK it is possible that drug companies might wish to predict which patients will potentially benefit from their drugs. This field is becoming even more complicated with the drive towards preventative methods in personalised medicine. With time, it is possible that these concerns may even go beyond territorial jurisdictions. In the Independent Commission for Whole Person Care (ICWPC) Report, 'data' sounds better reframed as a construct of 'information' for decisions owned by users of health and social care systems (ICWPC, 2014).

Collaborative leadership

Delivering more coordinated care requires a workforce that is flexible and able to work across traditional divides between health and social care, and mental health and physical health, and this inevitably requires a flexible workforce (Bickerstaffe, 2014). Leadership is widely recognised as an important ingredient in successful collaboration, and the formation and communication of a shared vision is clearly critical.

Collaborative leaders typically play a facilitative role, encouraging and enabling stakeholders to work together effectively. As provided by Archer and Cameron (2012) and Wilson (2013), there are considered to be a few defining aspects of 'collaborative leadership', such as:

» an ability to share control and decision-making processes

» consolidating 'shared intelligence' and 'shared knowledge'

» furthering trust and confidence

» maximising human resources

» sharing power and influence

» enabling innovation where necessary

» handling conflict

» building collaborative relationships.

Any healthcare setting is a complex network of communications and relationships and, much like other industries, has an idiosyncratic nature of organisational design (Litch, 2007). Health care is a very personal and service-oriented industry (Beckman and Katz, 2000). Coile (2000) relates that excellence in service is an achievable goal within today's healthcare services organisations, despite tight budgets and staffing. Collaboration permits a strengthening of social networks (interpersonal relationships), facilitating an environment of trust and granting access to diverse skill sets that can aid in nurturing creative problem-solving strategies (Uzzi and Dunlap, 2005). In his best-selling book *The Tipping Point* (2002), Malcolm Gladwell used the term 'connector' to describe individuals who have many ties to different social worlds. It is not the number of people they know that makes connectors significant, however; it's their ability to link people, ideas and resources that would not normally 'intersect'. According to Wilson (2013, p.336): 'In collaboration, job titles and professional affiliations take a back seat and people derive influence from their knowledge, networks and shared goals.'

In a pivotal article entitled 'Are you a collaborative leader?' Ibarra and Hansen (2011, p.73) state: 'Collaborative leadership is the capacity to engage people and groups outside one's formal control and inspire them to work toward common goals – despite differences in convictions, cultural values, and operating norms.' Collaborative (distributed) leadership might be beneficial for living well with dementia across physical care, mental health and social care. This is very much worth bearing in mind given the observations from Ibarra and Hansen (2011) on the nature of various different styles of leadership, taking into account ownership of information, authority of decisions, the basis of accountability and control.

I will return to the general issue of collaboration in Chapter 18 (my conclusion). One issue is, for example, what outcomes to align across sectors, both in service provision and in research. To illustrate this, it is known that people with dementia living in care homes often have complex mental health problems, disabilities and social needs, and it is appreciated that providing more comprehensive training for staff working in care home environments is a high national priority. It is important that this training is evidence-based and delivers improvement for people with dementia residing in these environments. The 'Wellbeing and Health for People with Dementia' (WHELD) initiative combines various approaches to develop a comprehensive but practical staff training intervention, and an overarching goal of this trial reported recently by Whitaker and colleagues (2014) is to determine whether this optimised WHELD intervention is more effective in improving quality of life and mental health than the usual care provided to people with dementia living in nursing homes.

Collaborative communication strategies promote an understanding of separate cultures, integration and interdependencies by sharing a common vision, values and business purposes (Atchison and Bujak, 2001). According to Kramer and Crespy (2011), skilled leaders can choose the level of collaboration they want and then communicate to achieve that level of collaboration in their various work groups, departments or committees. The management of knowledge across a firm's organisational silos is an important aspect of healthcare management that tends to be overlooked (Burns, 2005). De Meyer (2009) at the Judge Institute at Cambridge conceives that this knowledge management under a collaborative construct is a reaction to the 'command and control' ethos, and is more in keeping with the changing demands of modern society.

An important question is how exactly that leadership should be organised. In a report produced by the Independent Commission for Whole Person Care (2014, p.11), it is said:

> Such challenging times require each local health and care economy to provide collective system leadership to focus on whole person care. We believe revised and developed health and wellbeing boards, or analogous local arrangements, provide a locus for that leadership – which should include leading local providers.

I will return to collaboration at various points throughout the book, and in my final conclusion in Chapter 18.

Physical health conditions associated with dementia

Since dementia is frequently (but not exclusively) associated with older people, people with dementia most commonly present with additional co-existing medical conditions. I will return to co-morbidity once again in Chapter 18. Such co-morbidities may include diabetes, chronic obstructive pulmonary disorder, musculoskeletal disorders and chronic cardiac failure (Helvik *et al.*, 2014). People with dementia also have an increased risk of falling. Predisposing factors only tend to account for a small proportion of all falls. Eriksson and colleagues (2009) found that circumstances associated with an increased risk of falls, as shown by a short time to first fall, were anxiety, darkness, not wearing any shoes and, for women, urinary tract infection. Dementia aggravates age-related changes in sensory reception in the body, which can increase sensitivity to environmental conditions, and consequently the risk of falls (van Hoof *et al.*, 2010).

Dementia of the Alzheimer type may be a more important source of weight loss than previously recognised (Cronin-Stubbs *et al.*, 1997). The mechanisms linking dementia of the Alzheimer type and weight loss are uncertain (Wolf Klein and Silverstone, 1994). Lin and Albert (2014) also argue that the potential public health impact of hearing loss in the context of dementia is substantial given the high worldwide prevalence of hearing loss in older adults.

Pain is a very good example of the interaction between physical and mental health: brain imaging techniques demonstrate the cortical locations of sensory perception and the affective component of pain (Hobfauer *et al.*, 2001). Not treating pain medically is clearly unacceptable ethically and professionally in itself, and can lead to a plethora of many other problems such as sleep disruption, social isolation, difficult-to-understand behaviours and low mood.

Finally, as shown by Grant and colleagues (2013), compared with those without a dementia diagnosis, those with a dementia diagnosis have approximately three times the rate of diagnosis of urinary incontinence, and more than four times the rate of faecal incontinence, in UK primary care. Indeed, for the older age group of people living with dementia, it is still arguably true that one of the key messages of one of the first publications on the subject of geriatric medicine by George Day, whose *Diseases of Advanced Life* was published in 1849, holds true in the documentation of some modern-day 'geriatric giants' including incontinence (Scott, 1975, cited in Barton and Mulley, 2003).

Parity of esteem for mental health

Whole-person care is part of the long-standing debate about 'parity of esteem' between physical and mental health. In an interesting article in the *British Medical Journal*, Kroenke (2002) argued that medical care could be vastly improved with enhanced attention to psychological medicine. According to that article, in the general population at least 25–30% of general medical patients have co-existing depressive, anxiety, somatoform or alcohol-misuse disorders (Ormel *et al.*, 1994). Rather controversially, Sophia Bennett and Alan Thomas (2014, p.184) have even argued that:

> Overall there is convincing evidence to support both the notion that early life depression can act as a risk factor for later life dementia, and that later life depression can be seen as a prodrome to dementia. There is

also evidence to support both conditions showing similar neurobiological changes, particularly white matter disease, either indicating shared risk factors or a shared pattern of neuronal damage.

Clearly much more evidence is required to evaluate critically this bold claim.

According to a Royal College of Psychiatrists (2013) report, commissioners need to regard liaison services as essential. The report argues that NHS and social care commissioners should commission liaison psychiatry and liaison physician services to drive a whole-person, integrated approach to health care. The Mandate to Health Education England (HEE) recognises the importance of professional culture to achieving this parity. It tasks HEE with ensuring the mental health workforce has the skills and values to improve services, and to promote a culture of recovery and aspiration for their patients (Department of Health, 2014).

Care coordinators

Unfortunately, there is a general feeling that, while the vast majority of first diagnoses for possible dementia occur in primary care, this often occurs late in the illness or at a time of crisis, when the opportunities for the management of the condition to maximise quality of life have passed (Goodwin *et al.*, 2010). It is usually proposed in models of 'whole-person care' that individuals should have a designated care manager or care coordinator to support the implementation of the care plan, connect the patient to a range of appropriate services, coordinate multiple services, carefully monitor progress towards care plan goals including regular reviews, and adjust interventions as needed along the way. It is anticipated that the care plan is in fact a personalised, proactive care and support plan based on a person's 'needs, preferences and goals' (Department of Health, 2014).

Vollenberg, Schalk and Merks-Van Brunschot (2013) essentially argue that, in the context of the development towards a demand-driven organisation of care and active citizenship in the civil society through a community-focused organisation of health care, the demand of the patient should ideally determine the supply and therefore the provision of care instead of institutional determinants and constraints. It is helpful to look to the experiences of other jurisdictions in order to see what is happening there. Health care in the Netherlands is currently implementing a radical transformation (Merks-Van Brunschot, 2004).

The Dutch government increasingly relies on citizens taking up responsibility themselves (Schalk, van der Ham and Roozendaal, 2006). But commentators are uneasy about this transfer of 'responsibility', which can all too easily be equated with 'blame' when things go wrong. The Dutch government promotes community care with individualised support to promote fully fledged citizenship to enable people with disabilities to participate in the community by strengthening the control people have over their own situation (Merks-Van Brunschot, 2004). A care plan for a person with dementia might need a 'continuity of relationship', as unfamiliar people can cause distress to people with dementia. Continuity of relationship with their health professional should be offered for patients for whom it is important (KPMG and the Nuffield Trust, 2014). Named care coordinators are essential to support people with multiple health and social care problems. According to the report by Strategy& (2013, p.9), care collaborators might 'also include family members who provide backup assistance as needed, such as caring for an aging parent'; but further offloading of formal care requirements on to unpaid family carers is likely to remain a politically sensitive issue. A current review of the literature makes it clear that a care coordinator can have a plethora of different roles, but can be crucial in helping people with long-term conditions as they move between care settings (Manderson *et al.*, 2012). In a recent analysis of five case studies of care coordination programmes for people with long-term conditions, the role of the 'care coordinator' was considered to be a critical enabler of success of such programmes (Goodwin *et al.*, 2013).

Possible roles of a care coordinator are suggested in Box 10.3.

Box 10.3 Potential different roles of the 'care coordinator'

* Essentially non-medical entities
* Might involve very close friends, family, state agencies, occupational therapist, dietitian, physiotherapist, social care worker, faith groups, transport, translators, suppliers of assistive technology
* Manage care plan (including monitoring of progress of key contracts with key providers)
* Manage out-of-hospital support
* Manage discharge from hospitals
* Integration of information from different care settings
* Volunteering in other roles when required

In an occasional paper from the Royal College of Psychiatrists entitled 'Whole-person care: from rhetoric to reality. Achieving parity between mental and physical health' (2013), it is recommended that mental health service providers should provide all care coordinators with the training and support necessary to enable them to ensure that the 'medicines aspect' of a service user's care is attended to. From the organisational perspective, it is interesting to note that coordinated care might be more important than structurally integrated services (Bickerstaffe, 2014).

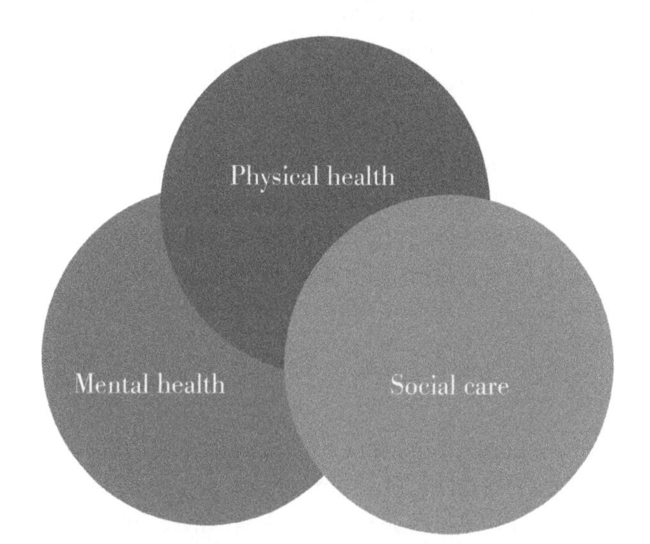

Access to intelligent technology
Access to justice
Community based resources, e.g. leisure and recreational facilities
Education and learning opportunities
Employment opportunities
Financial wellbeing
Housing
Social networks
The built environment, including shared open spaces
Transport

Figure 10.2 An 'integrated approach' to dementia post-diagnostic care and support

The role of the care coordinator is likely to be pivotal for dementia, as he or she will have oversight of all the care a person receives and will be able to work to ensure that transfers between settings are as seamless as possible (Department of Health, 2014).

Primary care

First and foremost, it is anticipated that there will be named, accountable general practitioners (GPs) with overall responsibility for care. It is hoped that a patient will also have access to a GP for phone consultations. A study by Mead and Bower (2002) sought to review all empirical studies to date that have investigated the relationship between measures of patient-centred consulting and outcomes in primary care, and to examine the methodological rigour of the studies. The pattern of associations was not clear or consistent. At GP practice level, regular reviews of outcomes will be fundamental to improving quality. GPs could review all emergency admissions to consider how the admission might have been avoided. This review will support practices to work with hospitals and other providers to improve processes for hospital admissions and discharges (Department of Health, 2014). Each area can develop local plans that set out how there will be better data sharing, seven-day services and joint assessments across health and social care.

Social care

There is currently a pilot programme of integrated care; this is an initiative funded by the Department of Health. The aim of this programme is to explore different ways of providing integrated services to help drive improvements in care and wellbeing – the pilots were evaluated from 2009 to 2011 (Bardsley *et al.*, 2013). In Bournemouth and Poole, there is a pilot project for structured care for people living with dementia. Also, the Better Care Fund offers a substantial opportunity to bring resources together to address immediate pressures on services and lay the foundations for a much more integrated system of health and social care delivered at scale and pace. But it will create risks as well as opportunities. The £3.8 billion is not new or additional money: £1.9 billion will come from clinical commissioning group (CCG) allocations (equivalent to around £10 million for an average CCG) in addition to NHS money already transferred to social care (Deloitte, 2014). For most CCGs, finding money for the Better Care Fund will involve redeploying funds from existing NHS services.

Furthermore, as described in the document 'Focus on social care for older people' (Health Foundation and Nuffield Trust, 2014), the Care Quality Commission's State of Health Care and Adult Social Care report for 2013 (CQC, 2013) summarises the results of inspection data for all types of social care providers. There were small increases in the percentage of providers meeting the various standards between 2011–12 and 2012–13. Taken overall, the data might be an indication that cuts in local authority funding have put pressure on providers' ability to retain staff. However, the CQC noted that other factors that were not possible to include in the analysis, such as the availability of GP and district nurse services, could also be important.

Self-management and self-care

There has been an impressive neglect of assessment of what people who have an early dementia can do, which means that there is a huge amount of research yet to be done about how people living well with dementia can embrace self-care. Barriers noted by Martin and colleagues (2013) included the fact that people with dementia are seen as 'passive recipients' of care and ideas that self-management is inappropriate. Disempowerment has been widely documented in dementia and acknowledged to lead potentially to further disablement (Kitwood, 1990). In contrast, working with the strengths and abilities of the person with dementia has seen significantly improved relationships between the person and their family member/carer (Peacock *et al.*, 2009).

The presumption that many people living well with dementia might be incapable of learning new skills relevant to self-care has proved incredibly hard to shift (Mountain, 2006), and new organisations such as Dementia Alliance International will now assume a key role in this policy plank. Furthermore, self-management is not based solely on the acquisition of new information and skills. Although skill acquisition can be important, other self-management work emphasises enjoyment and engaging in pleasurable activities (Moniz Cook and Manthorpe, 2009). Recent research has shown that people with moderate dementia may forget the details of an experience, but retain a positive feeling that impacts favourably on quality of life (Trigg, Skevington and Jones, 2007). There is, however, relatively little published research on self-management interventions for people living with dementia. Support groups, with an emphasis on social activities, sharing experiences with peers (Mather, 2006) and reciprocal support, have been shown to be valued and beneficial (Clare, Rowlands and Quin, 2008).

Gail Mountain (2006) notes the implications of policy neglect combined with a patchy evidence base and unrecognised service innovations. Ideally, the starting point of self-management and self-care should be healthy living, rather than containing the cost of healthcare budgets. A person with a chronic health condition often has to grapple with various challenges. Equipping the person with the long-term condition to cope with these challenges is at the heart of self-management. The available literature confirms the lack of research that has been undertaken to consider the needs and concerns of the person with the diagnosis of dementia. This is in comparison with the body of research into the needs of carers and the interventions that might support them (e.g. Fortinsky, Kercher and Burant, 2002; Thompson, Spilsbury and Barnes, 2003).

Self-management is conceptually thought to embrace a number of elements. The five core self-management skills, identified by Lorig and Holman (2003), are:

» undertaking problem solving

» decision making

» locating and using resources

» the creation of a partnership between the person and health professional

» making an action plan and taking action.

This schema is underpinned by an interpretation of needs on the part of the person with the chronic condition rather than by the professional. Weingarten *et al.* (2002) also identified a number of elements that might be included in a self-management programme. These are: education, feedback and reminders for both patients and healthcare providers, with financial incentives for patients who achieve treatment-related goals.

The whole population can be stratified according to 'risk'. For example, a 'unit' in primary care might be subdivided into three tiers:

» the top tier might be care for people with very complex needs and who are anticipated to require numerous hospital admissions for medical issues

» a middle tier might involve a geared-up, proactive primary care service to anticipate issues with long-term conditions, including living well with dementia

» a very low risk tier for those who will need access to primary care unpredictably at very short notice but who might benefit from high-quality advice about general health (e.g. nutrition) and preventative measures (e.g. falls avoidance, prevention of skin infections).

It is then important to understand how people with dementia see themselves and their surroundings, because this can influence how they manage their condition, how they relate to others and how they might respond to different kinds of services and support (Caddell and Clare, 2011). It is now widely recognised that the successful management of chronic illness depends on the active behavioural involvement of the patient (Lorig and Holman, 2003). Self-management of chronic illness involves both the adoption of new behaviours (e.g. blood glucose monitoring in diabetes, adherence to medication) and changes in existing behaviours (e.g. dietary modification).

The possibility of personal budgets in dementia care is discussed in Chapter 13. Beyond this, there is a general strand, loosely described as 'empowering people to make choices about their own health'. The quality and range of peer-reviewed evidence on self-management is poor, however, whether it is aimed at people themselves looking after their conditions or preventing these conditions from progressing. There is often very conflicting evidence on whether certain factors can prevent the onset of dementia at all (which was first introduced in this book in the context of the Blackfriars Consensus Statement, in Chapter 1).

Martin and colleagues (2013) were able to identify six main themes acting as barriers to self-care: the lived experience of dementia, diagnosis, role of carer/family, impact of healthcare professionals, organisation of health services and societal views. However, encouraging self-care at home for living well with dementia might involve a number of approaches (see Box 10.4).

Box 10.4 Encouraging self-care at home for living well with dementia

* A single point of contact, 'care coordinator', for care needs
* Access to other people with the same condition who can provide peer support
* Online access to own health and social care records including current medications
* A personalised care plan covering health and social care
* Advice about what welfare benefits might be available (e.g. from law centre or CAB)
* Information and access to assistive technologies which promote living well with dementia, and other advice from a community occupational therapist
* The option of a personal budget, if this is considered helpful
* Accurate professional advice from GPs or secondary care about aspects concerning physical or mental health (e.g. anxiety, depression, incontinence, falls, hearing impairment, or pain)
* Practical advice from a clinical or cognitive neuropsychologist about cognitive neurorehabilitation tools such as memory aids

* Advice about exercises which could be done at home, such as from a community physiotherapist

The overall framework of how services might be developed to support self-management has also been considered (Royal College of Physicians, 2004). Recently, the concept of self-management in the UK has been converted into self-care (Department of Health, 2005a, 2005b, 2005c). New models of enhanced self-care for people with dementia and their supporters are now being introduced and promulgated (Moniz Cook, De Lepeleire and Vernooij-Dassen, 2004). However, it is widely acknowledged that service provision has frequently failed to meet the needs of people with dementia, with a lack of investment in both research and service development (Heller and Heller, 2003). Apart from community nursing, there has been little investment in services to support people in their own homes (Pusey and Richards, 2001).

Assistive technology and ambient-assisted living

These were discussed comprehensively in Chapter 14 (assistive technology) and Chapter 15 (ambient-assisted living) of my book *Living Well with Dementia* (Rahman, 2014).

Living better with dementia: a 'year of care' for dementia?

Acute medicine is ideally suited to the medical model where a diagnosis is made on the basis of investigations, followed by the immediate implementation of a management plan. There should, of course, be prompt action on acute situations for people living with dementia, but this is rather different to the usual needs of a person trying to live better with dementia. A person with a long-term condition 'lives with the condition day by day for their whole life and it is the things they do or don't do that will make the difference to their quality of life and the long term outcomes they will experience' (Royal College of General Practitioners, 2011, p.9).

Shirley Ayres (2014, p.3) argues in her new 'provocation paper' entitled 'The Long-Term Care Revolution' that 'people in later life offer wisdom, experience, perspective and a wide range of skill sets and capacities', reflecting that long-term institutional care is not the correct setting for them. This argument also holds true, perhaps, for people living well with advanced dementia.

The burning question still remains, as it was in the genesis of the first English dementia strategy, as to how a framework of post-diagnostic support for people living with dementia could best take place in England. I believe firmly in the critical role of social care practitioners and clinical nursing specialists in a multi-disciplinary approach. It is also worth noting that the 'year of care' initiative has seen some crystallisation of the approach for living well. It offers a framework that supports delivery of Domain 2 of the NHS Outcomes Framework 'Enhancing quality of life for people with long-term conditions'. But this formulation is not set in stone, and should be prepared to evolve once weaknesses become known (such as in not adequately taking account of certain aspects of social care). Through this, it is hoped that 'far more people will have developed the knowledge, skills and confidence to manage their own health', but there are clear implications for the implementation of whole-person care, namely 'care which feels more joined-up to the users of services' and 'care [which] centres on the person as a whole, rather than on specific conditions' (Year of Care Partnerships, 2014).

There will always be the criticism that self-management, rather than having the prime goal of encouraging health and wellbeing, is meant as a 'cover' for essential services being cut. Possible key benefits of 'self-management' include a greater confidence of the patient and 'sense of control', prevention of avoidable hospital admissions, and better patient experiences in health and wellbeing (Royal College of General Practitioners (Clinical Innovation and Research Centre), 2011).

Indeed, this policy agenda has been slowly 'cooking' for some time. For example, a decade ago, the Department of Health (2005a, p.5) issued its document 'Supporting People with Long Term Conditions: An NHS and Social Care Model to Support Local Innovation and Integration: Improving Care, Improving Lives', in which it proposed a number of key priority areas – namely:

» To embed into local health and social care communities an effective, systematic approach to the care and management of patients with a long term condition.

» To reduce the reliance on secondary care services and increase the provision of care in a primary, community or home environment.

» Patients with long term conditions need high-quality care personalised to meet their individual requirements.

This follows on from an elegant analysis in one of Derek Wanless' numerous reports, this time called 'Securing our Future Health: Taking a Long-Term View'

(Public Enquiry Unit, 2002). This envisages one scenario for the future involving full public engagement.

It has become increasingly acknowledged that, under this approach, the 'care plan' is pivotal. The care plan 'should set out the patient's agreed health objectives and care needs, including what the individual can contribute towards their own self care, and what each professional and agency will do to help them meet these. It will include preventive and health promotion actions (such as avoiding accidents, reducing infection or nutrition)' (Department of Health, 2005a, p.18).

In a pamphlet from the King's Fund (2013), entitled 'Delivering better services for people with long-term conditions', the authors, Angela Coulter, Sue Roberts and Anna Dixon, describe a coordinated service delivery model – the 'house of care' – that incorporates learning from a number of sites in England that have been working to achieve these goals.

They describe that the 'house of care' model differs from others in two important ways:

» it encompasses all people with long-term conditions, not just those with a single disease or in high-risk groups

» it assumes an active role for patients, with collaborative personalised care planning at its heart.

(King's Fund, 2013, p.1)

This model is a system innovation, as applied to dementia, as it proposes a shift in power from professionals to persons living with dementia to play an active part in determining their own care and support needs. Such an approach, it is hoped, would respect autonomy and dignity, promote independence and offer maximum choice and control for help from the health and social care systems. The philosophy of 'whole-person care' moves the NHS towards an integrated health and social care system, which is concerned about individuals during health as well as disease.

Self-care is about individuals, families and communities taking responsibility for their own health and wellbeing. It includes actions people take in order to stay fit and maintain good physical and mental health, meet their social and psychological needs, prevent illness or accidents, and care more effectively for minor ailments and long-term conditions.

Both dementia and diabetes mellitus can be viewed as disabilities, and each may be a co-morbidity of the other. Sinclair and colleagues (2014) have outlined the key steps in an integrated care pathway for both elements of this clinical relationship, produced guidance on identifying each condition, dealt with the potentially risky issue of hypoglycaemia, and outlined important competencies required of healthcare workers in both medical/diabetes and mental health settings to enhance clinical care. In the overall construct, people living with a long-term condition, disability or a minor illness, as well as carers, can benefit enormously from being supported to self-care.

The 'Common core principles to support self care' aim to help health and social care services give people control over, and responsibility for, their own health and wellbeing, working in partnership with health and social care professionals (Skills for Care/Skills for Health, 2007).

Two critical principles in their list of seven are a drive to 'Support and enable individuals to access appropriate information to manage their self-care needs' and to 'Advise individuals how to access support networks and participate in the planning, development and evaluation of services'. A further principle promotes a healthy attitude to risk engagement, which is a theme which I return to in my conclusion (Chapter 18).

The National Institute for Health and Care Excellence 'Quality standard for supporting people to live well with dementia: information for the public' is intended to support people to live well with dementia. It sets out how high-quality social care services should be organised and what high-quality social care should include, so that the best support can be offered to people with dementia using social care services in England (NICE, 2013). This has provided a very useful yardstick against which services that purport to improve the quality of life of people with dementia can be judged. It is, further, reported that the 'Year of Care' (YOC) programme has been successful in implementing the key features of care planning in long-term conditions such as diabetes (Diabetes UK, 2011).

It is likely that the health and social care sectors will seek to engineer the 'best' solutions on offer for post-diagnostic support, within a framework of 'whole-person care'. Such solutions might include 'dementia advisers', 'clinical nursing specialists' or 'a year of care'. The solutions most appropriate for 'living better with dementia' might be drawn, for example, from best practice in other long-term conditions, such as diabetes or cancer. The quality of local commissioning, undoubtedly, is going to be pivotal in this. It will be a sensitive policy balance to make the argument that responsibilities of the State are not shunted across to the third sector in an unaccountable or unorthodox manner. But many will argue that there is a valid and crucial role for the third sector to play. Actually, the policy imperative for this could not be clearer: many persons living well with dementia report that they do not expect to see a professional until the end-of-life phase, having seen one for the initial diagnosis. This is clearly not acceptable if policy truly wishes to promote living better with dementia in England.

Conclusion

The opening salvo for whole-person care definitely comprises addressing needs of physical health, mental health and social care. The devil is, however, in the detail. It might be profoundly socialist, or it may be profoundly neoliberal. A full analysis will be completed with the entire suite of physical determinants of health, such as education, housing or income. It is no accident perhaps that some government departments in England in the past combined health and housing, for example. We may see, in time, history repeating itself. Inequalities or the 'social determinants of health' (or, even, 'social determinants of illness') constitute an important policy plank in public health, and intersect with age-friendly cities through the World Health Organization, for example. Chapter 11 provides an introduction to the social determinants of health, as relevant to dementia-friendly communities, and takes housing as its focus.

References

Aalten, P., van Valen, E., Clare, L., Kenny, G. and Verhey, F. (2005) Awareness in dementia: a review of clinical correlates. Aging and Mental Health, 9, 5, 414–22.

Archer, D. and Cameron, A. (2012) Collaborative Leadership. Training Journal, June, 35–8. Available at www.trainingjournal.com (accessed 6 December 2014).

Atchison, T.A. and Bujak, J.S. (2001) Leading Transformational Change: The Physician–Executive Partnership. Chicago, IL: Health Administration Press.

Ayres, S. (2014) The Long-Term Care Revolution: A Provocation Paper Commissioned by Innovate UK. Available at https://connect.innovateuk.org/documents/15494238/0/LTCRprovocationPaper.pdf/45cf1947-c477-4f21-913e-4eb3f9061aa0 (accessed 6 December 2014).

Balint, E. (1969) The possibilities of patient-centred medicine. Journal of the Royal College of General Practitioners, 17, 269–76.

Bardsley, M., Steventon, A., Smith, J. and Dixon, J. (Nuffield Trust) (2013) Evaluating integrated and community-based care. How do we know what works? Available at www.nuffieldtrust.org.uk/sites/files/nuffield/publication/evaluation_summary_final.pdf (accessed 6 December 2014).

Barton, A. and Mulley, G. (2003) History of the development of geriatric medicine in the UK. Postgraduate Medical Journal, 79, 930, 229–34; quiz 233–4.

Beckman, S.L. and Katz, M.L. (2000) The business of health care concerns us all: an introduction. California Management Review, 43, 1, 9.

Bennett, S. and Thomas, A.J. (2014) Depression and dementia: cause, consequence or coincidence? Maturitas, 79, 2, 184–90.

Bickerstaffe, S. (Institute for Public Policy Research) (2014) Towards whole person care. Available at www.ippr.org/assets/media/images/media/files/publication/2013/11/whole-person-care_Dec2013_11518.pdf (accessed 6 December 2014).

Buck, H.G. (2006) Spirituality: concept analysis and model development. Holistic Nursing Practice, 20, 288–92.

Burns, L.R. (2005) The Business of Healthcare Innovation. New York, NY: Cambridge University Press.

Butler, M., Kane, R.L., McAlpin, D., Kathol, R.G. *et al.* (2008) Integration of mental health/substance abuse and primary care no. 173 (prepared by the Minnesota Evidence-based Practice Center under Contract No. 290-02-0009), AHRQ Publication No. 09-E003. Rockville, MD: Agency for Healthcare Research and Quality.

Byrne, P. and Long, B. (1976) Doctors Talking to Patients. London: HMSO.

Caddell, L.S. and Clare, L. (2011) Interventions supporting self and identity in people with dementia: a systematic review. Aging and Mental Health, 15, 7, 797–810.

Care Quality Commission (CQC) (2013) The State of Health Care and Adult Social Care in England. London: The Stationery Office. Available at www.cqc.org.uk/sites/default/files/documents/cqc_soc_report_2013_lores2.pdf (accessed 6 December 2014).

Cassel, E.J. (1982) The nature of suffering. New England Journal of Medicine, 306, 639–45.

Charles, C., Gafni, A. and Whelan, T. (1997) Shared decision making in the medical encounter: what does it mean? Social Science and Medicine, 44, 681–92.

Clare, L., Rowlands, J.M. and Quin, R. (2008) Collective strength: the impact of developing a shared social identity in early-stage dementia. Dementia, 7, 9–30.

Clarke, A. (2000) Using biography to enhance the nursing care of older people. British Journal of Nursing, 9, 429–33.

Coile, R.C. (2000) New Century Healthcare: Strategies for Providers, Purchasers, and Plans. Chicago, IL: Health Administration Press.

Collins, C., Hewson, D.L., Munger, R. and Wade, T. (2010) Evolving Models of Behavioural Health Integration in Primary Care. New York, NY: Milbank Memorial Fund.

Cronin-Stubbs, D., Beckett, L.A., Scherr, P.A., Field, T.S. *et al.* (1997) Weight loss in people with Alzheimer's disease: a prospective population based analysis. British Medical Journal, 314, 7075, 178–9.

de Haes, H. (2006) Dilemmas in patient centeredness and shared decision making: a case for vulnerability. Patient Education and Counseling, 62, 3, 291–8.

De Meyer, A. (2009) Cambridge Judge Business School. Working Paper Series (5/2009): Collaborative leadership. Available at www.jbs.cam.ac.uk/fileadmin/user_upload/research/workingpapers/wp0905.pdf (accessed 6 December 2014).

Deloitte (The Deloitte Centre for Health Solutions) (2014) Better care for frail older people: Working differently to improve care. Available at https://www2.deloitte.com/content/dam/Deloitte/uk/Documents/life-sciences-health-care/deloitte-uk-better-care-for-frail-older-people.pdf (accessed 18 May 2015).

Department of Health (2005a) Supporting People with Long Term Conditions: An NHS and Social Care Model to Support Local Innovation and Integration. Improving Care, Improving Lives. London: The Stationery Office.

Department of Health (2005b) Self Care: A Real Choice. London: The Stationery Office.

Department of Health (2005c) Self Care Support: A Compendium of Practical Examples Across the Whole System of Health and Social Care. London: The Stationery Office.

Department of Health (2010) Equity and Excellence: Liberating the NHS. London: The Stationery Office.

Department of Health (2014) Transforming Primary Care: Safe, Proactive, Personalised Care for Those Who Need it Most. London: The Stationery Office.

Diabetes UK (2011) Year of Care: report of findings from the pilot programme (June 2011). Available at www.diabetes.org.uk/upload/Professionals/Year%20of%20Care/YOC_Report.pdf (accessed 6 December 2014).

Dixon-Fyle, S., Gandhi, S., Pellathy, T. and Spatharou, A. (McKinsey and Co.) (2012) Changing patient behavior: the next frontier in health care value. Available at www.networks.nhs.uk/nhs-networks/commissioning-for-long-term-conditions/systematisation-of-self-care-and-self-management/self-care-resources/HI12_64-73%20PatientBehavior_R8.pdf/view (accessed 6 December 2014).

Edvardsson, D., Winblad, B. and Sandman, P.O. (2008) Person-centred care of people with severe Alzheimer's disease: current status and ways forward. Lancet Neurology, 7, 4, 362–7.
Ennis, E.M. and Kazer, M.W. (2013) The role of spiritual nursing interventions on improved outcomes in older adults with dementia. Holistic Nursing Practice, 27, 2, 106–13.
Eriksson, S., Strandberg, S., Gustafson, Y. and Lundin-Olsson, L. (2009) Circumstances surrounding falls in patients with dementia in a psychogeriatric ward. Archives of Gerontology and Geriatrics, 49, 1, 80–7.
Fortinsky, R.H., Kercher, K. and Burant, C.J. (2002) Measurement and correlates of family caregiver efficacy for managing dementia. Aging and Mental Health, 6, 2, 153–60.
Friedson, E. (1970) Profession of Medicine: A Study of the Sociology of Applied Knowledge. New York, NY: Harper & Row.
George, L.K. (2010) Still happy after all these years: research frontiers on subjective well being in later life. Journal of Gerontology: Social Sciences, 65B, 331–9.
Gladwell, M. (2002) The Tipping Point: How Little Things Can Make a Big Difference. London: Abacus.
Goffman, E. (1968) Stigma: Notes on the Management of Spoiled Identity. Harmondsworth: Penguin.
Goodwin, N., Curry, N., Naylor, C., Ross, S. and Duldig, W. (2010) Managing people with long-term conditions: an Inquiry into the Quality of General Practice in England. London: King's Fund. Available at www.kingsfund.org.uk/sites/files/kf/field/field_document/managing-people-long-term-conditions-gp-inquiry-research-paper-mar11.pdf (accessed 14 May 2015).
Goodwin, N., Smith, J., Davies, A., Perry, C. *et al.* (2012) Integrated Care for Patients and Populations: Improving Outcomes by Working Together. London: King's Fund and Nuffield Trust.
Goodwin, N., Sonola, L., Thiel, V. and Kodner, D.L. (2013) Co-ordinated Care for People with Complex Chronic Conditions: Key Lessons and Markers for Success. London: King's Fund.
Grant, R.L., Drennan, V.M., Rait, G., Petersen, I. and Iliffe, S. (2013) First diagnosis and management of incontinence in older people with and without dementia in primary care: a cohort study using the Health Improvement Network primary care database. PLoS Medicine, 10, 8, e1001505.
Harris, M., Greaves, F., Patterson, S., Jones, J. and Majeed, A. (2012) The North West London Integrated Care Pilot: innovative strategies to improve care coordination for older adults and people with diabetes. Journal of Ambulatory Care Management, 35, 3, 216–25.
Health Foundation and Nuffield Trust (2014) Focus on social care for older people. Available at www.nuffieldtrust.org.uk/sites/files/nuffield/publication/140326_qualitywatch_focus_on_social_care_older_people_0.pdf (accessed 11 February 2015).
Heller, T. and Heller, L. (2003) First among equals? Does drug treatment for dementia claim more than its fair share of resources? International Journal of Social Research and Practice, 2, 1, 7–19.
Helvik, A.S., Engedal, K., Benth, J.S. and Selbæk, G. (2014) A 52 month follow-up of functional decline in nursing home residents – degree of dementia contributes. BMC Geriatrics, 14, 45.
Herman, P.M. (2013) Evaluating the economics of complementary and integrative medicine. Global Advances in Health and Medicine, 2, 2, 56–63.
Hobfauer, R.K., Rainville, P., Duncan, G.H. and Bushnell, M.C. (2001) Corticol representation of the sensory dimension of pain. Journal of Neurophysiology, 86, 402–11.
Ibarra, H. and Hansen, M.T. (2011) Are you a collaborative leader? Harvard Business Review, 89, 7–8, 68–74.
Iliffe, S. and Manthorpe, J. (2014) Barker & Burstow's care packages for England. British Medical Journal, 29, 349, g5879.
Independent Commission for Whole Person Care (ICWPC) (2014) One person, one team, one system. Available at www.yourbritain.org.uk/uploads/editor/files/One_Person_One_Team_One_System.pdf (accessed 6 December 2014).

Jansen, S.J.T., Kievit, J., Nooij, M.A., de Haes, J.C.J.M., Overpelt, I.M.E. and van Slooten, H. (2001) Patients' preferences for adjuvant chemotherapy in early-stage breast cancer: is treatment worthwhile? British Journal of Cancer, 84, 1577–85.

Kaufmann, E.G. and Engel, S.A. (2014) Dementia and wellbeing: a conceptual framework based on Tom Kitwood's model of needs. Dementia (London), Jun 19, pii: 1471301214539690 [Epub ahead of print].

Kelly, J.F. and Coons, H.L. (2012) Integrated health care and professional psychology: is the setting right for you? Professional Psychology: Research and Practice, 43, 6, 586–95.

King's Fund (authors: Angela Coulter, Sue Roberts and Anna Dixon) (2013) Delivering better services for people with long-term conditions. Available at www.kingsfund.org.uk/sites/files/kf/field/field_publication_file/delivering-better-services-for-people-with-long-term-conditions.pdf (accessed 6 December 2014).

Kitwood, T. (1990) The dialectics of dementia, with particular reference to Alzheimer's disease. Ageing and Society, 10, 177–96.

Koch, T. and Iliffe, S. (EVIDEM-ED Project) (2010) Rapid appraisal of barriers to the diagnosis and management of patients with dementia in primary care: a systematic review. BMC Family Practice, 11, 52.

KPMG and the Nuffield Trust (2014) The primary care paradox – new designs and models. Available at www.kpmg.com/global/en/issuesandinsights/articlespublications/primary-care-paradox/pages/default.aspx (accessed 6 December 2014).

Kramer, M.W. and Crespy, D.A. (2011) Communicating collaborative leadership. Leadership Quarterly, 22, 1024–37.

Kroenke, K. (2002) Psychological medicine. British Medical Journal, 324, 7353, 1536–7.

Lane, L. (2000) Client-centred practice: is it compatible with early discharge hospital-at-home policies? British Journal of Occupational Therapy, 63, 7, 310–15.

Lin, F.R. and Albert, M. (2014) Hearing loss and dementia – who is listening? Aging and Mental Health, 18, 6, 671–3.

Litch, B.K. (2007) The marriage of form and function: creating a healing environment. Healthcare Executive, 22, 4, 20–7.

Locadia, M., van Grieken, R.A., Prins, J.M., de Vries, H.J.C., Sprangers, M.A.G. and Nieuwkerk, P.T. (2006) Patients' preferences regarding the timing of highly active antiretroviral therapy initiation for chronic asymptomatic HIV-1. Antiviral Therapy, 11, 335–41.

Lorig, K.R. and Holman, H. (2003) Self-management education: history, definition, outcomes, and mechanisms. Annals of Behavioral Medicine, 26, 1, 1–7.

Manderson, B., McMurray, J., Piraino, E. and Stolee, P. (2012) Navigation roles support chronically ill older adults through healthcare transitions: a systematic review of the literature. Health and Social Care in the Community, 20, 2, 113–27.

Martin, F., Turner, A., Wallace, L.M., Choudhry, K. and Bradbury, N. (2013) Perceived barriers to self-management for people with dementia in the early stages. Dementia (London), 12, 4, 481–93.

Mather, L. (2006) Memory Lane Cafe: follow-up support for people with early stage dementia and their families and carers. Dementia: The International Journal of Social Research and Practice, 5, 290–3.

Maxwell, J., Tobey, R., Barron, C., Bateman, C. and Ward, M. (2014) National Approaches to Whole-Person Care in the Safety Net. Prepared for the Blue Shield of California Foundation. San Francisco, CA: John Snow, Inc. Available at www.jsi.com/JSIInternet/Inc/Common/_download_pub.cfm?id=14261&lid=3 (accessed 25 May 2014).

McCormack, B. (2004) Person-centredness in gerontological nursing: an overview of the literature. International Journal of Older People Nursing, 13, 31–8.

McEwen, M. (2005) Spiritual nursing care: state of the art. Holistic Nursing Practice, 19, 161–8.

Mead, N. and Bower, P. (2000) Patient-centredness: a conceptual framework and review of the empirical literature. Social Science and Medicine, 51, 7, 1087–110.

Mead, N. and Bower, P. (2002) Patient-centred consultations and outcomes in primary care: a review of the literature. Patient Education and Counseling, 48, 1, 51–61.

Merks-Van Brunschot, I. (2004) Organisational Dynamics in the Care Sector. Groningen: Wolters-Noordhoff.

Moniz Cook, E. and Manthorpe, J. (2009) Introduction: Personalising Psychosocial Interventions. In E. Moniz Cook and J. Manthorpe (eds) Early Psychosocial Interventions in Dementia: Evidence-Based Practice. London: Jessica Kingsley Publishers.

Moniz Cook, E., De Lepeleire, J. and Vernooij-Dassen, M. (2004) Chronic disease management – what can be learned from dementia management? British Medical Journal, 328, 99, 7453, 1396-d.

Morris, B.W., Kleist, V.F., Dull, R.B. and Tanner, C.D. (2014) Secure information market: a model to support information sharing, data fusion, privacy, and decisions. Journal of Information Systems, 28, 1, 269–85.

Mount, B. and Kearney, M. (2003) Healing and palliative care: charting our way forward. Palliative Medicine, 17, 657–8.

Mountain, G.A. (2006) Self-management for people with early dementia: an exploration of concepts and supporting evidence. Dementia, 5, 3, 429–46.

Mulley, A. (2009) Inconvenient truths about supplier induced demand and unwarranted variation in medical practice. British Medical Journal, 339, b4073.

National Institute for Health and Care Excellence (NICE) (2013) Quality standard for supporting people to live well with dementia: information for the public. Available at www.nice.org.uk/guidance/qs30 (accessed 6 December 2014).

NHS England (2015) The care.data programme – collecting information for the health of the nation. Available at www.england.nhs.uk/ourwork/tsd/care-data (accessed 10 June 2015).

Ormel, J., Von Korff, M., Ustun, T.B., Pini, S., Korten, A. and Oldehinkel, T. (1994) Common mental disorders and disability across cultures. Results from the WHO Collaborative Study on Psychological Problems in General Health Care. Journal of the American Medical Association, 272, 22, 1741–8.

Parsons, T. (1951) The Social System. Glencoe, IL: Free Press.

Peacock, S., Forbes, D., Markle-Reid, M., Hawranik, P. *et al.* (2009) The positive aspects of the caregiving journey with dementia: using a strengths based perspective to reveal opportunities. Journal of Applied Gerontology, 29, 5, 640–59.

Peisah, C., Brodaty, H. and Quadrio, C. (2006) Family conflict in dementia: prodigal sons and black sheep. International Journal of Geriatric Psychiatry, 21, 5, 485–92.

Pinkston, E.M. and Linsk, N.L. (1984) Care of the Elderly: A Family Approach. New York, NY: Pergamon.

Poline, J.B., Breeze, J.L., Ghosh, S., Gorgolewski, K. *et al.* (2012) Data sharing in neuroimaging research. Frontiers in Neuroinformatics, 6, 9.

Public Enquiry Unit (2002) Securing our Future Health: Taking a Long-Term View. Final Report (author: Derek Wanless). Available at http://si.easp.es/derechosciudadania/wp-content/uploads/2009/10/4.Informe-Wanless.pdf (accessed 6 December 2014).

Pusey, H. and Richards, D. (2001) A systematic review of the effectiveness of psychosocial interventions for carers of people with dementia. Aging and Mental Health, 5, 2, 107–19.

PwC (2011) Old data learns new tricks: managing patient privacy and security on a new data-sharing playground. Available at www.pwc.com/us/en/health-industries/publications/old-data-learns-new-tricks.jhtml (accessed 6 December 2014).

Rahman, S. (2014) Living Well with Dementia: The Importance of the Person and the Environment for Wellbeing. Oxford: Radcliffe Health.

Royal College of General Practitioners (Clinical Innovation and Research Centre) (authors: Nigel Mathers, Sue Roberts, Isabel Hodkinson and Brian Karet) (2011) Care Planning: Improving the Lives of People with Long Term Conditions. Available at www.impressresp.com/index.php?option=com_docman&task=doc_view&gid=75&Itemid=70 (accessed 6 December 2014).

Royal College of Physicians (2004) Clinicians, Services and Commissioning in Chronic Disease Management in the NHS. London: Royal College of Physicians.

Royal College of Psychiatrists (2013) Whole-person care: from rhetoric to reality. Achieving parity between mental and physical health. Occasional paper OP88 March 2013. Available at www.rcpsych.ac.uk/pdf/OP88summary.pdf (accessed 6 December 2014).

Schalk, R., van der Ham, K. and Roozendaal, M. (2006) De WMO komt! [The WMO is Coming!] Amsterdam: Kluwer.

Schultz, M. and Valentina, E. (2013) Twelve essential tools for living the life of whole person. Permanente Journal, 17, 4, e155–7.

Scott, C.J. (1975) George Day and diseases of advanced life. The Practitioner, 214, 832–6.

Sinclair, A.J., Hillson, R. and Bayer, A.J./National Expert Working Group (2014) Diabetes and dementia in older people: a Best Clinical Practice Statement by a multidisciplinary National Expert Working Group. Diabetic Medicines, 31, 9, 1024–31.

Skills for Care/Skills for Health (2007) Common core principles to support self care: a guide to support implementation. Available at www.skillsforcare.org.uk/document-library/skills/self-care/commoncoreprinciples.pdf (accessed 6 December 2014).

Stechl, E., Lämmler, G., Steinhagen-Thiessen, E. and Flick, U. (2006) Subjektive Wahrnehmung und Bewältigung der Demenz im Frühstadium. Eine qualitative Interviewstudie mit Betroffenen und ihren Angehörigen [article in German]. Zeitschrift für Gerontologie und Geriatrie, 40, 20, 71–80.

Stott, N. and Davis, R. (1979) The exceptional potential in every primary care consultation. Journal of the Royal College of General Practitioners, 29, 201–5.

Strategy& (formerly Booz & Company) (2013) Healthcare for complex populations: the power of whole-person care models. Available at www.strategyand.pwc.com/media/file/Strategyand_Healthcare-for-Complex-Populations.pdf (accessed 6 December 2014).

Thompson, C.A., Spilsbury, K. and Barnes, C. (2003) Information and support interventions for carers of people with dementia (protocol). Cochrane Database of Systematic Reviews, 4, CD004513.

Trigg, R., Skevington, S.M. and Jones, R.W. (2007) How can we best assess the quality of life of people with dementia? The Bath Assessment of Subjective Quality of Life in Dementia (BASQID). Gerontologist, 47, 789–97.

Unison (2013) FOIs show 73% of councils still commissioning 15 minute homecare visits (press release, 17 June 2013). Available at www.unison.org.uk/local-government/fois-show-73-of-councils-still-commissioning-15-minute-homecare-visits (accessed 6 December 2014).

Uzzi, B. and Dunlap, S. (2005) How to build your network. Harvard Business Review, 83, 12, 53–60.

van Hoof, J., Kort, H., Duijnstee, M., Rutten, P. and Hensen, J. (2010) The indoor environment and the integrated design of homes for older people with dementia. Building and Environment, 45, 5, 1244–61.

Vollenberg, M., Schalk, R. and Merks-Van Brunschot, I. (2013) How to coordinate care for people with dementia? A case study of a region in the Netherlands. Dementia (London), 12, 5, 513–22.

Weingarten, S.R., Henning, J.M., Badamgarav, E., Knight, K. *et al.* (2002) Interventions used in disease management programmes for patients with chronic illness – which ones work? Meta-analysis of published reports. British Medical Journal, 325, 7370, 925.

Whitaker, R., Fossey, J., Ballard, C., Orrell, M. *et al.* (2014) Improving wellbeing and health for people with dementia (WHELD): study protocol for a randomised controlled trial. Trials, 15, 1, 284.

Wilson, S.N. (2013) Collaborative leadership: it's good to talk. British Journal of Healthcare Management, 19, 7, 335–7.

Wolf Klein, G.P. and Silverstone, F.A. (1994) Weight loss in Alzheimer's disease: an international review of the literature. International Psychogeriatrics, 6, 135–42.

Woods, B. (1999) Promoting well-being and independence for people with dementia. International Journal of Geriatric Psychiatry, 14, 2, 97–105; discussion 105–9.

Year of Care Partnerships (2014) Policy. Available at www.yearofcare.co.uk/policy-0 (accessed 6 December 2014).

Chapter 11

INEQUALITIES AND LIVING BETTER WITH DEMENTIA

A Focus on Housing

'Everyone has an equal right to inequality.'

John Ralston Saul (b. 1947)

Introduction

Humans are social beings. A typical social science approach to identifying inequalities or the social determinants of health is to analyse the correlation between the variations of social environment and those of the health outcomes. Welfare states are important determinants of health. Comparative social epidemiology has almost invariably concluded that population health is enhanced by the relatively generous and universal welfare provision of the Scandinavian countries (Bambra, 2011). The reduction of health inequalities is not achieved by a competitive market. While in other illnesses there may be a simple association between health-related quality of life (HRQL) and an easily measurable clinical variable, in dementia this had not been so; there are now elegant instruments available with which to measure disease-specific HRQL directly in clinical trials and other studies that can yield informative data (Banerjee *et al.*, 2009).

For a whole host of reasons, inequalities vary from country to country, and this can impact on dementia policy. Both lack of health care and low educational level in rural settings in China may thus explain further the relatively low detection rates of dementia and depression associated with low socioeconomic status (Chen *et al.*, 2013). Previous studies in high-income countries do not tend to show a significant association between low socioeconomic status and the risk of undetected dementia. Lawton and Nahemow have articulated a relationship through the 'environmental docility hypothesis' (Lawton, 1986), which indicates that the less competent the person, the greater the effects of environmental factors on that person.

In the 1850s, the destructive effect of living conditions on the health of the poor in Denmark came into focus and the first initiatives to improve these conditions were made (Diderichsen *et al.*, 2012). Research on adult chronic diseases has traditionally focused on identifying opportunities to intervene to improve health in the population, whether via clinical treatments, behavioural interventions or policy changes (Liu, Jones and Glymour, 2010). Since the Victorian public health acts in England, the now-named 'environmental health practitioner' has been pivotal in providing healthier housing through a range of policy initiatives and legislative requirements (Stewart and Bourn, 2013).

Some important universal policies with great potential effect on health inequalities, implemented on a national level, may therefore be overlooked (e.g. maternal and child health services). However, local governments have certain competences in a number of sectors from which they can contribute in the reduction of socioeconomic health inequalities (Collins and Hayes, 2010).

Housing as a social determinant of health

Housing is especially important.

Health inequalities tend to be greater in urban areas with disadvantaged and poor populations, affecting, as a result, all city residents (WHO-UNHABITAT, 2010). However, for many households on low incomes living in owner-occupied and privately rented housing, the situation is inequitable and, for many, has negative health effects. In a report entitled 'Housing improvements for health and associated socioeconomic outcomes' (a Cochrane Review) (Thomson *et al.*, 2013), data from studies of warmth and energy efficiency interventions suggested that improvements in general health, respiratory health and mental health are possible. Studies that targeted those with inadequate warmth and existing chronic respiratory disease were most likely to report health improvement (Thomson *et al.*, 2013). Living in poorer-quality housing has been associated with poorer mental health and higher rates of infectious diseases, respiratory problems and injuries (Krieger and Higgins, 2002).

Introduction to public health and social determinants

On the WHO website, the following introduction is given to the social determinants of health:

> Health inequities are *avoidable* inequalities in health between groups of people within countries and between countries. These inequities arise from inequalities within and between societies. Social and economic conditions and their effects on people's lives determine their risk of illness and the actions taken to prevent them becoming ill or treat illness when it occurs.

It was reported a decade ago that much has been known about these determinants from national and international projects and research, but even now the knowledge is still too fragmentary. That knowledge needs to be more fully developed and widely shared so that it can be utilised more effectively (Jong-Wook, 2005). Over the last 40 years, a new paradigm has emerged in public health, demonstrating that social factors such as housing, employment, education and the urban environment are the strongest influences on a population's health (Wilkinson and Marmot, 2003). In effect, both the biological and social sciences have identified contributing factors to human health. However, health outcomes are unlikely to equal a simple sum of these identified factors (Shi and Zhong, 2014). Debates around concepts of wellbeing were initially precipitated within the philosophy of ethics, particularly around moral ways of conducting oneself and how this might assist in leading a 'happy' or 'satisfying' means of existence (La Placa and Knight, 2014).

Every aspect of government and the economy has the potential to affect health and health equity – finance, education, housing, employment, transport and health, to name just six. While health may not be the main aim of policies in these sectors, they have a strong bearing on health and health equity. Recently it has been suggested that minorities (African American, Hispanic/Latino, Native American and Pacific Islander) are disproportionately affected, resulting in poorer health outcomes compared with non-minority (white) populations, perhaps due to multiple inequality factors including inadequate and unsafe housing (Thomas, 2014).

The concept of wellbeing is intrinsic to the current modernisation of the public health structure in England and elsewhere. It is being linked to broader concepts around 'democratic legitimacy' and 'involvement', as well as stronger participation by individuals and local communities in the very structures that define and implement policies and initiatives around their lives (La Placa and Knight, 2014). A decade ago, Marmot (2005) identified a theme that relates to the question of how one can tell if a population is thriving, in relation to 'health status'.

Lalonde (1974) elaborated a concept of the social determinants of health, as shown in Figure 11.1. It is said by Lewis and colleagues (2008) that he was building on studies of morbidity and mortality in Canadians by Thomas McKeown to identify four fields: biology, lifestyle, environment and health care.

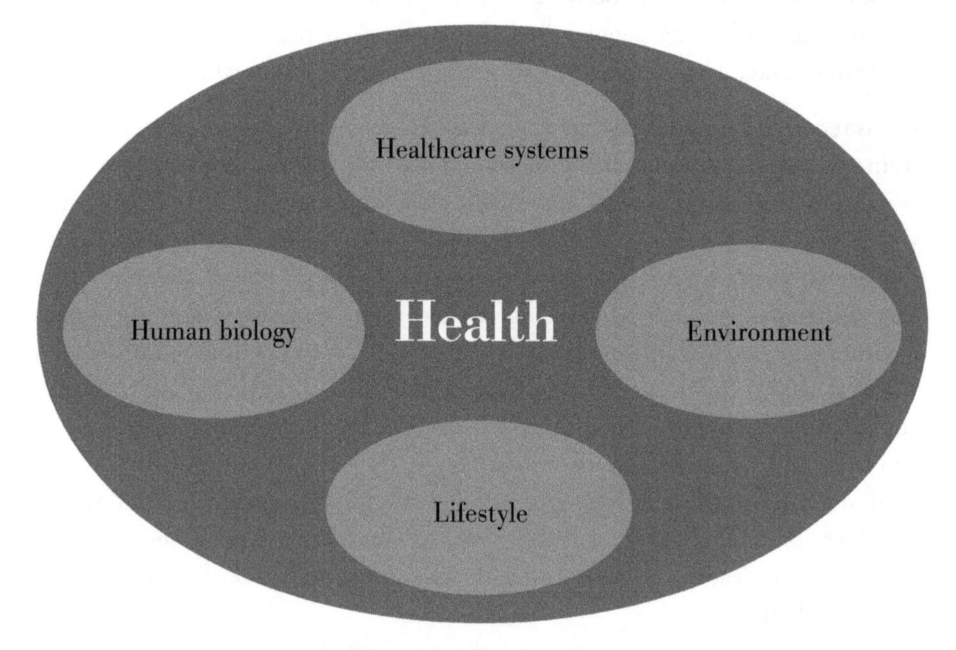

Figure 11.1 Lalonde's 'health field concept'

Source: Adapted from Lalonde, 1974

An alternative view is given in Figure 11.2. This famous model – Dahlgren and Whitehead's 'health rainbow' (1991) – aims to stimulate discussion as to how health is affected at different levels.

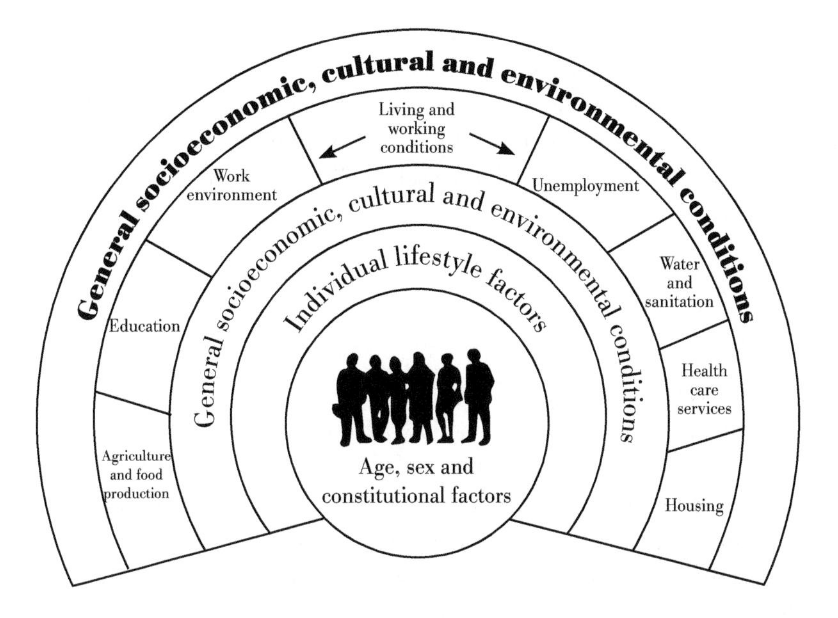

Figure 11.2 Dahlgren and Whitehead's 'health rainbow'

Source: Dahlgren and Whitehead, 1991 (reproduced by kind permission of the Institute for Futures Studies, Stockholm, Sweden)

For an excellent and succinct introduction to this field, the reader is strongly urged to consult Chapter 2H of *Mastering Public Health: A Postgraduate Guide to Examinations and Revalidation* by Geraint Lewis and colleagues (2008).

Supporting action to create cohesion and resilience at the local level is essential, through a whole-of-society approach. At the local level, this approach encourages the development of partnerships with those affected by inequity and exclusionary processes by working with civil society and a range of civic partners. Central to this approach is empowerment – putting in place effective mechanisms that give those affected a real say in decisions that affect their lives and recognising their fundamental human rights, including the right to health (Marmot *et al.*, 2012).

Health equity depends vitally on the empowerment of individuals to challenge and change the unfair and steeply graded distribution of social resources to which everyone has equal claims and rights. Inequity in power interacts across four main dimensions – political, economic, social and cultural – together constituting a continuum along which groups are, to varying degrees, excluded or included. The World Health Organization's Commission on Social Determinants of Health has called for health equity impact assessments (HEIAs) of all economic agreements, market regulation and public policies (WHO, 2008).

There are, however, a few 'blind spots' in research on this topic, such as a lack of studies on tertiary prevention, especially with regard to prevention and health promotion service use among men, as well as general studies on health promotion among men and women. There is also a lack of published intervention studies demonstrating how to better reach the socially disadvantaged (Janßen, Sauter and Kowalski, 2012).

Policy

The global context affects how societies prosper through its impact on international relations and domestic norms and policies. Despite a dramatic growth in social determinants of health/health equity (SDH/HE) public policy research and demonstrated government interest in promoting equity in health policies, health inequities continue to grow among some populations and there is little evidence that 'healthy public policies' are being adopted and implemented (Embrett and Randall, 2014). Using a 'policy analysis lens' to help identify why healthy public policies are typically not being adopted is an important step towards moving beyond advocacy to understanding and addressing some of the political barriers to reforms (Embrett and Randall, 2014). WHO defines governance for health as 'the attempts of governments or other actors to steer communities, whole countries, or even groups of countries in the pursuit of health as integral to wellbeing through both a whole-of-society and a whole-of-government approach' (Kickbusch and Gleicher, 2012, p.vi). Drawing on public policy studies, I recommend a number of strategies to increase the efficacy of current interventions. More broadly, the notion has emerged that up-stream interventions need to be 'fit for purpose', and cannot be easily replicated from one context to the next (Carey, Crammond and Keast, 2014).

Implementation of policy locally

Health inequalities can be tackled with appropriate health and social policies, involving all community groups and governments, from local to global (Pons-Vigués *et al.*, 2014). In Germany, one approach has been to determine whether differences in the use of prevention and health promotion services can be attributed to health inequality between different social status groups measured by education, occupation and income, and where certain improvements can be made in health promotion through reducing inequality (Janßen *et al.*, 2012).

Extra care housing and well-being

A starting point for the development of the 'Enriched Opportunities Programme' followed on from the experience of taking a group of extra care housing residents with dementia on an 'Activity Challenge week' where people experienced canoeing, abseiling, swimming, hot-air ballooning and a host of other exciting activities (Bradford Dementia Group, 2009). The levels of wellbeing that people showed on these short breaks have been apparently striking in this sustained initiative (Brooker, 2001; Brooker *et al.*, 2011). Once back in the nursing home setting, however, levels of wellbeing reverted to 'normal'. The provision of extra care housing is increasingly put forward as a means of improving the quality of life of those individuals requiring support while maintaining their independence and rights of tenancy or home ownership (Royal Commission on Long Term Care, 1999). Within this policy emphasis, it is envisaged that mainstream planning and provision of extra care housing schemes will be inclusive of people with dementia, older people with learning disabilities and those needing intermediate care.

It seems that residents can experience significant problems associated with dementia and depression (Brooker, Argyle and Clancy, 2009). Without proactive strategies in place, it is difficult to assess in the longer term what will happen to people who develop significant cognitive disabilities or other mental health problems within extra care housing. Furthermore, as is the case with community-dwelling individuals, it could be that the sense of belonging that comes with living in an extra care housing scheme could enhance feelings of wellbeing and mental health (Bailey and McLaren, 2005).

Dutton (2010) summarised the findings from a number of studies in this area and found strong evidence that certain aspects of extra care housing have a positive impact on the wellbeing of residents with dementia. These included person-centred care, maximising dignity and independence, effective communication and meaningful social interactions. A scoping review by O'Malley and Croucher (2005) explored the evidence base for housing provision for people with dementia and identified a number of gaps. This revealed a significant number of research gaps in the UK context, most notably in relation to end-of-life care for people with dementia and the effectiveness of integrated and segregated facilities. Hoof, Kort and Waarde (2009) have helpfully reported on trends in the provision of housing and care for people with dementia in the Netherlands, where there has been a move towards small-scale group accommodation. Key elements in the provision of care are facilitating the involvement of family carers, the use of technology and making modifications to the living environment.

Care homes

Institutional care models for persons with dementia continue to evolve.

The change in approach to care over the course of the past several decades, from institutional to home-like care, can be seen as a progressive shift in the culture of long-term care facilities (Robinson, Reid and Cooke, 2010). Care homes provide residential care for people with long- or short-term health conditions, older people, disabled people, people with learning disabilities or people with drug or alcohol problems. Some care homes also provide nursing care.

The Care Quality Commission (CQC) (2014) very recently produced a document entitled 'What standards you have a right to expect from the regulation of your care home'. This is intended for members of the general public and their friends and family to know what the legally enforceable standards of quality and safety of care homes are. The CQC monitors, inspects and regulates services to make sure they meet fundamental standards of quality and safety. They also protect the interests of vulnerable people, including those whose rights are restricted under mental health legislation.

These rights are stated in Box 11.1.

Box 11.1 Standards expected of care homes by the Care Quality Commission

* You can expect to be respected, involved and told what's happening at every stage
* You can expect care, treatment and support that meets your needs
* You can expect to be safe
* You can expect to be cared for by staff with the right skills to do their jobs properly
* You can expect your care home routinely to check the quality of its services

Source: Care Quality Commission, 2014 (pp.4–8) (reproduced under the Open Government Licence v3.0)

As reviewed by Manthorpe and Samsi (2014), the Mental Capacity Act 2005 currently provides the legal framework in England and Wales for how decisions are made. It forms a critical legal basis for the work of care home staff. In the years since the Mental Capacity Act 2005 was implemented in England and Wales (from 2007), training and associated resources have been provided for all those working with people whose decision-making capacity may be impaired or diminishing (Stanley *et al.*, 2007).

Investigating how residents in a dementia care setting navigate and participate within social groups is critical as the therapeutic benefits of social engagement are unequivocal (Doyle, de Medeiros and Saunders, 2011). Ageing in place – the ability of individuals to remain in their home in the community – is a consistent wish and expectation of middle-aged and older people (AARP, 2003). The concept of nested social groups refers to the clusters of residents who were frequently observed in close proximity to each other and interacting with one another. The concept of nesting was borrowed from the social ecology model (Bronfenbrenner, 1977). Relationships among people are nested within the local cultures of the setting and both levels interact and influence each other (Bronfenbrenner, 1979). Best practice requires the development, continuation and ongoing management of social relations that are meaningful not only to the person with dementia but also to the family and the institutional staff who care for that person (Nolan, Keady and Aveyard, 2001). Ericsson, Hellström and Kjellstrom (2011) advised, on the basis of their 31 observation sessions using a standpoint of 'social interaction theory', that sensitivity is required to interpret individuals' expressions of desire not to participate, while simultaneously it is important to try to interpret why they want to refrain.

Campo and Chaudhury (2012) reported a study of informal social interaction among residents with dementia in special care units. The authors were particularly interested in exploring the role of the physical and social environments. Their findings appear to suggest that social factors, such as staff work roles and resident group size, and physical factors, such as a non-institutional character, the nursing station location and adequate seating and sightlines, are influential for prompting or supporting informal social interactions. Design recommendations are provided with the intent to create physical environments that foster informal social interactions among people in dementia care environments. This framework predicts that meaningful informal social interaction is a result of a dynamic interplay between physical and social environment, one's past history and situational factors, and individual-level factors including functional and cognitive abilities.

Architectural considerations in dementia-friendly housing

Marquardt and Schmieg (2009) reported a fascinating cross-sectional study that evaluated the association between environment and functioning at home in older adults with dementia using space syntax methods. They further found that increased convexity of a place – meaning that the spatial system is broken up into various convex spaces – was associated with increased functional dependency in basic activities of daily living of the inhabitant.

The development of dementia cottages is a recent effort to effectively accommodate the care needs of residents with dementia (Robinson *et al.*, 2010). Central to the concept of a dementia cottage is the incorporation of home-like attributes, which have been put forth in the research literature as a necessary condition of optimal dementia care (Chappell and Reid, 2000). There is a plethora of various evidence-based ways of improving the design of housing to assist people living with dementia proposed in an outstanding document from the Dementia Services Development Centre from the University of Stirling (2013), entitled 'Improving the design of housing to assist people with dementia'. These include making reasonable adjustments for those with impairments of old age in sight, hearing, circadian rhythm and musculoskeletal problems, and impairments from the dementia including impaired learning and memory, impaired planning and visuospatial problems. These key design features are proposed for external areas – lighting, floors in hallways, stairs, doors, signs and lifts, for example. Despite the fact that half of those who live in their own home live alone, the home can be the best place for someone to manage the consequences of dementia (National Housing Federation, 2013).

A picture of where people live is provided in Figure 11.3.

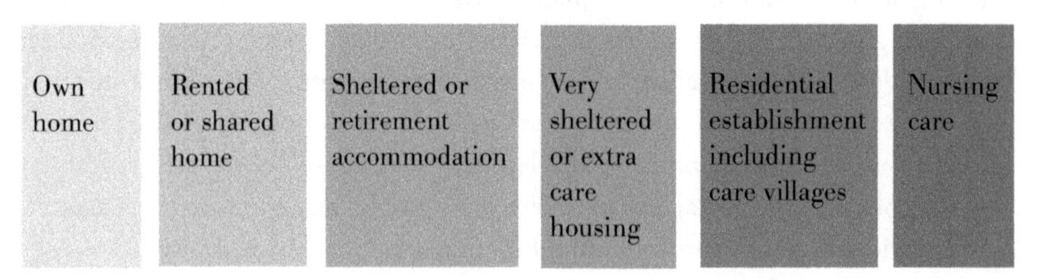

Figure 11.3 Types of accommodation for people living with dementia

Source: Housing Learning and Improvement Network, 2012 (p.3) (reproduced by kind permission of the Housing Learning and Improvement Network. For further information about their work please refer to www.housinglin.org.uk)

The wellbeing and behaviour of people living well with dementia in care homes is strongly determined by the design of their environment in these homes across all jurisdictions. Housing conditions can severely impede the ability of people to remain independent. Sometimes this is because a house becomes less useable so that bathroom and kitchen designs restrict use. Poorly insulated houses can be badly heated and cause illness; well-heated homes can bring the anxiety of paying fuel bills. If people live in challenging neighbourhoods, this may cause stress and a fear of leaving home (Housing Learning and Improvement Network, 2012). Local authorities, housing providers, home improvement agencies, GPs and NHS Trusts should work in partnership to develop support services for people with dementia (National Housing Federation, 2013).

Spatial disorientation is a prime reason for transfer into residential settings. The autonomy of the residents and their quality of life, however, is strongly linked with their ability to reach certain places within their nursing home. The physical environment has a great potential for supporting a resident's wayfinding abilities. Results from Marquardt and Schmieg (2009) confirm that people with advancing dementia are increasingly dependent on a compensating environment. The significant factors include a small number of residents per living area, the straight layout of the circulation system without any changes in direction, and the provision of only one living/dining room. These and additional results were transformed into architectural guidelines. The work of Care and Repair England is showcased by the National Housing Federation (2013). Care and repair services work with health and social care providers to identify those at risk of losing their independence or experiencing a decline in their health and wellbeing due to housing shortcomings.

Guidance on the top ten housing adaptations is shown in Box 11.2.

Box 11.2 Top ten housing adaptations

* Double the usual levels of lighting in the home
* Pay attention to acoustics and reduce noise pollution
* Use contrast of tone (rather than colour) to differentiate between walls, skirting boards and floors. Ensure that floors are of a consistent tone.
* Ensure there is good signage mounted low enough for poor eyesight
* Use contrast of colour or tone to make switches and objects easily visible

* Ensure that people can see important rooms such as the toilet, that furniture and fittings give strong clues to the purpose of the room and that there are clear signs
* Ensure that kitchens and bathrooms are easy to understand; avoid new designs for things such as taps or kettles
* Give strong clues to the purpose of the room and that there are clear signs
* Place illuminated clocks in each room indicating whether it is a.m. or p.m.
* All doors should be visible on entering the dwelling; cupboards should be glass fronted or open

---

Source: National Housing Federation, 2013 (p.11)
(copyright © Dementia Services Centre, Stirling)

I should, however, like to emphasise that the considerations for housing as a whole in dementia-friendly communities are broader in scope than simply the design features in Chapter 13 and the built environment in Chapter 16 of my book *Living Well with Dementia* (Rahman, 2014). I did consider the design of homes and wards. Where housing staff are appropriately trained in dementia, they have the ability to support people with a range of housing choices that can contribute to a better quality of life (Housing Learning and Improvement Network, 2012). When the transition from mainstream to specialist housing is required, it is important that people with dementia maintain their links to their community and can participate in new friendships and activities.

Extra care housing has the capacity to support a good quality of life for people with dementia (Housing Learning and Improvement Network, 2012). However, some people describe feeling isolated or cite a lack of acceptance from other residents.

A robust notion is emerging that a dementia-friendly community must be inclusive of people with dementia and their carers, no matter what care setting they live in. Therefore, an important aspect is ensuring that housing schemes are also integrated with health and social care services and involved in the local community (Alzheimer's Society, 2013). Care homes also need to ensure that residents with dementia can maintain relationships and interests within the immediate environment and the broader community. An important shift is needed to move away from the perception of care homes as a 'last resort' and to build positive and active profiles in the community (Mason, 2012).

For housing to be both inclusive and dementia-friendly, it also needs to address sensory and cognitive challenges (Housing Learning and Improvement Network, 2012). But new design literature, published in the last decade or so, seeks to promote therapeutic and supportive environments that enhance residents' wellbeing, strengths and abilities, and meet residents' physical, emotional and psychological needs (Housing Learning and Improvement Network, 2012). The EVOLVE evaluation tool was developed from research on extra care housing and was not specifically designed to make these dementia-friendly. There are a number of important ethical considerations within the framework that formed the basis for the design of the research methods, as well as the basis for choosing the devices to be tried out (Bjørneby *et al.*, 2004).

British government policy for older people focuses on a vision of active ageing and independent living within the community, even for those with significant health problems (Department of Health, 2006). This has led to a growing interest in extra care housing schemes (or assisted living schemes, as they are more popularly known in North America) as a potentially more 'homely' alternative to residential and nursing home care (Heywood, Oldman and Means, 2002). Independence is one of the most important elements of quality of life for people with dementia living in extra care housing. A range of factors in the physical, social and care environments should be considered in order to maximise independence. Good design of individual apartments and communal areas, the provision of appropriate activities and the availability of flexible care and support were all found to be important (Evans *et al.*, 2007).

The wish to remain living independently, regardless of the condition of housing, neighbourhood and health, is often a personal choice (Gitlin, 2003), but it is influenced by the personal disablement process or health status of a partner, and more specifically the objective and subjective burdens of care experienced by the partner (van Hoof *et al.*, 2010). The importance of the own-home environment as a setting for the provision of (dementia) care was already acknowledged at least two decades ago by Pynoos, Cohen and Lucas (1989). Governments and patient/healthcare organisations have the important task to supply information regarding environmental interventions to individuals with dementia and their informal carers.

Research that investigates the built environment for people with dementia is feasible and may help guide planning policies likely to enhance independent community living for this group (Sheehan, Burton and Mitchell, 2006). Future research in the area should involve subjects across the full range of dementia severity, should concentrate on specific design features in the public environment that may be amended (e.g. signs), and should involve larger numbers of subjects to avoid the risk of erroneous observations. It may be most fruitful to research areas with larger concentrations of older people, among whom dementia will be more common (Sheehan *et al.*, 2006).

Reducing risk is a major consideration driving policy. Waugh (2009) has warned against being engulfed in the notion of risk, and urged for a balancing of safety and human rights – as well as risk – in all interventions. I will return to risk engagement in Chapter 13 when discussing personal budgets, and in my concluding chapter (Chapter 18).

Conclusion

This chapter has taken as its focus the housing environment of the person aspiring to live better with dementia. But what happens when a person living with dementia leaves their home environment? Chapter 12 considers whether there is a beneficial role to be played by 'global positioning systems'; this topic inevitably raises strong emotions, despite fairly succinct legal and ethical arguments.

References

AARP (2003) These Four Walls: Americans 45+ Talk About Home and Community. Washington, DC: AARP. Available at http://assets.aarp.org/rgcenter/il/four_walls.pdf (accessed 28 February 2015).

Alzheimer's Society (2013) Building dementia-friendly communities. Available at www.alzheimers.org.uk/site/scripts/documents_info.php?documentID=2283 (accessed 6 December 2014).

Bailey, M. and McLaren, S. (2005) Physical activity alone and with others as predictors of sense of belonging and mental health in retirees. Aging and Mental Health, 9, 1, 82–90.

Bambra, C. (2011) Health inequalities and welfare state regimes: theoretical insights on a public health 'puzzle'. Journal of Epidemiology and Community Health, 65, 9, 740–5.

Banerjee, S., Samsi, K., Petrie, C.D., Alvir, J. *et al.* (2009) What do we know about quality of life in dementia? A review of the emerging evidence on the predictive and explanatory value of disease specific measures of health related quality of life in people with dementia. International Journal of Geriatric Psychiatry, 24, 1, 15–24.

Bjørneby, S., Topo, P., Cahill, S., Begley, E. *et al.* (2004) Ethical considerations in the ENABLE project. Dementia, 3, 3, 297–312.

Bradford Dementia Group (2009) 'The Enriched Opportunities Programme: a cluster randomised controlled trial of a new approach to living with dementia and other mental health issues in ExtraCare housing schemes and villages. Available at www.extracare.org.uk/media/32600/pdf%20for%20dementia%20link_eop_%20final_%20report_%202009.pdf (accessed 6 December 2014).

Bronfenbrenner, U. (1977) Toward an experimental ecology of human development. American Psychologist, 32, 7, 513–31.

Bronfenbrenner, U. (1979) The Ecology of Human Development: Experiments by Nature and Design. Cambridge, MA: Harvard University Press.

Brooker, D. (2001) Enriching lives: evaluation of the ExtraCare activity challenge. Journal of Dementia Care, 9, 3, 33–7.

Brooker, D., Argyle, E. and Clancy, D. (2009) Mental health needs of people living in extra care housing. Journal of Care Services Management, 3, 3, 295–309.

Brooker, D., Argyle, E., Scally, A.J. and Clancy, D. (2011) The Enriched Opportunities Programme for people with dementia: a cluster-randomised controlled trial in 10 extra care housing schemes. Aging and Mental Health, 15, 8, 1008–17.

Campo, M. and Chaudhury, H. (2012) Informal social interaction among residents with dementia in special care units: exploring the role of the physical and social environments. International Journal of Social Research and Practice, 11, 3, 401–423

Care Quality Commission (2014) What standards you have a right to expect from the regulation of your care home. Available at www.cqc.org.uk/sites/default/files/documents/standards_to_expect_carehome.pdf (accessed 20 February 2015).

Carey, G., Crammond, B. and Keast, R. (2014) Creating change in government to address the social determinants of health: how can efforts be improved? BMC Public Health, 14, 1087.

Chappell, N.L. and Reid, R.C. (2000) Dimensions of care for dementia sufferers in long term care institutions: are they related to outcomes? Journals of Gerontology: Social Sciences, 55, S234–44.

Chen, R., Hu, Z., Chen, R.L., Ma, Y., Zhang, D. and Wilson, K. (2013) Determinants for undetected dementia and late-life depression. British Journal of Psychiatry, 203, 3, 203–8.

Collins, P.A. and Hayes, M.V. (2010) The role of urban municipal governments in reducing health inequities: A meta-narrative mapping analysis. International Journal for Equity in Health, 9, 13.

Dahlgren, G. and Whitehead, M. (1991) Policies and Strategies to Promote Social Equity in Health. Stockholm, Sweden: Institute for Futures Studies.

Dementia Services Development Centre (2013) Improving the design of housing to assist people with dementia. Available at www.cih.org/resources/PDF/Scotland%20general/Improving%20the%20design%20of%20housing%20to%20assist%20people%20with%20dementia%20-%20FINAL.pdf (accessed 6 December 2014).

Department of Health (2006) Our Health, Our Care, Our Say: A New Direction for Community Services, Cm 6737. London: Department of Health.

Diderichsen, F., Andersen, I., Manuel, C. and the Working Group of Danish Review on Social Determinants of Health (2012) Health inequality: determinants and policies. Scandinavian Journal of Public Health, 40 (8 Suppl), 12–105.

Doyle, P.J., de Medeiros, K. and Saunders, P.A. (2011) Nested social groups within the social environment of a dementia care assisted living setting. Dementia, 11, 3, 383–99.

Dutton, R. (2010) People with dementia living in extra care housing: learning from the evidence. Working with Older People, 14, 1, 8–11.

Embrett, M.G. and Randall, G.E. (2014) Social determinants of health and health equity policy research: exploring the use, misuse, and nonuse of policy analysis theory. Social Science and Medicine, 108, 147–55.

Ericsson, I., Hellström, I. and Kjellstrom, S. (2011) Sliding interactions: an ethnography about how persons with dementia interact in housing with care for the elderly. Dementia, 10, 523.

Evans, S., Fear, T., Means, R. and Vallehy, S. (2007) Supporting independence for people with dementia in extra care housing. Dementia, 6, 144–50.

Gitlin, L.N. (2003) Next Steps in Home Modification and Assistive Technology Research. In N. Charness and K.W. Schaie (eds) Impact of Technology on Successful Aging. New York, NY: Springer Publishing Company.

Heywood, F., Oldman, C. and Means, R. (2002) Housing and Home in Later Life. Buckingham: Open University Press.

Hoof, J., Kort, H.S.M. and Waarde, H. (2009) Housing and care for older adults with dementia: a European perspective. Journal of Housing and the Built Environment, 24, 3, 369–90.

Housing Learning and Improvement Network (2010) EVOLVE Tool – Evaluation of Older People's Living Environments. Available at www.housinglin.org.uk/Topics/type/resource/?cid=7997 (accessed 6 December 2014).

Housing Learning and Improvement Network (2012) Breaking New Ground: The Quest for Dementia Friendly Communities, Viewpoint 25. Available at www.housinglin.org.uk/_library/Resources/Housing/Support_materials/Viewpoints/Viewpoint25_Dementia_Friendly_Communities.pdf (accessed 6 December 2014).

Janßen, C., Sauter, S. and Kowalski, C. (2012) The influence of social determinants on the use of prevention and health promotion services: results of a systematic literature review. Psychosocial Medicine, 9, doi: 10.3205/psm000085.

Jong-Wook, L. (2005) Public health is a social issue. Lancet, 365, 1005–6.

Kickbusch, I. and Gleicher, D. (2012) Governance for Health in the 21st Century. Geneva: World Health Organization. Available at www.euro.who.int/__data/assets/pdf_file/0019/171334/RC62BD01-Governance-for-Health-Web.pdf (accessed 28 February 2015).

Krieger, J. and Higgins, D. (2002) Housing and health: time again for public health action. American Journal of Public Health, 92, 758–68.

La Placa, V. and Knight, A. (2014) Wellbeing: its influence and local impact on public health. Public Health, 128, 1, 38–42.

Lalonde, M. (1974) A new perspective on the health of Canadians: a working document. Available at www.phac-aspc.gc.ca/ph-sp/pdf/perspect-eng.pdf (accessed 6 December 2014).

Lawton, M.P. (1986) Environment and Aging. Albany, NY: Center for the Study of Aging.

Lewis, G.H., Sheringham, J., Kalim, K. and Crayford, T.J.B. (2008) Mastering Public Health: A Postgraduate Guide to Examinations and Revalidation. London: CRC Press.

Liu, S., Jones, R.N. and Glymour, M.M. (2010) Implications of lifecourse epidemiology for research on determinants of adult disease. Public Health Reviews, 32, 2, 489–511.

Manthorpe, J. and Samsi, K. (2014) Care homes and the Mental Capacity Act 2005: changes in understanding and practice over time. Dementia (London), pii: 1471301214542623 [Epub ahead of print].

Marmot, M. (2005) Social determinants of health inequalities. Lancet, 365, 9464, 1099–104.

Marmot, M., Allen, J., Bell, R., Bloomer, E. and Goldblatt, P./Consortium for the European Review of Social Determinants of Health and the Health Divide (2012) WHO European review of social determinants of health and the health divide. Lancet, 380, 9846, 1011–29.

Marquardt, G. and Schmieg, P. (2009) Dementia-friendly architecture: environments that facilitate wayfinding in nursing homes. American Journal of Alzheimer's Disease and Other Dementias, 24, 4, 333–40.

Mason, M. (2012) Care Home Sweet Home. London: International Longevity Centre.

National Housing Federation (published by the National Housing Federation, the Dementia Services Development Centre, the Housing Learning and Improvement Network, and Foundations) (2013) Dementia: finding housing solutions. Available at www.housing.org.uk/publications/browse/dementia-finding-housing-solutions.pdf (accessed 22 May 2015).

Nolan, M., Keady, J. and Aveyard, B. (2001) Relationship-centred care is the next logical step. British Journal of Nursing, 10, 12, 757.

O'Malley, L. and Croucher, K. (2005) Housing and dementia care – a scoping review of the literature. Health and Social Care in the Community, 13, 6, 570–7.

Pons-Vigués, M., Diez, È., Morrison, J., Salas-Nicás, S. *et al.* (2014) Social and health policies or interventions to tackle health inequalities in European cities: a scoping review. BMC Public Health, 14, 198.

Pynoos, J., Cohen, E. and Lucas, C. (1989) Environmental coping strategies for Alzheimer's caregivers. American Journal of Alzheimer's Disease and Other Dementias, 4, 6, 4–8.

Rahman, S. (2014) Living Well with Dementia: The Importance of the Person and the Environment for Wellbeing. Oxford: Radcliffe Health.

Robinson, C.A., Reid, C. and Cooke, H.A. (2010) A home away from home: the meaning of home according to families of residents with dementia. Dementia, 9, 4, 490–508.

Royal Commission on Long Term Care (1999) With Respect to Old Age: Long Term Care – Rights and Responsibilities. London: The Stationery Office.

Sheehan, B., Burton, E. and Mitchell, L. (2006) Outdoor wayfinding in dementia. Dementia, 5, 2, 271–81.

Shi, Y. and Zhong, S. (2014) From genomes to societies: a holistic view of determinants of human health. Current Opinion in Biotechnology, 28, 134–42.

Stanley, N., Lyons, C., Manthorpe, J., Rapaport, J. *et al.* (2007) Mental Capacity Act 2005. Acute Hospitals Training Set. London: Department of Health.

Stewart, J. and Bourn, C. (2013) The environmental health practitioner: new evidence-based roles in housing, public health and wellbeing. Perspectives in Public Health, 133, 6, 325–9.

Thomas, B. (2014) Health and health care disparities: the effect of social and environmental factors on individual and population health. International Journal of Environmental Research and Public Health, 11, 7, 7492–507.

Thomson, H., Thomas, S., Sellstrom, E. and Petticrew, M. (2013) Housing improvements for health and associated socio-economic outcomes. Cochrane Database of Systematic Reviews, 28, 2, CD008657.

van Hoof, J., Kort, H., Duijnstee, M., Rutten, P. and Hensen, J. (2010) The indoor environment and the integrated design of homes for older people with dementia. Building and Environment, 45, 5, 1244–61.

Waugh, F. (2009) Where does risk feature in community care practice with older people with dementia who live alone? Dementia, 8, 205–22.

WHO (2008) Commission on Social Determinants of Health (CSDH) Final Report. Closing the Gap in a Generation: Health Equity through Action on the Social Determinants of Health. Geneva: World Health Organization.

WHO/UN-HABITAT (2010) Hidden Cities: Unmasking and Overcoming Health Inequities in Urban Settings. Geneva: World Health Organization. Available at www.who.int/kobe_centre/publications/hiddencities_media/who_un_habitat_hidden_cities_web.pdf (accessed 20 April 2015).

Wilkinson, R. and Marmot, M. (2003) Social Determinants of Health: The Solid Facts. Copenhagen: World Health Organization.

Chapter 12

DOES GPS TRACKING HAVE A ROLE TO PLAY IN LIVING BETTER WITH DEMENTIA?

'A lonely kite
lost in flight –
someone once
had flown.'

From 'The Wanderer' by Lang Leav

Introduction

We live in a 'surveillance society'.

If you log in on Facebook, Facebook can identify your location exactly and then offer you a choice of cheap hotels there. The idea that GPS (global positioning system), as a tracker, can identify you where you are feels like an invasion of privacy.

Tracking for people with dementia raises strong emotions, not helped when some of the discussion takes place at the extremes – such as a hypothermic person with dementia found in a ditch due to a GPS tracker. But the conflation of 'tracking' with 'tagging', as per frequent offenders in the criminal law, is an unfortunate one. The word 'tracking' itself, however, is a misnomer, in that these trackers do not actively 'follow' people, but can pinpoint someone's location through the method of 'trilateration'.

The question is whether someone can consent to doing himself or herself harm – exercising his or her own ethical right to autonomy – and a clear definition of consent depends on a clear definition of capacity. A human right to privacy, which is inalienable, albeit qualified, may transcend capacity, causing further disquiet in legal circles. The term 'wandering' may inadvertently lay blame on innocent people.

Primary ethical considerations

According to DuBois and Miley (2005), ethics generate standards that direct one's conduct. In other words, 'ethics represents values in action' (p.110). They identify three levels as follows:

» microethics: those standards and principles that direct practice

» macroethics: those concerned with organisational arrangements and values as well as those that underlie and guide social policies

» ethical behaviour: actions that uphold moral obligations and comply with standards for practice as prescribed by ethical codes.

(DuBois and Miley, 2005, p.110)

Today, as research in the application of technologies continues to evolve (Westphal, Dingjan and Attoe, 2010), possibilities are emerging for using new technologies to provide individualised aid to people with dementia. Such technologies, including devices based on standard telephone communications, simple monitors and video cameras, can be used to transmit basic vital information (Hudson and Cohen, 2010). Furthermore, it is likely that the ethical debate about tracking or other electronic monitoring devices is likely to become intense. Hughes and Baldwin (2006) discussed in a fascinating way how electronic tracking might come under the umbrella of 'covert coercion' or 'cajoling'. The authors remarked that, while coercion invalidates valid consent, 'cajoling' does occur, for example, when a carer strongly urges a person living with dementia to attend a day centre or respite care. Electronic monitoring or tracking might possibly represent an example of the cusp between autonomy and coercion.

Is 'wandering' the most appropriate term?

> 'I am a person living well with dementia. If I then go on a long walk, will I then be known as a "wanderer"?'
>
> Kate Swaffer, advocate for people living with dementia

'Wandering' is not a trivial policy issue. The problem with the word 'wandering' is that it is often used synonymously with the term 'difficult behaviour' or 'challenging behaviour'. It can be interpreted as a rather pejorative label that seeks to blame the 'wanderer', and therefore can impose a moralistic judgment inadvertently or intentionally with terms such as 'nuisance'. Where it is used in this chapter, it will adopt the various definitions given in the papers cited. But the lack of consensus is problematic. Jan Dewing (2006, p.239) noticed: 'People with dementia may think and feel differently about wandering, as will be suggested in this paper. The voices of those who have experiential expertise of dementia and wandering need to be included in the debate on wandering to influence both nursing research and practice.'

'Wandering' is a complex behaviour involving walking-type movements that include rummaging, walking around the home and going outdoors (Dewing, 2005). People who wander are typically younger, have a greater level of cognitive impairment, are more commonly male, have a higher incidence of sleep problems and had a more active lifestyle prior to the onset of the dementia illness (Lai and Arthur, 2003). 'Wandering' in long-term care settings is associated with a variety of negative outcomes including falls, injuries and untimely death (Shinoda-Tagawa *et al.*, 2004). It is also a cause of admissions in medical and psychiatric units (Hughes and Louw, 2002). Studies have suggested substantial risks are posed by getting lost, including death, injury, dehydration and hypothermia (Koester and Stooksbury, 1995; Rowe and Bennett, 2003; Rowe and Glover, 2001). Although widely discrepant estimates of its prevalence have been reported, wandering behaviour is also considered a significant problem for carers (Logsdon *et al.*, 1998) and may lead to a premature move to a care home (Algase *et al.*, 2010). Molinari and colleagues (2008, p.748) argue that 'psychiatric wanderers may be conceptualised better as exhibiting ambulatory concomitants of unremitted neurological/psychiatric symptoms or medication side effects of their treatment. Findings have implications for addressing treatable causes of wandering.'

Researchers in France found that 12.6% of 571 dementia patients engaged in some level of wandering (Rolland *et al.*, 2003). Wandering can be a potentially life-threatening behaviour for older people with dementia. They are at higher risk for getting lost, falling and being involved in road traffic accidents (McShane *et al.*, 1998), and being found injured, suffering from exposure or dead (Kibayashi and Shojo, 2003). The demands on family carers are considerable enough, even if you consider the additional pressures posed by 'wandering' (Dodds, 1994).

But it is important to note that even getting lost with a tracker can be very distressing for a person with dementia who is classed in the literature as a 'wanderer'. White and Montgomery (2014) highlight that further research might be warranted to assess whether carers, when anticipating the consequences of getting lost, have a heightened awareness of the risks posed by getting lost relative to the risks posed by the technology to a person's liberty. There is clearly a balance to be struck here between risk pursuant to liberty and safety.

Spatial navigation

It is clear that people who are prone to 'wander' are more than merely 'lost'.

Getting lost is not just common in dementia of the Alzheimer type, but it is one of its earliest clinical manifestations (Henderson, Mack and Williams, 1989). Cushman, Stein and Duffy (2008) have previously characterised navigational impairments, which are indicative of cognitive ageing or Alzheimer's disease, by means of real-world navigational tests. Such tests can, however, be time-consuming and difficult to conduct. They, therefore, hypothesised that a virtual-reality test could provide an alternative method of identifying navigational deficits. Episodes of topographical disorientation were reported in patients residing in a community (Pai and Jacobs, 2004).

Moreover, almost 90% of patients with dementia of the Alzheimer type had their first incident of disorientation in familiar surroundings (Tu and Pai, 2006). This reflects a deficit in spatial memory, generally defined as the ability to encode, store and retrieve spatial information in order to build an internal representation of the environment (a 'cognitive map') (O'Keefe and Nadel, 1978). Passini and colleagues (2000) make the distinction between aimless wandering and wayfinding, and state that in the former the person walks without having a destination in mind and without knowing where he or she is. However, potential consequences of not being able to reach a desired destination include diminishing activities of daily living, wandering and becoming lost, mistakenly going into the rooms of other residents (leading to resident-to-resident aggression) and interference with other residents in the public spaces of the unit (Mahoney, Volicer and Hurley, 2000).

Owing to Lawton's 'environmental docility hypothesis', first introduced in Chapter 11, modification of the physical environment is considered an important focus for intervention to address wandering and other dementia-related behaviours – from securing boundaries to incorporating specific internal and external design features (Lawton and Simon, 1968). Algase and colleagues (2010) reported on the influences of the physical environment on the behaviour of persons who 'wander'. In all, 80% of wandering occurred in the residents' own rooms, day rooms, hallways or dining rooms.

Tagging and tracking

In electronic tagging, the tag is usually a wristband. The circuitry in the tag may either set off a boundary alarm or emit a radio signal that allows the wearer to be tracked down by means of a hand detector (Hughes and Louw, 2002). At face value, these technologies may be a way of creating a more secure environment (Welsh *et al.*, 2003) and offer the potential to increase freedom of movement and independence. However, it is not these technologies themselves that pose the problem, but failure to question the ethics around their use (Eltis, 2005).

GPS location allows a receiver on earth to 'listen' to the positions of various satellites, using information about where that person is in relation to those satellites. GPS uses information from at least three satellites, in a process known as 'trilateration', in order to calculate an object's latitude, longitude and altitude (see Figure 12.1).

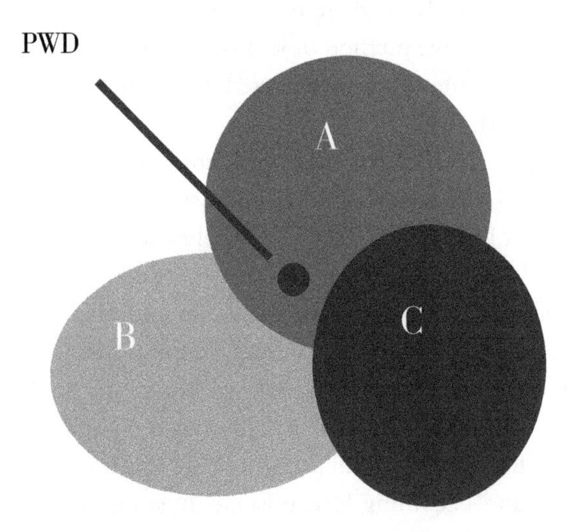

Figure 12.1 The process of 'trilateration'

SOURCE: ADAPTED FROM HUTCHINS, 2007 (P.417)

Although GPS location has been promoted to facilitate safe walking, reduce carers' anxiety and enable people with dementia to remain at home, there is little high-quality evidence about its acceptability, effectiveness or cost-effectiveness. An observational study by Milne and colleagues (2014) explored the feasibility of recruiting and retaining participants, and the acceptability of outcome measures, to inform decisions about the feasibility of a randomised controlled trial (RCT). The data in this hugely influential study suggest that an RCT will be hard to implement, not least because widespread enthusiasm for GPS among social care staff may challenge recruitment. Time spent searching (if this could be accurately captured) and days until long-term admission are potentially suitable outcomes. However, in the English jurisdiction, influential support has been given. If tracking is found to be successful, it would be the least restrictive and most preferred method of dealing with wandering in dementia (House of Lords Select Committee on Science and Technology, 2005).

Electronic tracking through GPS can locate a person at any given moment by positioning the device through satellite technology and sending the information via the mobile phone network to a personal computer, a call centre or a mobile phone (Kearns and Fozard, 2007). Accuracy of GPS tracking ranges from 5 to 100 metres (Miskelly, 2004; Shimizu, Kawamura and Yamamoto, 2000). GPS tracking does not prevent the person from wandering or getting lost, but it enables a carer to locate the person with dementia at any given moment. Two systematic reviews of interventions for wandering behaviour conclude that there is insufficient research evidence to make recommendations about the use of GPS technology (Hermans, Htay and Cooley, 2007; Robinson *et al.*, 2006).

Using GPS technology, the geographical position of a tracking device can be determined with considerable accuracy. In recent years, advanced technologies, such as GPS and radio frequency identification (RFID), have been developed that allow researchers to log and track human spatial activity. These can also be employed to measure wandering behaviour in people with dementia, and to intervene to manage that behaviour. Electronic tracking devices may enhance the personal safety of older people by alerting carers to potential dangers or adverse events that might threaten their health and safety (Robinson *et al.*, 2007).

Dignity is seen as an essential need, fundamental right and inherent quality of each human being (Tranvåg, Petersen and Nåden, 2014). I will return to dignity in the sphere of human rights in Chapter 13. Opinions have varied: while some research underlines dignity as a crucial foundation for quality of life (Manthorpe *et al.*, 2010) and essential in caring for older adults (Andersberg *et al.*, 2007), others criticise the concept of dignity as vague (Billings, 2008, cited in Tranvåg *et al.*, 2014). It is important, at least, to acknowledge a fundamental issue of education and policy to reduce or eliminate physical restraint of persons with dementia to overcome identified barriers at the individual, cultural and organisational levels

(De Bellis *et al.*, 2013). No evidence exists that 'subjective barriers' – such as patterns on the floor, mirrors, curtains or other forms of camouflage on doors – reduce wandering, but the possibility of harm, particularly psychological distress, cannot be excluded (Price, Hermans and Grimley Evans, 2001). Certain physical restraints have the potential to cause serious injury and death, and locked doors and bean bags, which are also physical restraints, are anathema to some (Parker and Miles, 1997).

Intriguingly, some carers describe informal GPS tracking, using mobile phone technology, as being beneficial. Frank Miskelly wrote a very helpful letter in *Age and Ageing* (2005) to describe how GPS phones were linked to a mobile phone service via the GSM (Global System for Mobile Communications) network, and were registered to a central computer based at the London Borough of Ealing Control Centre. Each participant had a relative or carer who was taught how to use the phone and given a manual. The relative or carer was responsible for ensuring that the phone was set up correctly and that the participant wore it correctly every day. Landau and colleagues (2009) later found there was considerable variation in the attitudes of their sample family and professional carers towards the use of advanced electronic tracking such as GPS and RFID for elderly people with dementia. The study revealed four principal findings, but most striking is the finding that professionals appear to have greater reservations about electronic tracking than carers.

First, carers' views ranged from feeling obligated to use the tracking device for the sake of patients' safety, through support of the use of the device for the sake of the carers' peace of mind and restricted support, to objection to the use of the device and respect for a person's autonomy. 'Autonomy' is critical in clinical ethics, and a patient wishing to establish autonomy or 'self-determination' can be in conflict with the desire of GPs to establish beneficence (Bremberg and Nilstun, 2000). This might be understood in two different ways: 'as expressing respect for the patient or as indifference to his or her medical needs' (Bremberg and Nilstun, 2000, p.128). It is worth noting that assessing the autonomy of a person with dementia requires an assessment of an individual's competence or capacity to understand the relevant options and consequences of a particular task or decision in light of one's own values, and yet judgments of competence in a specific area are routinely made informally by attending physicians, other healthcare professionals and family members. Second, family carers showed higher support for the use of GPS and RFID both for their own peace of mind and for the safety of the person in their care. Professionals attached higher value to respect for a person's autonomy and restricted support for using GPS and RFID. Third, both family and professional carers agreed that the decision on tracking dementia patients should be an intra-family issue. Fourth, family carers attached more importance to the tracking device's characteristics and design, thus emphasising that the tracking device must be considered by them as 'user-friendly'. The implications of the results for social work are also discussed.

According to Landau and colleagues (2009), professional carers saw the spouse and the patient as the most appropriate decision makers. Although professional carers' support for the patient's participation in the decision-making process is significantly higher than the support of the family carers, it ranks second to their rating of the spouse as the key decision maker. This position suggests that, while they respect patients' autonomy, professionals are aware of the fact that patients living with dementia may be incompetent to make the decision in this context. This is discussed further in Landau and Werner (2012). Professional carers in both community and care homes/institutions should be more actively involved in making important decisions for their patients' life, including deciding whether to use GPS. Moorman, Hauser and Carr (2009) have collected empirical evidence that family carers predict the end-of-life treatment preferences of their relatives incorrectly in about one-third of cases. Spouses may face difficulty in making hard decisions in end-of-life issues due to their own poor health (Lautrette *et al.*, 2006). In addition, in practice, family carers tend to promote the safety of people with dementia over their autonomy. For all these reasons, decision making in advance by the patient, together with family and professionals, appears important.

This overall narrative, however, perhaps appears consistent with a literature where patients should be initially asked for their consent, as suggested in the literature regarding the participation of persons with dementia in research (Petersen and Wallin, 2003; Sugarman *et al.*, 2007). In the next stage, perhaps the decision should be considered as a process involving both the patients and their family members, as suggested by Fisk, Beattie and Donnelly (2007), and include advance treatment planning, as suggested by Defanti *et al.* (2007). White and Montgomery (2014) reported on a thorough review of the literature and an original study. This article examined ethical issues associated with use of electronic tracking in a domestic setting. The qualitative study consisted of in-depth interviews with ten carers who were using it. The study explored the values, beliefs and contextual factors that motivated carers to use electronic tracking.

Dewing's process of obtaining consent

Consent in the context of cognitive impairment adds complexity to use of electronic tracking in dementia care. The right of a competent person to make decisions has been afforded protection across legal systems in Western Europe and North America. While legislation on capacity exists in most jurisdictions, it is beyond the scope of this book to review the diversity of legislative models. Cases where the person with dementia fully understands the implications of electronic tracking and readily consents to use are unproblematic. However, this may not typically be the case. Wandering appears to be most common in the moderate to severe stages of dementia (Hope *et al.*, 2001). At this stage, capacity to make decisions is likely to be diminished and to fluctuate over time. This calls into question difficulties associated with borderline capacity (Nuffield Council on Bioethics, 2009).

A major methodological concern has been the inclusion of people with dementia in research on such matters, due to the difficulties in consent. Whilst not without limitations, this method for process consent does seem to offer a valid and acceptable way for researchers to go about including a greater number of persons with dementia in research, from which they otherwise might have been excluded.

Jan Dewing (2007) offers an excellent structured approach to resolve this vexing methodological and ethical issue.

1. Background and preparation

The first element in the method sets the scene by prompting the researcher to check they are not taking short cuts.

2. Establishing the basis for capacity

In the second element of the method the researcher is primarily concerned with establishing the basis for capacity to consent and how this has been achieved.

3. Initial consent

By the third element of the method, the researcher should be feeling confident enough to seek an initial consent for the specific research. Thus the consent process moves from what is known about consent and assent in general terms to its translation into the specific situation. The exact way of achieving this will vary.

4. Ongoing consent monitoring

In element four, the focus is on ensuring initial consent is revisited and re-established on every occasion or even within the same occasion. This emphasises consent as a process rather than an abrupt event.

5. Feedback and support

Element five of the method asks the researcher to consider feedback and support. In some situations it may be necessary for the researcher to consider providing staff with some feedback about the person's wellbeing or on a particular concern.

Borderline capacity does not sit comfortably in a legal framework that constructs capacity as dichotomous, present or absent. In response to this challenge, the Nuffield Council on Bioethics (2009) proposed a joint decision-making model, involving trusted family members, as an interim measure for when the person is not fully able to make decisions but is not yet at a stage where a system of total proxy decision making is required.

Are persons with cognitive impairment able to make consistent choices (Feinberg and Whitlatch, 2001)? As discussed by Landau and Werner (2012), a proxy decision on using assistive technologies, such as GPS tracking, might be based on the prior attitudes and values of the person with dementia. They cite Becker and Kahana (1993), who emphasise that in the early stages of dementia the carers need to anticipate possible future situations and determine in advance the disposition of the person with dementia in such situations.

Human rights

The nub of the legal issue over tracking can be found in the legal doctrine of proportionality, which many comparative lawyers agree can be found in the German jurisdiction (Cohen-Eliya and Porat, 2010).

The legal doctrine of proportionality is essentially this: if you pursue an end, you must use a means that is helpful, necessary and appropriate. It is out of proportion to use a means that does more than necessary – for example, a means which is more harmful or more expensive than necessary. It is equally out of proportion to use a means that is inappropriate because, even though it is necessary, by using it you do more harm than the end is worth or you spend more than you gain. In addition to the need to weigh personal safety against autonomy and privacy, the question of capability of people with impaired cognitive ability to exercise their will is also of importance.

Furthermore, tracking technology raises human rights concerns in the framework of equality and dignity (Eltis, 2005). Article 8 of the European Convention for the Protection of Human Rights and Fundamental Freedoms (1950) outlined the right to private life, which has been adopted into law in many jurisdictions. Article 8 is a qualified right, so in certain circumstances public authorities can interfere with the private and family life of an individual. These circumstances are set out in Article 8(2). Such interference must be proportionate, in accordance with law, and necessary to protect national security, public safety or the economic wellbeing of the country, to prevent disorder or crime, to protect health or morals, or to protect the rights and freedoms of others. Electronic tracking by its very nature infringes on the privacy of the person with dementia by enabling another person to check their whereabouts at any given moment. This is most problematic for a device attached to the person in a way that prevents them from removing it.

The Equality and Human Rights Commission state the following about Article 8 on their website:

> Not enough is done to protect the dignity and autonomy of people who use health and social care services. Article 8 protects dignity and autonomy. Though these concepts are not mentioned in the article itself, they have developed through case law. (2014)

Likewise, the 'Fourth Amendment' of the United States is as follows:

> The right of the people to be secure in their persons, houses, papers, and effects, against unreasonable searches and seizures, shall not be violated, and no warrants shall issue, but upon probable cause, supported by oath or affirmation, and particularly describing the place to be searched, and the persons or things to be seized.

The situation in which the State can intervene is therefore highly dependent on the word 'unreasonable'.

In Katz v. United States, 389 U.S. 347 (1967), the Court considered whether a warrantless wiretapping of a public phone booth violated the unreasonable search and seizure clause of the Fourth Amendment to the United States Constitution. By a 7–1 vote, the US Supreme Court agreed with Katz and held that placing a warrantless wiretap on a public phone booth constituted an unreasonable search in violation of the Fourth Amendment. In the case of Olmstead v. United States (1928), the Supreme Court had, however, held that the warrantless wiretapping of phone lines did not constitute an unreasonable search under the Fourth Amendment.

But is tracking any more an invasion of privacy than surveillance by a carer? Surveillance by a carer, normatively deemed appropriate, could also be experienced as an intrusion on privacy (McShane, Hope and Silkinson, 1994). Debate within the medical profession around the ethics of tagging and tracking has been fierce. On the one hand, opinions have been expressed that tagging technology may increase the liberty and dignity of people with dementia by leading to a timely debate on the restrictions that locked-door facilities place on residents (Bail 2003; Hughes and Louw, 2002). On the other hand, others suggest that tagging should be limited to babies in maternity units, convicted criminals and animals (O'Neill, 2003), and that while technologies other than tagging clearly have a role to play in dementia care, tagging is unacceptable because it removes personhood and infringes human rights (Cahill, 2003).

The College of Occupational Therapists' Code of Ethics and Professional Conduct (2010, p.7) clearly states: 'You should enable individuals to preserve their individuality, self-respect, dignity, privacy, autonomy and integrity' (rule 2.2.1).

Stigma

As articulated by Hughes and Louw (2002, p.848), 'being lost and half dressed in the middle of the night near a dual carriageway is hugely stigmatising, and electronic tagging may avoid this'. Stigma can compound depersonalisation of the individual (Innes, 2009). A small qualitative study by Robinson and colleagues (2007) found people with dementia associated electronic tracking with surveillance and as having overtones of 'big brother'.

Any conflation of living well with dementia and the criminal law is bound to be extremely concerning. One person living well with dementia urged me never to call the GPS device 'a tag'; it is 'a tracker': 'As far as I know, Shibley, I have never been convicted of dementia.'

Conclusion

The central tenet of my thesis is that dementia-friendly communities are best promoted through a due regard to the autonomy and dignity of a person living with dementia. Human rights have been a major consideration in the analysis of global positioning systems for certain people living with dementia. This is very closely related to the onrunning thrust of English dementia policy, about choice and control. It can be argued that budgets can give you choice and control, but so can rights-based approaches. Which wins out may depend somewhat on who determines the political ideological weather at any particular time.

Chapter 13 will sample some of the current policy climate. You may conclude at the end of it, however, that there may be trouble ahead.

References

Algase, D.L., Beattie, E.R., Antonakos, C., Beel-Bates, C.A. and Yao, L. (2010) Wandering and the physical environment. American Journal of Alzheimer's Disease and Other Dementias, 25, 4, 340–6.

Andersberg, P., Lepp, M., Berglund, A.L. and Segesten, K. (2007) Preserving dignity in caring for older adults: a concept analysis. Journal of Advanced Nursing, 59, 635–43.

Bail, M. (2003) Devices may be preferable to locked doors (Letter). British Medical Journal, 326, 281.

Becker, D. and Kahana, Z. (1993) Informed consent in demented patients: a question of hours. Medicine and Law, 12, 271–6.

Billings, J.A. (2008) Dignity. Journal of Palliative Medicine, 11, 138–9.

Bremberg, S. and Nilstun, T. (2000) Patients' autonomy and medical benefit: ethical reasoning among GPs. Family Practice, 17, 2, 124–8.

Cahill, S. (2003) Technologies may be enabling. British Medical Journal, 326, 281.

Cohen-Eliya, M. and Porat, I. (2010) American balancing and German proportionality: the historical origins. International Journal of Constitutional Law, 263, 271–3.

College of Occupational Therapists (2010) Code of Ethics and Professional Conduct. Available at www.cot.co.uk/sites/default/files/publications/public/Code-of-Ethics2010.pdf (accessed 6 December 2014).

Cushman, L.A., Stein, K. and Duffy, C.J. (2008) Detecting navigational deficits in cognitive aging and Alzheimer disease using virtual reality. Neurology, 71, 12, 888–95.

De Bellis, A., Mosel, K., Curren, D., Prendergast, J., Harrington, A. and Muir-Cochrane, E. (2013) Education on physical restraint reduction in dementia care: a review of the literature. Dementia (London), 12, 1, 93–110.

Defanti, C.A., Tiezzi, A., Gasparini, M., Gasperini, M. *et al.* for the Bioethics and Palliative Care in Neurology Study Group of the Italian Society of Neurology (2007) Ethical questions in the treatments of subjects with dementia. Part I. Respecting autonomy: awareness, competence and behavioural disorders. Neurological Sciences, 28, 216–31.

Dewing, J. (2005) Screening for wandering among older persons with dementia. Nursing Older People, 17, 3, 20–4.

Dewing, J. (2006) Wandering into the future: reconceptualizing wandering 'a natural and good thing'. International Journal of Older People Nursing, 1, 4, 239–49.

Dewing, J. (2007) Participatory research: a method for process consent with persons who have dementia. Dementia, 6, 1, 11–25.

Dodds, P. (1994) Wandering: a short report on coping strategies adopted by informal carers. International Journal of Geriatric Psychiatry, 9, 9, 751–6.

DuBois, B. and Miley, K.K. (2005) Social Work: An Empowering Profession, 5th edition. New York, NY: Pearson.

Eltis, K. (2005) Society's Most Vulnerable Under Surveillance: The Ethics of Tagging and Tracking Dementia Patients with GPS Technology: A Comparative View. Oxford University Comparative Law Forum. Available at http://ouclf.iuscomp.org/articles/eltis.shtml (accessed 11 February 2015).

Equality and Human Rights Commission (2014) Article 8: the right to respect for private and family life, home and correspondence. Available at www.equalityhumanrights.com/about-us/our-work/human-rights/human-rights-review-2012/articles/article-8 (accessed 6 December 2014).

Feinberg, L.F. and Whitlatch, C.J. (2001) Are persons with cognitive impairment able to state consistent choices? Gerontologist, 41, 3, 374–82.

Fisk, J.D., Beattie, B.L. and Donnelly, M. (2007) Ethical considerations for decision making for treatment and research participation. Alzheimer's and Dementia, 3, 4, 411–17.

Henderson, V.W., Mack, W. and Williams, B.W. (1989) Spatial disorientation in Alzheimer's disease. Archives of Neurology, 46, 4, 391–4.
Hermans, D., Htay, U.H. and Cooley, S.J. (2007) Non-pharmacological interventions for wandering of people with dementia in the domestic setting. Cochrane Database of Systematic Reviews, 1, CD005994.
Hope, T., Keene, J., McShane, R.H., Fairburn, C.G., Gedling, K. and Jacoby, R. (2001) Wandering in dementia: a longitudinal study. International Psychogeriatrics, 13, 2, 137–47.
House of Lords Select Committee on Science and Technology (2005) Science and Technology: First Report. London: House of Lords.
Hudson, D.L. and Cohen, M.E. (2010) Intelligent agents in home healthcare. Annals of Telecommunications – Annales de Telecommunications, 65, 693–700.
Hughes, J.C. and Baldwin, C. (2006) Ethical Issues in Dementia Care: Making Difficult Decisions. London: Jessica Kingsley Publishers.
Hughes, J.C. and Louw, S.J. (2002) Electronic tagging of people with dementia who wander. British Medical Journal, 325, 7369, 847–8.
Hutchins, R.M. (2007) Tied up in Knotts? GPS technology and the Fourth Amendment. UCLA Law Review, 55, 409–65. Available at www.uclalawreview.org/pdf/55-2-3.pdf (accessed 6 December 2014).
Innes, A. (2009) Dementia Studies. London: Sage.
Kearns, W.D. and Fozard, J.L. (2007) Technologies to Manage Wandering. In A.L. Nelson and D.L. Algase (eds) Evidence-Based Protocols for Managing Wandering Behaviors. New York, NY: Springer Publishing Company.
Kibayashi, K. and Shojo, H. (2003) Accidental hypothermia in elderly people with Alzheimer's disease. Medicine, Science and the Law, 43, 2, 127–31.
Koester, R. and Stooksbury, D. (1995) Behavioural profile of possible Alzheimer's disease subjects in search and rescue incidents in Virginia. Wilderness and Environmental Medicine, 6, 34–43.
Lai, C.K.Y. and Arthur, D.G. (2003) Wandering behaviour in people with dementia. Journal of Advanced Nursing, 44, 2, 173–82.
Landau, R. and Werner, S. (2012) Ethical aspects of using GPS for tracking people with dementia. International Psychogeriatrics, 24, 3, 358–66.
Landau, R., Werner, S., Auslander, G.K., Shoval, N. and Heinik, J. (2009) Attitudes of family and professional care-givers towards the use of GPS for tracking patients with dementia: an exploratory study. British Journal of Social Work, 39, 4, 670–92.
Lautrette, A., Ciroldi, M., Ksibi, H. and Azoulay, E. (2006) End-of-life family conferences: rooted in the evidence. Critical Care Medicine, 34, S364–72.
Lawton, M.P. and Simon, F. (1968) The ecology of social relationships in housing for the elderly. Gerontologist, 8, 2, 108–15.
Logsdon, R.G., Teri, L., McCurry, S.M., Gibbons, L.E., Kukull, W.A. and Larson, E.B. (1998) Wandering: a significant problem among community-residing individuals with Alzheimer's disease. Journals of Gerontology Series B: Psychological Sciences and Social Sciences, 53, 5, 294–9.
Mahoney, E.K., Volicer, L. and Hurley, A.C. (2000) Management of Challenging Behaviors in Dementia. Baltimore, MD: Health Professions Press.
Manthorpe, J., Iliffe, S., Samsi, K., Cole, L. *et al.* (2010) Dementia, dignity and quality of life: nursing practice and its dilemmas. International Journal of Older People Nursing, 5, 235–44.
McShane, R., Gedling, K., Kenward, B., Kenward, R., Hope, T. and Jacoby, R. (1998) The feasibility of electronic tracking devised in dementia. International Journal of Geriatric Psychiatry, 13, 556–63.
McShane, R., Hope, T. and Silkinson, J. (1994) Tracking patients who wander: ethics and technology. Lancet, 343, 8908, 1274.

Milne, H., van der Pol, M., McCloughan, L., Hanley, J. *et al.* (2014) The use of global positional satellite location in dementia: a feasibility study for a randomised controlled trial. BMC Psychiatry, 14, 160.

Miskelly, F. (2004) A novel system of electronic tagging in patients with dementia and wandering. Age and Ageing, 33, 3, 304–6.

Miskelly, F. (2005) Electronic tracking of patients with dementia and wandering using mobile phone technology (Research letter). Age and Ageing, 34, 497–9.

Molinari, V., King-Kallimanis, B., Volicer, L., Brown, L. and Schonfeld, L. (2008) Wandering behavior in veterans with psychiatric diagnoses residing in nursing homes. International Journal of Geriatric Psychiatry, 23, 7, 748–53.

Moorman, S.M., Hauser, R.M. and Carr, D. (2009) Do older adults know their spouses' end of life treatment preferences? Research on Aging, 31, 463–91.

Nuffield Council on Bioethics (2009) Dementia: Ethical Issues. A Guide to the Report. London: Nuffield Council on Bioethics. Available at http://nuffieldbioethics.org/wp-content/uploads/2014/07/Dementia-short-guide.pdf (accessed 6 December 2014).

O'Keefe, J. and Nadel, L. (1978) The Hippocampus as Cognitive Map. Oxford: Oxford University Press.

O'Neill, D.J. (2003) Tagging should be reserved for babies, convicted criminals and animals. British Medical Journal, 326, 281.

Pai, M.C. and Jacobs, W.J. (2004) Topographical disorientation in community-residing patients with Alzheimer's disease. International Journal of Geriatric Psychiatry, 19, 3, 250–5.

Parker, K. and Miles, S. (1997) Deaths caused by bedrails. Journal of the American Geriatrics Society, 45, 797–802.

Passini, R., Pigot, H., Rainville, C. and Tetreault, M.H. (2000) Wayfinding in a nursing home for advanced dementia of the Alzheimer's type. Environment and Behavior, 32, 5, 684–710.

Petersen, G. and Wallin, A. (2003) Alzheimer disease ethics: informed consent and related issues in clinical trials: results of a survey among the members of the research ethic committees in Sweden. International Psychogeriatrics, 15, 2, 157–70.

Price, J.D., Hermans, D.G. and Grimley Evans, J. (2001) Subjective barriers to prevent wandering of cognitively impaired people. Cochrane Database of Systematic Reviews, 4, CD001932.

Robinson, L., Hutchings, D., Corner, L., Beyer, F. *et al.* (2006) Wandering in dementia: a systematic literature review of the effectiveness of non-pharmacological interventions to prevent wandering in dementia and evaluation of the ethical implications and acceptability of their use. Health Technology Assessment, 10, 26, 1–124.

Robinson, L., Hutchings, D., Corner, L., Finch, J. *et al.* (2007) Balancing rights and risks: conflicting perspectives in the management of wandering in dementia. Health, Risk and Society, 9, 4, 389–406.

Rolland, Y., Gillette-Guyonnet, S., Nourhashemi, F., Andrieu, S. *et al.* (2003) Wandering and Alzheimer's disease: descriptive study. REAL.FR program on Alzheimer's disease and field of care. Revue de Médecine Interne, 24, Suppl. 3, S333–8.

Rowe, M.A. and Bennett, V. (2003) A look at deaths occurring in persons with dementia lost in the community. American Journal of Alzheimer's Disease and Other Dementias, 18, 6, 343–8.

Rowe, M.A. and Glover, J.C. (2001) Antecedents, descriptions and consequences of wandering in cognitively-impaired adults and the safe return (SR) program. American Journal of Alzheimer's Disease and Other Dementias, 16, 6, 344–52.

Shimizu, K., Kawamura, K. and Yamamoto, K. (2000) Location system for dementia wandering. Engineering in Medicine and Biology Society, 2000. Proceedings of the 22nd Annual International Conference of the IEEE, 2, 1556–1559. Chicago, IL: IEEE.

Shinoda-Tagawa, T., Leonard, R., Pontikas, J., McDonough, J.E., Allen, D. and Dreyer, P.I. (2004) Resident-to-resident violent incidents in nursing homes. Journal of the American Medical Association, 291, 591–8.

Sugarman, J., Roter, D., Cain, C., Wallace, R., Schmechel, D. and Weish-Bohmer, K.A. (2007) Proxies and consent discussions for dementia research. Journal of the American Geriatrics Society, 55, 4, 556–61.

Tranvåg, O., Petersen, K.A. and Nåden, D. (2014) Crucial dimensions constituting dignity experience in persons living with dementia. Dementia (London), Apr 17 [Epub ahead of print].

Tu, M.C. and Pai, M.C. (2006) Getting lost for the first time in patients with Alzheimer's disease. International Psychogeriatrics, 18, 3, 567–70.

US Courts (1967) Katz v. United States, 389 U.S. 347 (1967). Available at www.uscourts.gov/educational-resources/get-involved/constitution-activities/fourth-amendment/wiretaps-cell-phone-surveillance/facts-case-summary.aspx (accessed 6 December 2014).

US Supreme Court (1928) Olmstead v. United States, 277 U.S. 438 (1928). Available at http://caselaw.lp.findlaw.com/scripts/getcase.pl?court=US&vol=277&invol=438 (accessed 6 December 2014).

Welsh, S., Hassiotis, A., O'Mahoney, G. and Deahl, M. (2003) Big brother is watching you – the ethical implications of surveillance measures in the elderly with dementia and in adults with learning difficulties. Aging and Mental Health, 7, 5, 372–5.

Westphal, A., Dingjan, P. and Attoe, R. (2010) What can low and high technologies do for late-life mental disorders? Current Opinions in Psychiatry, 23, 510–15.

White, E.B. and Montgomery, P. (2014) Electronic tracking for people with dementia: an exploratory study of the ethical issues experienced by carers in making decisions about usage. Dementia (London), 13, 2, 216–32.

Chapter 13

RIGHTS-BASED APPROACHES, PERSONAL BUDGETS AND LIVING BETTER WITH DEMENTIA

> 'The philosopher and disability activist Judith Snow says: The gift of disability is the fact that the disabled person really needs help from another human.'
>
> Simon Duffy, Tizard Memorial Lecture (4 March 2011)

Introduction

Under international law, the UN Convention on the Rights of Persons with Disabilities exists to protect citizens with disabilities. The Preamble begins:

> The States Parties to the present Convention,
>
> (a) Recalling the principles proclaimed in the Charter of the United Nations which recognize the inherent dignity and worth and the equal and inalienable rights of all members of the human family as the foundation of freedom, justice and peace in the world... (United Nations General Assembly, 2006)

The Equality Act 2010 in England and Wales makes discrimination against persons living with disabilities unlawful. Dementia is a disability. On 6 December 2014, the BBC news website ran an article entitled 'Disabled people's access to High Street "shocking", audit finds' (BBC News, 2014), which described discrimination against people living with disabilities. According to the report, accessibility experts DisabledGo visited all of the 30,000 venues in person to assess them, in the largest ever audit of its kind in the UK. They found one-fifth of shops had no wheelchair access, only 15% of restaurants and shops had hearing loops, and three-quarters of restaurants did not cater for those with visual impairments (BBC News, 2014). If we are shocked about this lack of access for people who are physically disabled, we should be equally shocked by the lack of accessibility for people with cognitive or behavioural problems as a result of living with dementia.

Swaffer (2014) compares the medical and the social responses to the event that is the disclosure of the dementia diagnosis:

> Misguided and preconceived misconceptions about the symptoms of dementia are used to support telling us to give up living our pre-diagnosis lives. Instead, the recognition of the symptoms as disabilities would assist with a more equitable and dementia-friendly experience for the person with dementia after diagnosis. In contrast to the medical model, the disAbility model of care is positive and supports continued engagement with our prediagnosis lives.

The different ways in which a person might progress after a diagnosis are shown in Figure 13.1.

I introduced parity of esteem in Chapter 10 on whole-person care. For the sake of parity of esteem – in other words, not treating mental health as inferior to physical health – we need to apply the same rigour for 'reasonable adjustments' for cognitive or behavioural interventions as for physical ones. Equality law recognises that bringing about equality for disabled people may mean changing the way in which employment is structured, the removal of physical barriers and/or providing extra support for a disabled worker (see, for example, Equality and Human Rights Commission, 2014). Early dementia of the Alzheimer type is characterised by problems in learning and memory, including in spatial navigation (Serino and Riva, 2013). People with such cognitive disabilities will benefit from specialist design as a reasonable adjustment (Habell, 2013).

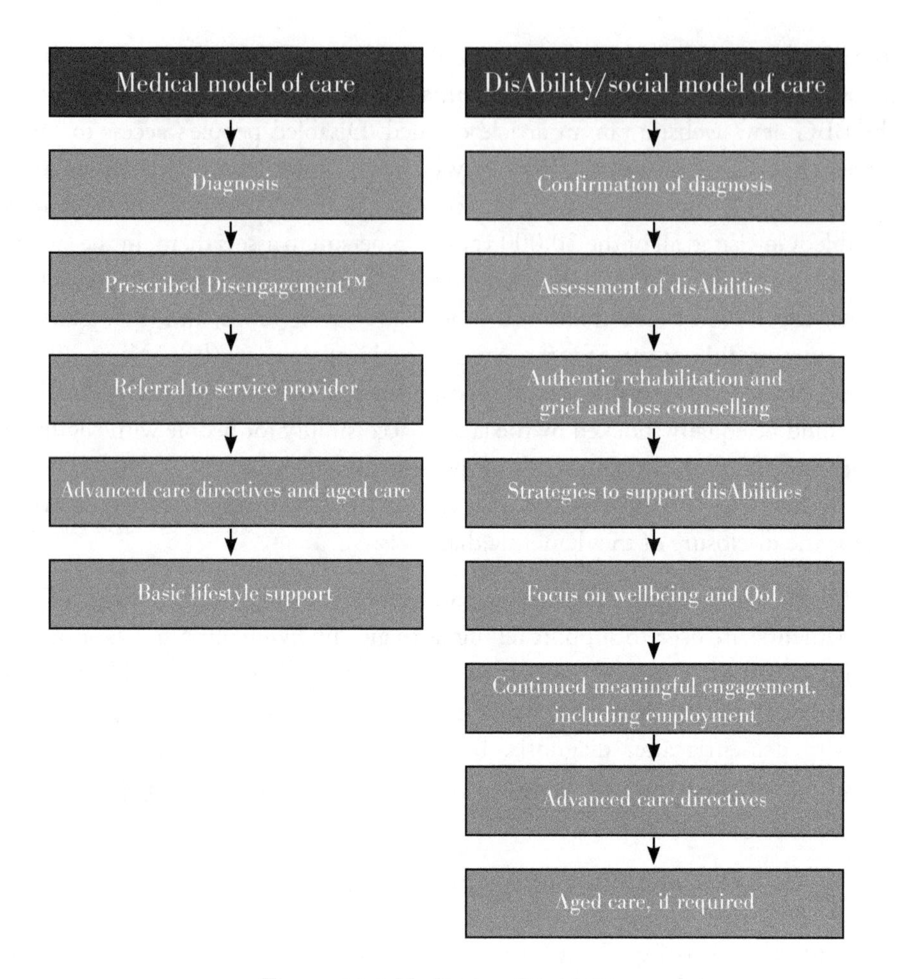

Figure 13.1 Medical vs DisAbility model

SOURCE: SWAFFER, 2014 (REPRODUCED BY KIND PERMISSION FROM KATE SWAFFER)

Promoting autonomy and dignity and the Deprivation of Liberty Safeguards policy

Promoting dignity for people trying to live better with dementia means a culture free from abuses of human rights, free from discrimination, and free from any other abuse. The Social Care Institute for Excellence (SCIE) Law Practice Guide 9 entitled 'Promoting dignity within the law' (2008) outlines the context in which dignity applies to health and social care. The philosophy is that human rights principles are very closely related to other principles of good professional practice, and share an ethical basis of concern with the autonomy, privacy and dignity of people using services. And the law is continuing to evolve, both in the UK and abroad, at a very fast pace. The Care Act 2014 received Royal Assent (became law) in May 2014. This is the most significant reform of adult social care for more than 60 years, replacing a wide range of existing legislation with a single statute and introducing many new principles and procedures. For example, the introduction of the principle of the promotion of 'wellbeing' as the basis for any action or decision taken in relation to meeting someone's social care needs, or for service planning.

Human rights law applies to all 'public authorities'. No public authority must act in a way that is incompatible with human rights; 'public authorities' include local authorities and their staff, health boards and hospital staff, general practitioners, sheriffs, tribunals and others carrying out public functions (see, for example, Mental Welfare Commission for Scotland, n.d.). The human rights approach starts from the principle of human autonomy. I have discussed the notion of autonomy in some considerable detail, particularly in Chapter 9 of my book *Living Well with Dementia* (Rahman, 2014), in relation to advocacy, choice and control.

Deprivation of liberty should be 'exceptional, objectively justified and of no longer duration than absolutely necessary' (Macovei, 2002, p.6). The aim is to secure rights for individuals. Although a private care home is not a public authority (even though it may be providing care under contract to the local authority), Lady Hale in the House of Lords in YL v Birmingham City Council and others [2007] provided the key finding:

> Given the approach of the Strasbourg court in Storck v Germany (2005) 43 EHRR 96, it is perhaps unlikely that the United Kingdom would be absolved from responsibility for deprivations of liberty taking place in private care homes. (Paragraph 70)

The Deprivation of Liberty Safeguards (DoLS) were intended to provide a level of protection to people who lacked capacity to make decisions about care and treatment. The safeguards are intended to protect people who lack mental capacity from being detained when this is not in their best interests, to prevent arbitrary detention, and to give people the right to challenge a decision. Whether someone has been deprived of their liberty depends on the particular circumstances of each case.

The safeguards apply to people in care environments including hospitals and care homes. Both self-funded and publicly funded residents are covered by the safeguards. The Code of Practice also includes a list of factors that have been taken into account by the European Court of Human Rights and UK courts when deciding what amounts to deprivation of liberty.

These are only factors and not conclusive on their own. It will be a question of degree or intensity. It has been known for some time that the DoLS are fundamentally a human rights issue (Tingle, 2012). These safeguards were not, in fact, part of the original Mental Capacity Act in 2005. Introduced as amendments via the Mental Health Act 2007 in response to the findings of the European Court of Human Rights in the 'Bournewood case' and enacted in 2009, they are often seen as entirely separate from the rest of the Act. The European Court of Human Rights found that UK law did not give adequate protection to people who lacked mental capacity to consent to care or treatment, and who needed limits on their liberty to keep them safe. The change in the law introducing the Deprivation of Liberty Safeguards was necessary following the decision of the European Court of Human Rights in HL v United Kingdom (2004), concerning the deprivation of liberty of a man with autism and a profound learning disability. The Deprivation of Liberty Safeguards continue to attract much interest (Griffith, 2014).

At clause 254 of a recent House of Lords publication entitled 'Select Committee on the Mental Capacity Act 2005: Report of Session 2013–14 on Mental Capacity Act 2005: Post-Legislative Scrutiny' (2014), Toby Williamson of the Mental Health Foundation, and former co-chair of the Making Decisions Alliance, a campaign in support of the introduction of mental capacity legislation at the time the Act was passed, is reported as saying: 'We wanted a relatively simple legislative solution that met the requirements of the European court's findings on the case, something that reflected the elegant simplicity of the Mental Capacity Act.'

The recent law has added some clarity. The Supreme Court gave judgment on 19 March 2014 in two linked appeals: (1) P v Cheshire West and Chester Council and another; and (2) P and Q v Surrey County Council [2014] UKSC 19. Both appeals were brought by the Official Solicitor, who had acted as litigation friend for all of them. This case concerned the living arrangements of three adults without capacity to consent to their residence and care arrangements. The question was whether the arrangements amounted to a deprivation of liberty. Paragraph 45 of the judgment by Lady Hale is striking as it emphasises the universality of human rights. The judgment of Storck v Germany (2005) outlines the three tests of whether there has been a deprivation of liberty. Critically, section 64(5) of the Mental Capacity Act (2005) states: 'In this Act, references to deprivation of a person's liberty have the same meaning as in Article 5(1) of the Human Rights Convention.'

And reading the relevant clauses of the European Convention on Human Rights (ECHR) is indeed a helpful start:

> Article 5: The right to liberty and security
>
> 1. Everyone has the right to liberty and security of person. No one shall be deprived of his liberty save in the following cases and in accordance with a procedure prescribed by law:
>
> (a) the lawful detention of a person after conviction by a competent court;
>
> ...
>
> (e) the lawful detention of persons for the prevention of the spreading of infectious diseases, of persons of unsound mind, alcoholics or drug addicts or vagrants...

While human rights law recognises that in certain specified situations (e.g. following the commission of a criminal offence) a person may be deprived of this right, this should only be for sufficiently weighty and pressing reasons, justifiable under the ECHR doctrines of 'necessity' and 'proportionality'. The legal doctrine of proportionality is pivotal to our law. Crucially, it states in Article 5(4) of the ECHR:

> Everyone who is deprived of his liberty by arrest or detention shall be entitled to take proceedings by which the lawfulness of his detention shall be decided speedily by a court and his release ordered if the detention is not lawful.

At the time of writing, the UK Government, in the face of some significant opposition, intends to repeal the Human Rights Act (1998), but the international legal instruments still remain in force; critically, it remains to be determined whether the UK will voluntarily remain a signatory of the European Convention of Human Rights.

The Supreme Court judgments in the cases of P v Cheshire West and Chester Council and another, and P and Q v Surrey County Council [2014], are widely considered to be highly significant. These very significant judgments have provided clarification on the definition of a deprivation of liberty and have reduced the widespread confusion that service users, their representatives and professionals have been grappling with over the past few years. The Supreme Court found that there is a deprivation of liberty for the purposes of Article 5 of the European Convention on Human Rights in the following circumstances: the person is under continuous supervision and control and is not free to leave, and the person lacks capacity to consent to these arrangements.

Personal budgets and self-directed support

The roll-out nationally of personal budgets and 'self-directed support' cannot ever, of course, be compulsory, as this would defy the ethos of choice and control in avoiding being forced to do anything.

A personal budget is the funding available for a person's care and support needs, in line with an agreed support plan, and can be received as:

» a direct (cash) payment

» a fund managed by the local authority or a third-party provider on the person's behalf

» a combination of the two.

In 2009, in the face of some opposition and scepticism (e.g. from the public service union Unison, the British Medical Association, the Royal College of General Practitioners and the Royal College of Nursing, as well as many doctors and nurses), a three-year pilot programme for personal health budgets began (Policy Research Unit in Commissioning and the Healthcare System, 2013). A year later, in an influential report, the Health Foundation concluded that there was not enough evidence at the time to say whether personal budgets improve health outcomes (Health Foundation, 2010). Most of the international evidence about this had come from the US and suggests that some improvements are possible, but the literature is far from conclusive and studies are small and open to criticism. In spite of the low take-up of personal budgets to meet mental health social care needs, the Government has piloted personal health budgets for long-term conditions in England (Department of Health, 2009).

Personal health budgets aim to enhance choice and control over health care but, unlike social care personal budgets, are not means-tested. Notwithstanding that, the Nuffield Trust (2013) has argued that bringing personal health budgets together with personal budgets in social care to create integrated individual budgets potentially offers a new route to service integration at the level of the user and carer. The evaluation of personal health budgets showed promising findings and they were particularly cost-effective for people with mental health problems (Forder *et al.*, 2012). Consequently, the Government has begun to introduce them into the NHS in England, with plans to make them available in mental health services in 2015. Despite the policy rhetoric, there is limited evidence about outcomes of personal budgets for people with mental health problems (Health Foundation, 2010).

Webber and colleagues (2014) have conducted a systematic review of the international literature on the effectiveness of personal budgets for people with mental health problems. It has found generally positive outcomes for mental health service users in terms of choice and control, impact on quality of life, service use and cost-effectiveness. However, methodological limitations make these findings rather unreliable and insufficient to inform policy and practice. There is a need for large, high-quality experimental studies in this key policy area to inform personal budget policy and practice with people with mental health problems. There are, furthermore, conspicuous gaps in the literature. When carers and people using services are asked about the qualities they value in social care workers, their replies invariably highlight the nature of the relationship between them (Beresford, 2012; Beresford *et al.*, 2005).

Traditionally, people have been offered little choice over either the kind of support provided or the time it is delivered. Indeed, Victoria Hart, an experienced social care practitioner with extensive experience in working with people with dementia, remarked recently, 'I'm loath to critique what is inherently the great policy aim of involving people in choice and more flexible care, not least because there has been an agenda from policymakers to lay much of the blame for poor implementation on disgruntled practitioners' (Hart, 2014, p.112). In 2007, the Government published *Putting People First*, a concordat between central government, local government and the social care sector. In this, personalisation was linked to adult social care to 'create a new, high quality system which is fair, accessible and responsive to the individual needs of those who use services and their carers' (Department of Health, 2007, p.2). Social care funding is means-tested, and even where NHS and social care services are integrated, personal budgets require financial assessments and separate funding arrangements from NHS care (Audit Commission, 2010). Additionally, it has been proposed that there is a pervasive tension in mental health care between safeguarding against risk and the provision of user-directed care, which often involves some risk taking (Carr, 2010). Consequently, mental health practitioners sometimes see people with enduring mental health problems as incapable of managing personal budgets (Carr, 2011; Taylor, 2008).

The implementation of the personalisation changes detailed in *Putting People First* was seen as key to delivering Objective 6 of the National Dementia Strategy (Department of Health, 2009). This set out the Government's intention to improve community personal support services by providing an appropriate range of flexible and reliable services to support people with dementia living at home, responsive to the personal needs and preferences of each individual. Most of the support provided to people with disabilities and long-term illnesses living at home is given by family members, friends and neighbours. However, there is also a wide range of community care services available through health and social work services, all aimed at helping people stay independent and in their own homes (Alzheimer Scotland, 2010). Self-directed support is envisaged as a process of involving the individual and carer in decisions about care and support, where they are at the centre of decision making.

As observed by Rogers (2011), many commentators have observed that an increasingly significant force in the welfare systems of most modern developed societies is that of consumerism. Broadly, this term refers to a view of public services as commodities and increasing attention being paid to protecting and satisfying the individual needs and wishes of those who use, or 'consume', such services. Governments have responded to this demand by adapting, to varying degrees, many State-run public services, in attempts to offer greater responsiveness and greater choice. The Coalition Government elected in 2010 was quick to produce plans for change in the NHS, in the white paper 'Equity and Excellence' (Department of Health, 2010b).

Indeed, it was mooted that personal health budgets could motivate the NHS to produce more effective patient information systems and resources (2009, p.6). In addition, the NHS Confederation noted: '...they would require health leaders to be more transparent over the cost of treatments. Several social care interviewees noted that this had been an unexpected benefit of personal budgets – it "disciplined" their departments by having to publicly reconsider services which were costly yet unpopular.'

Potential barriers to implementation of 'self-directed support' are summarised in Box 13.1.

Box 13.1 Barriers to implementation of personal budgets/self-directed support

* A personal budgets system that has not yet adapted to the needs of people with dementia and their carers, and is overly complex and burdensome
* Lack of knowledge and awareness of self-directed support among people with dementia, carers and families
* Ineligibility for care funding long before the time of crisis

* local authority concerns about the use of self-directed support by people with dementia and general lack of enthusiasm
* Challenging financial climate and funding pressures on local authorities
* A lack of tailored and accessible information for people with dementia and their carers, leading to a lack of understanding about personal budgets and direct payments and concerns about their use
* Lack of addressing of real carer and family concerns about managing self-directed support
* Local markets that are not yet sufficiently developed to deliver a wide range of different types of dementia service
* Insufficient overall levels of funding in the system
* The cultural attitudes of health and social care professionals who are operating in 'silos'
* Mechanisms for direct payments for people who lack capacity
* Safeguarding concerns about using self-directed support
* Overcomplicated monitoring and regulatory systems
* Concerns about obtaining criminal record checks and reliable references for personal assistants

---

A long-standing concern has been whether NHS funds should be 'misspent on treatments that lacked an evidence base', including 'laptops and travel passes' (Limb, 2012, p.1). The Dutch have had personal budgets since 1997 for long-term care but they exclude medical and alternative therapies (Chinthapalli, 2012). For example, the introduction of personal health budgets was not embraced by clinicians in the pilots (Limb, 2012). Direct payments for care recipients are not new, of course. Within the social care sector initiatives to transfer resources to disabled people as direct payments began in the 1980s, and were given legal endorsement in the Community Care (Direct Payments) Act 1996 (Glasby and Littlechild, 2009). Direct payments were generally taken up by younger disabled people, and numbers were relatively small. Although they were known to potentially benefit from direct payments (Clark, 2006), attitudes of both social workers and older people themselves posed significant barriers (Ellis, 2007; Glendinning *et al.*, 2008). Other barriers to implementation include the increased levels of bureaucracy that have accompanied personal budgets (Jacobs *et al.*, 2013) and concern among service users about managing personal budgets, and about the quality of support provided to help them with this (Newbronner *et al.*, 2011; NHS Confederation, 2011). Professor Clare Gerada is also reported as asking, when Chair of the Royal College of General Practitioners, 'Should we be spending taxpayers' money in cash strapped systems on gardening or aromatherapy that may make people feel better, but for which there is no evidence that it actually makes them better?' (White, 2011).

Participants who took part in the study by Gridley, Brooks and Glendinning (2014, p.822) stressed the importance of ongoing professional support – for example, from a specialist key worker or case manager – to coordinate diverse services and ensure good practice at an organisational level. While much has been made of 'vested interests', it is striking that the authors of this paper argue that 'despite the recent move to shift power from professionals to service users, people with the most complex needs still value support from professionals and appropriate organisational support' (p.588).

According to Goodchild (2011), one local authority reported that the recovery model of specialist mental health services has established an organisational culture that is not conducive to the needs of people with dementia. This is an extremely odd claim given how the recovery model of dementia as a disability has gained traction in recent times. In common with other sensitive areas of health policy in England, political leadership was also reported as being a significant enabler to implementing personal budgets across all care groups, including dementia. Interviewees reported that 'a strong political drive locally can make a significant difference and if an elected member is championing personal budgets for people with dementia then implementation is likely to develop at a faster pace' (Goodchild, 2011, p.12).

There are genuine concerns as to whether personal health budgets offend the founding principle of universality for the NHS. Professor Peter Beresford, a social policy professor who heads Brunel University's Centre for Citizen Participation, has commented that 'they tend to work for the most confident, assertive, more experienced and able people' (Limb, 2014, p.1). He said that claims being made in support of the policy were selective and ignored the experience of most people with personal budgets, whose outcomes had not improved. Beresford said that extending the policy in England was not consistent with an NHS based on universal principles. Beresford further warned of greater commercialisation, saying that large multinational companies would move in to offer services, edging out smaller community providers and leaving people who needed care 'to try to work the market on their own' (Limb, 2014, p.1). This indeed tallies with Professor Martin McKee's concern (2013) that 'at some point in the future each of us will be allocated a fixed amount to purchase insurance, with the requirement to top up anything that is not covered'. At the time of writing, Slasberg, Beresford and Schofield (2012) had deduced that the evidence in this paper of the failures of the Government's self-directed support strategy could well have been a further indication of the early warnings discernible from the evaluation of the individual budget pilots (Glendinning *et al.*, 2008).

Genetic discrimination

The issue of genetic discrimination has been recognised at an international level for some time.

> No one shall be subjected to discrimination based on genetic characteristics that is intended to infringe or has the effect of infringing human rights, fundamental freedoms and human dignity.
>
> Article 6 of the Universal Declaration on the Human Genome and Human Rights (UNESCO, 1997)

Genetic discrimination is defined as 'differential treatment, denial of rights, privileges or opportunities or other adverse treatment, based solely on genetic information, including a family history' (Goh *et al.*, 2013, p.115). Discrimination can also happen to individuals who have a genetic diagnosis, but who are asymptomatic or who will never become significantly impaired (Billings *et al.*, 1992). Recent developments in genetic technology have resulted in an increasing number of tests becoming available to detect genes associated with disease (Mainsbridge, 2002). The Human Genome Project began in 1990 as a concerted international scientific research project to produce detailed maps of the 23 pairs of human chromosomes and to sequence the three billion nucleotide bases that make up the human genome. This mammoth project has allowed neuroscientists to use patterns of brain structure and function, as revealed by neuroimaging, to identify neural correlates of disease and predict an individual's predisposition to future disease.

Genetic testing involves examining a person's DNA (deoxyribonucleic acid), RNA (ribonucleic acid) or associated proteins for the purpose of determining the existence of or predisposition to a particular disease. In some instances, genetic information may be used for diagnostic purposes, to make or confirm a conclusion about the condition of a person who is already exhibiting symptoms. Genetic information can also be used for predictive purposes, to determine the possibility that a person who currently has no symptoms of a particular disorder may develop the disorder at some time in the future. However, many genetic disorders are multi-factorial in nature – that is, they are the result of a complex interaction between genes and environmental and lifestyle factors. The argument for genetic factors can be overstated; for example, it has been reported that approximately 60% of persons with dementia of the Alzheimer type do not have a family history of the disease (Shastry and Giblin, 1999).

Genetic information is not an absolute indicator that symptoms will develop. From an employer's perspective, there are clear economic incentives associated with the use of genetic information about employees and potential employees. Such information offers employers an opportunity to exclude from the workforce individuals who have been identified as being at risk of developing a genetic condition that may affect their future capacity for work. There have been concerns in a number of jurisdictions about whether people with a strong family history of inherited disease have been discriminated against either in the workplace or for private insurance purposes. It is crucial to note what is actually happening in real time in response to people knowing about the genetic basis of their conditions. Goh and colleagues (2013) recently reported on the 'Perception, experience, and response to genetic discrimination in Huntington's disease: the Australian results of the International RESPOND-HD Study'. They found that 68% of participants reported feeling 'great benefit' from knowing their genetic test results. The reported benefits of knowledge included planning for the future and making decisions, and many individuals found meaning in active participation in the Huntington's disease (HD) community and in advocating for themselves or families at risk for HD. People also found personal meaning in the ability to participate in research. Despite these positive feelings toward gene testing, results demonstrated that 33% of participants perceived that they had experienced genetic discrimination, which occurred repeatedly and caused great self-reported distress.

Genetic discrimination has potentially serious consequences, not only for individual employees but also for society as a whole. First, it raises the spectre of a 'genetic underclass' of individuals who are deemed to be unemployable because genetic tests have revealed that they have a susceptibility to a particular disease. This class of people, sometimes referred to as the 'asymptomatic ill', may be denied employment throughout their lives, yet never actually develop the condition for which they have a higher than normal risk. Society is denied the benefit of the contributions that such individuals could make in their productive years. A second problem is that genetic discrimination has the capacity to spill over into and support other forms of discrimination, particularly race discrimination. Some conditions are known to be more prevalent in some races and ethnicities than others. Third, the threat of genetic discrimination by employers may act as a powerful deterrent to people obtaining genetic information that could provide them with potential health benefits.

In May 2008, in the US jurisdiction, the Genetic Information Non-discrimination Act (GINA) was signed into law. This long-awaited statute paved the way for individuals to take full advantage of the promise of personalised medicine without fear of discrimination on the basis of genetic information acquired by employers. GINA is wide-ranging, but Title II makes it unlawful for employers and employer organisations to discriminate on the basis of genetic information. It is clearly going to be necessary for NHS England and the legislature to allow for similar legislation in the English jurisdiction if it wishes to pursue personalised medicine. GINA forbids an employer from discharging or refusing or failing to hire an employee because of genetic information. It also makes it unlawful for an employer to discriminate against any employee with 'respect to compensation, terms, conditions, or privileges of employment' because of genetic information (see the article in *Vanderbilt Law Review*: authors undisclosed, 2012). This directly mirrors the legislation of the Equality Act 2010 where 'prohibited behaviour' is outlawed against a 'protected characteristic': section 4 outlines the protected characteristics (age; disability; gender reassignment; marriage and civil partnership; pregnancy and maternity; race; religion or belief; sex; sexual orientation); genetic genotype is not a protected characteristic at the time of writing.

Under the guidance for the Equality Act 2010, 'a disability can arise from a wide range of impairments which can be...progressive, such as motor neurone disease, muscular dystrophy, and forms of dementia'. While 'this list, however, is not exhaustive', this clearly opens the door to new case law in the England and Wales jurisdiction for various offences under the Equality Act 2010 which are protected behaviours, including direct and indirect discrimination, against people living with dementia. This could well include the situation in which employers do not make reasonable adjustments for their staff under the main body and Schedules of legislation under the Equality Act 2010. This shifts the terrain of dementia-friendly communities, in specific scenarios, from aspiration to legal obligation in England and Wales. Similar principles will apply to equality in other jurisdictions, according to whether dementia falls under disability. For example, there are two main equality laws in Ireland: the Equal Status Acts 2000–11 and the Employment Equality Acts 1998–2011.

Rights-based approaches

'Rights' in a number of jurisdictions have been viewed as operating not just at a structural level but also at a personal level, in the explicit use of human rights principles of respect for family life and privacy (McDonald, 2010). For example, *Standards of Care for Dementia in Scotland: Action to Support the Change Programme* (Scottish Government, 2011) is a key part of Scotland's National Dementia Strategy (2013–16). It followed on from the Charter published in 2009 (Scottish Government, 2009).

Box 13.2 Charter of Rights for People with Dementia and their Carers in Scotland

In pursuance of the Human Rights Act 1998 and The Scotland Act 1998 the rights contained within this charter are based on internationally agreed human rights and are intended to promote the respect, protection and fulfilment of all human rights of people with dementia and their carers, as guaranteed in the European Convention of Human Rights, the Universal Declaration of Human Rights, the International Covenants on Economic, Social and Cultural Rights and Civil and Political Rights, and the Convention on the Rights of Persons with Disabilities, the key principles of which are:

* respect for inherent dignity, individual autonomy including the freedom to make one's own choices, and independence of persons;
* non-discrimination;
* full and effective participation and inclusion in society;
* respect for difference and acceptance of persons with disabilities as part of human diversity and humanity;
* equality of opportunity;
* accessibility;
* equality between men and women.

The Charter also reflects other legal provisions and in particular the principles of the Adults with Incapacity (Scotland) Act 2000; the Mental Health (Care and Treatment) (Scotland) Act 2003, and the Adult Support and Protection (Scotland) Act 2007.

The Charter was guided by a human rights-based approach (known as the **'PANEL'** approach, endorsed by the United Nations). It emphasises the rights of everyone to:

Participate in decisions which affect their human rights.

Accountability of those responsible for the respect, protection and fulfilment of human rights.

Non-discrimination and equality.

Empowerment to know their rights and how to claim them.

Legality in all decisions through an explicit link with human rights legal standards in all processes and outcome measurements.

SOURCE: SCOTTISH GOVERNMENT, 2009 (P.4) (REPRODUCED BY KIND PERMISSION OF ALZHEIMER SCOTLAND)

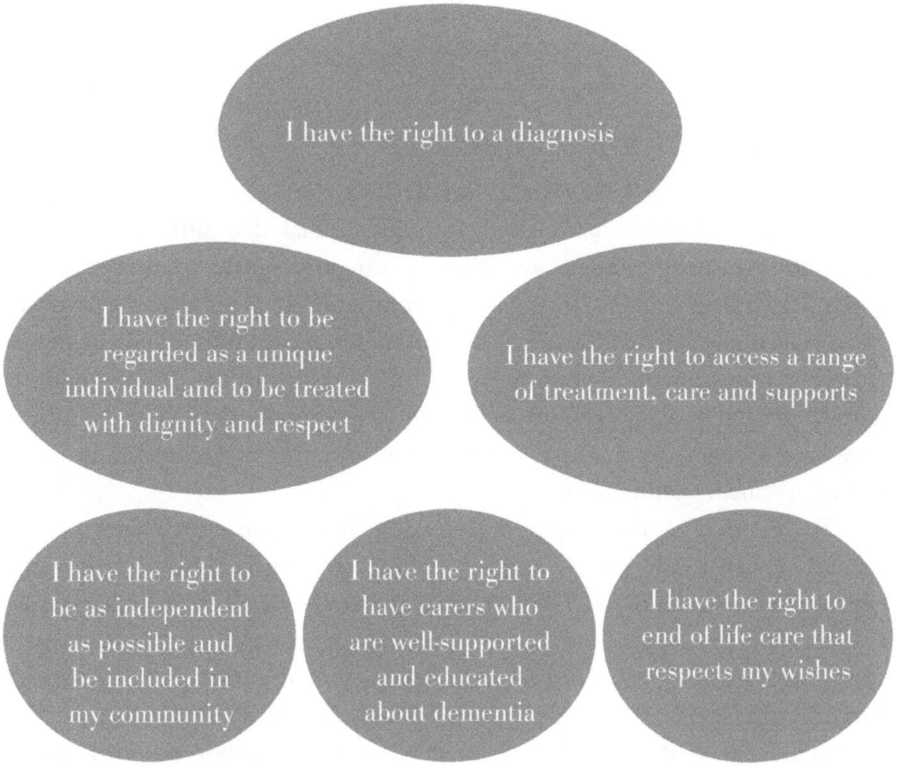

I have the right to a diagnosis

I have the right to be regarded as a unique individual and to be treated with dignity and respect

I have the right to access a range of treatment, care and supports

I have the right to be as independent as possible and be included in my community

I have the right to have carers who are well-supported and educated about dementia

I have the right to end of life care that respects my wishes

Figure 13.2 Rights of persons with dementia in Scotland

SOURCE: SCOTTISH GOVERNMENT 2011 (P.5) (REPRODUCED BY KIND PERMISSION OF THE SCOTTISH GOVERNMENT)

People with dementia retain the same rights as anyone else in society, but the nature of their illness means that they often have great difficulty in protecting their own rights. There is still stigma and discrimination against people with dementia, and they and their carers often feel, with some justification, that they are treated with less respect, dignity and understanding than other members of society. These standards relate to everyone with a diagnosis of dementia in Scotland regardless of where they live, their age, the supports they receive or the severity of their illness. There is predictably going to be concern about whether these standards of care are merely aspirational or in any way enforceable (Scottish Government, 2011). There has been quite intense concern about whether or not the Mental Capacity Act 2005, as implemented, truly encourages a rights-based approach; the paper by Anne McDonald (2010) argues that 'social workers operating under the MCA may, to some extent, have abandoned, or feel that they have abandoned, a rights-based approach in favour of risk-based legalistic and actuarial approaches' (p.1243).

Disability and dementia

Andrew Power recently identified complexities involved in facilitating active community connection for persons with intellectual disabilities and revealed important cautionary lessons for other jurisdictions where community living policy has arguably been moving away from communal services towards self-managed supports in 'real' communities through personal budgets in an effort to remove barriers to participation (Power, 2013). Power further critically reflected upon the rapid pursuit for transformation in personalised adult social care in government policy, arguing that the process of fostering meaningful community inclusion will and should take time.

During this time, the concept of 'belonging' has filtered into the international lexicon of social care policy, arguably taking the concept of social inclusion beyond narrow definitions. 'Belonging' in now understood not only in terms of the increased presence of marginalised persons in society, but also in terms of such people returning to or beginning to occupy valued social roles within society and community life (CLBC, 2009; Kendrick and Sullivan, 2009). This thinking has been crystallised in the 2007 United Nations Convention on the Rights of Persons with Disabilities (CRPD), which mandates that States Parties must ensure that 'the full enjoyment by persons with disabilities of their human rights and fundamental freedoms and of full participation by persons with disabilities will result in their enhanced sense of belonging' (United Nations General Assembly, 2006, preamble). Here the emphasis is on meaningful engagement and reciprocal relationships within the community and policies to address the inequalities faced by people with disabilities. Article 19 of the Convention states:

> Article 19 – Living independently and being included in the community
>
> State Parties to this Convention recognize the equal right of all persons with disabilities to live in the community, with choices equal to others, and

> shall take effective and appropriate measures to facilitate full enjoyment by persons with disabilities of this right and their full inclusion and participation in the community, including by ensuring that:
>
> (a) Persons with disabilities have the opportunity to choose their place of residence and where and with whom they live on an equal basis with others and are not obliged to live in a particular living arrangement;
>
> (b) Persons with disabilities have access to a range of in-home, residential and other community support services, including personal assistance necessary to support living and inclusion in the community, and to prevent isolation or segregation from the community;
>
> (c) Community services and facilities for the general population are available on an equal basis to persons with disabilities and are responsive to their needs.

In an outstanding talk for the Alzheimer Europe conference held in Glasgow in 2014, entitled 'The UN Disability Convention as an instrument for people with dementia and their carers', Gráinne McGettrick, currently policy and research manager for Acquired Brain Injury Ireland, argued the following:

> This international treaty promotes and protects the rights of the person with a disability. It aims to ensure their enjoyment of human rights and equality under the law. If we view dementia as a 'disability' then the Disability Convention has significant relevance and meaning and can shape the field of dementia at the global and local levels. Firstly, it provides a framework to rethink and re-imagine dementia as rights, a social justice and an equality issue and helps us to reframe how we talk dementia (and who does that talking).
>
> Secondly, it can act as a catalyst for change as we begin to move towards the social/rights-based model of dementia. People with dementia in this model are themselves the change agents. There is also a major shift in the power dynamics and stakeholder relationships.
>
> Thirdly, it promotes us utilising a specific human rights based approach (HRBA) in our work. Using human rights based approaches impacts on how policy gets shaped, how services are provided, what research gets done, how we advocate, fundraise and communicate in the public spheres.
>
> (McGettrick, 2014, reproduced by kind permission)

While meaningful social inclusion is not new within the disability literature, the recent generation of policy mechanisms that purport to endorse belonging has arguably become more pervasive, whilst simultaneously promoting an agenda of increased 'choice' and personalisation in the form of personal budgets and self-managed support. The international focus on personalisation approaches is now evident across a range of countries including Canada, England, many states in the US and, more recently, Ireland, and is increasingly endorsed as a mechanism which can facilitate greater community inclusion (Bigby and Frawley, 2010).

Dignity

In September 2014, Rosa Kornfeld-Matte, a UN Independent Expert on the enjoyment of all human rights, called on Member States across the globe to do more to protect older people affected by dementia from stigmatisation, discrimination, victimisation and neglect (DNA Web Team, 2014). Speaking ahead of World Alzheimer's Day 2014, Kornfeld-Matte called for concerted action to ensure that people living with dementia can fully enjoy their human rights in all circumstances.

There has been a relative paucity of published studies dealing with the subjective experience of individuals with early-stage dementia as a 'lived experience' (De Boer *et al.*, 2007; The, 2013). However, more recently there has been an increased awareness of the importance of taking into account the beliefs, concerns, needs and expectations of these individuals (Clare, 2003). Qualitative studies can potentially provide much-needed insights into the personal perspectives of those living well with dementia. By doing so, these studies are invaluable in understanding the dynamics involving people living well with dementia and those closest to them (Dröes *et al.*, 2006).

In the hospital care setting, 'enforcement' of autonomy is intimately bound up with clinical governance mechanisms (Bowman, 2001). Rapaport and colleagues (2005) are amongst a few to have drawn and articulated helpfully the relationship between autonomy and capacity. Autonomy is bound strongly with the notion of 'competency'. Competency refers to a person's ability to make responsible decisions on matters that affect different areas of his or her life and involve assuming risks; the critical argument is that an individual must make an informed decision freely and without being influenced (Alvaro, 2012).

It is strongly felt that adherence to human rights and equalities legislation should be reflected in policy and in practice (see, for example, Social Care Institute for Excellence, 2010). The Charter of Fundamental Rights of the European

Union (2000) places dignity at the heart of human rights (Article 1), stating that: 'Human dignity is inviolable. It must be respected and protected.' It goes on to make particular reference to older people, who have 'a right to lead a life in dignity and independence and to participate in social and cultural life' (Article 25), and workers: 'Every worker has the right to working conditions which respect his or her health, safety and dignity' (Article 31). The ethics and values that underpin good practice in social care, such as autonomy, privacy and dignity, are at the core of human rights legislation. There are ongoing tensions between adherence to these values and the need to protect people from abuse, neglect and harm. For example, someone with dementia may want to do something that presents a risk to themselves or others, and in such a case workers would need to consider whether this decision has been made with capacity.

Dignity is a key concept for living well with dementia (Gastmans, 2013). The Nuffield Foundation's report *Dementia: Ethical Issues* also underlines the importance of person-centred care, stating that treating a patient with dignity is a matter of showing respect for the personhood of the individual, recognising his or her value as a person, equal to anyone without dementia (Nuffield Council on Bioethics, 2009). Heggestad, Nortvedt and Slettebø (2013) argue that what matters most to maintaining the dignity of the residents, according to the relatives, is that the residents were seen and taken seriously as relational human beings.

Nordenfelt (2004) presents dignity as a complex phenomenon constituted within four varieties. Dignity as merit is a manifestation of dignity based on formal position and social rank; dignity as moral stature is based on personal moral values; and dignity of identity embraces dimensions of autonomy, integrity and self-respect. These three notions of dignity are changeable and violable, and may therefore vary from situation to situation or time to time. Nordenfelt's fourth dimension, *Menschenwürde* (human dignity), is, however, unchangeable, inviolable and constituted by the intrinsic worth of each human being.

Risk

In Chapter 11 of my book *Living Well with Dementia* (2014) I considered a particular interest of mine: how decisions are made by people living with dementia, and how they interface with the English law. I feel that active risk engagement is a pivotal strand in our English policy – so much so that I will return to this topic in my conclusion (Chapter 18). Decisions are fundamental to our lives. Decision making is a fundamental and complex skill which is crucial at any age. We all have to face decisions regarding our health care, medical treatment, retirement, housing, transport and finances, for example. We not only have to consider the benefit of a decision for our current living situation, but must also anticipate the consequences of decisions of such actions in the near and more distant future. We need to hold the decision in our memory for long enough to think strategically through the options, and be able to action an outcome. Everyday life requires numerous and fast decisions. Often these decisions have an uncertain result. Wrong decisions may thus have severe consequences in several domains.

Disturbances in a person's ability to make decisions or to anticipate the possible consequences of decisions can result in massive problems. In cognitive neuroscience and cognitive neurology in the last decade, there has been an increasing interest in investigating the neural basis of decision-making abilities and disturbances, both in healthy subjects and in people where there has been some disruption. An assessment of cognitive deficits in neurodegenerative diseases has focused so far almost entirely on memory, language, attention, visuospatial perception and executive functioning (Gleichgerrcht *et al.*, 2010). In the past decade, however, the study of decision making in these conditions has increased, prompting the development of new tasks that have enabled this cognitive process to be readily assessed. In clinical practice, it is not uncommon to find persons with early behavioural variant frontotemporal dementia (bvFTD) who, to a considerable extent, are intellectually unimpaired, while relatives and carers depict a strikingly different picture: they claim that these patients show severe changes in their behaviour and real-life decision-making skills (e.g. Manes *et al.*, 2011; Rahman *et al.*, 1999).

The literature has been able to identify the orbitofrontal, anterior cingulate and dorsolateral prefrontal cortices as being critical to decision making (Rosenbloom, Schmahmann and Price, 2012). A schematic view of the important neural substrates proposed by Rahman and colleagues (2001) is shown in Figure 13.3.

Various independent models of decision-making converge upon the critical importance of the orbitofrontal cortex especially in stimulus encoding. The 'somatic marker hypothesis' provides that somatosensory perception is important for arriving at decisions. However, it is overall felt that there are three main systems especially involved in decision-making: a stimulus encoding system (orbitofrontal cortex), an action selection system (anterior cingulate cortex) and an expected reward system (striatum and amygdala). Currently it is arguably not possible to specific exact neuroanatomical and functional relationships, and the schematic diagram shown reflects this. The picture does, however, embrace evidence from the current literature.

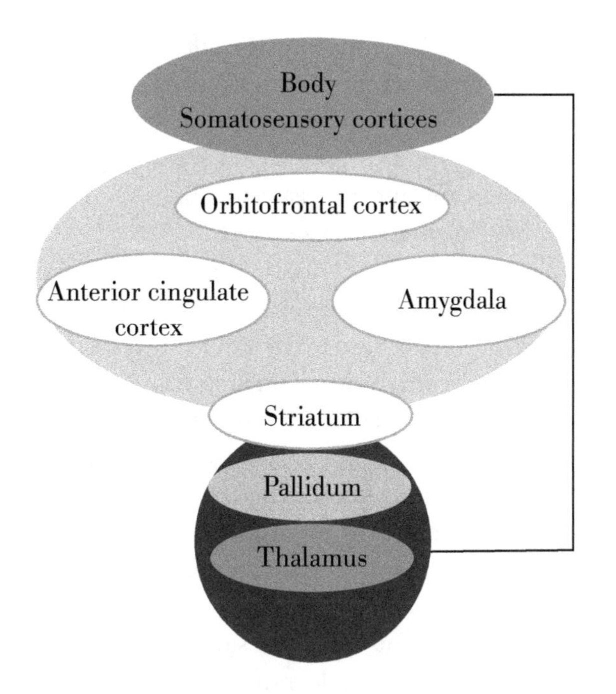

Figure 13.3 A neuroanatomical model of decision making

SOURCE: ADAPTED FROM GLEICHGERRCHT ET AL., 2010; RAHMAN ET AL., 2001; HOLLAND AND KENSINGER, 2010

Rahman and colleagues (1999) showed that patients with bvFTD exhibited a profile of risk taking but not impulsive behaviour in decision making, suggestive of dysfunction in the ventromedial prefrontal or orbitofrontal cortex. Kloeters and colleagues (2013), 12 years later, published results showing that atrophy in the orbitofrontal cortex and amygdala correlated with performance on the Iowa Gambling Task used in their study to examine decision making.

A large proportion of human cognitive social neuroscience research has focused on the issue of decision making. Impaired decision making is a symptomatic feature of a number of neurodegenerative diseases, but the nature of these decision-making deficits depends on the particular disease. Each person with dementia will have a cognitive profile detailing how far the condition has progressed and the extent to which functional problems are perceived. This might depend on the likely diagnostic category in which a patient living with dementia finds himself or herself. Examining the qualitative differences in decision-making impairments associated with different neurodegenerative diseases provides potentially valuable information regarding the underlying neural basis of decision making.

A good account of decision making in different neurological conditions, including dementia, is provided by Brand, Labudda and Markowitsch (2006). According to the authors, the model suggests a possibility to decide advantageously on the basis of rational or cognitive strategies alone. They also propose that the optimal way of decision making in 'risky situations' is to use both cognitive strategies as well as biasing emotional signals.

The comparison of the profiles of decision making in different conditions are arguably helpful in predicting what the person with dementia might expect. Several studies have reported altered decision making in Parkinson's disease (Perretta, Pari and Beninger, 2005) and pathological gambling has been found in Parkinson's disease patients with L-Dopa medication (Weintraub *et al.*, 2006), attributing a key role to the chemical dopamine in taking risky decisions. Recent studies also investigated decision making in Huntington's disease and found that learning and memory processes, rather than motivational processes, are responsible for decision-making deficits in this group (Busemeyer and Stout, 2002). Hampton and O'Doherty (2007), some time ago, were amongst several international neuroscience groups to publish on the neural substrates of reward-related decision making with functional MRI. They identified that the combined signals from three specific brain areas (anterior cingulate cortex, medial prefrontal cortex and ventral striatum) were found to provide all of the information sufficient to decode subjects' decisions out of all the regions studied. These findings appear to implicate a specific network of regions in encoding information relevant to subsequent behavioural choice. Evidence for the important role of the orbitofrontal cortex and the amygdala in decision making, particularly under ambiguous conditions, comes from a recent study by Hsu and colleagues (2005).

Dementia of the Alzheimer type (DAT), the cause of the most cases of dementia worldwide, is characterised by typical structural, neurochemical and cognitive changes as the disease progresses. Pathological changes in mild DAT affect primarily the medial temporal lobes and limbic structures (e.g. entorhinal cortex, hippocampus) and then extend to the association cortices of the frontal, temporal and parietal lobes (Braak and Braak, 1991). Ha and colleagues (2012) have argued that the changes in DAT fundamentally alter the frames of reference for making decisions. The study by Delazer and colleagues (2007) further highlighted important differences in decision making between patients with mild DAT and healthy controls. Findings from the study by Sinz and colleagues (2008) are consistent with the notion that decisions under ambiguity as well as decisions under risk are impaired in mild DAT. It may thus be expected that patients with mild DAT have difficulties in taking decisions in everyday life situations, both in cases of ambiguity (information on probability is missing or conflicting, and the expected utility of the different options is incalculable) and in cases of risk (outcomes can be predicted by well-defined or estimable probabilities).

The legal instrument currently used to assess capacity through the Mental Capacity Act 2005 is intended to be practical, but perhaps a greater sophisticated analysis of decision-making abilities is needed for improved risk mitigation of certain people living with dementia. It is likely that the implementation of the Mental Capacity Act will come under increasing scrutiny, in parallel with advances in decision-making research in cognitive neuroscience and cognitive neurology.

Risk engagement and living better with dementia

Much has been written on the subject of risk (e.g. Brearley, 1982; Kemshall and Pritchard, 1996). Risk can be linked with the concepts of harm or danger, or as a chance to gain benefits in a situation where harm is also possible. The way we define risk and assess its impact changes over time and in different contexts (Green, 2008). Alaszewski and Manthorpe's (2000) research on how agencies respond to risk concludes that explicit risk policy and practice is still limited, and Kemshall and Pritchard (1996) agree that the issue of risk assessment and management remained under-researched. Risk enablement is based on the idea that the process of measuring risk involves balancing the positive benefits from taking risks against the negative effects of attempting to avoid risk altogether.

However, research commissioned by the Department of Health, but conducted predominantly through Professor Jill Manthorpe and Jo Moriarty of the Social Care Workforce Research Unit, King's College London, arguably put risk engagement for people living well with dementia firmly on the map with *Nothing Ventured, Nothing Gained: Risk Guidance for Dementia* (Department of Health, 2010a). Developing systems for enabling and managing risk is one of the most important ways of allowing people with dementia to retain as much control over their lives as possible. Risk enablement takes a tailored approach to risk by acknowledging that dementia affects different people in different ways. A more person-centred approach to risk and dementia concentrates on identifying risky situations for individuals with dementia rather than viewing every person with dementia as being at equal risk.

According to the document from the Department of Health (2012) entitled *Personal Health Budgets Guide. Integrating Personal Budgets – Myths and Misconceptions*, it is argued: 'A variety of potential risks need to be taken into account when supporting people with health and social care needs, including financial, clinical and personal risks' (p.16). There needs to be a shared plan and shared responsibility, in a coordinated way and consistently, with people with health and social care needs, in order to identify risks and manage them in such a way as to promote good safeguarding practice. The main types of risk mentioned by family carers have included dealing with heating, falling, managing money, road safety, getting lost and cooking. There is a view that resources and support are needed to enable professionals, families and people with dementia to achieve a sense of shared negotiated responsibility for risk taking (Gilmour, Gibson and Campbell, 2003). Gilmour and colleagues (2003) also, interestingly, found that priorities of risk management tended to vary amongst the disciplines. For example, responses from paid workers tended to emphasise the importance of locality in terms of assessing and managing risk.

I resume my discussion of risk and uncertainty in my conclusion (Chapter 18).

Conclusion

Coming to terms with life after a diagnosis of one of the dementias is bound to be a demanding experience. It is after all a life-changing event for that person, his or her friends and/or his or her family. Risk engagement is a valuable component of an approach to life for a person to live better with dementia and is intimately related to a personal achievement of choice and control which has been pervasive in English policy. The narrative from a biomedical model will tend to drift in the direction of 'here's what you cannot do now that you could do six months ago'. Some people who have faced the diagnosis of dementia have found positive aspects to the experience, such as finding a corpus of sincere friends who are very supportive. In some cases, the dementia itself might unlock abilities in art or wellbeing through music. This is considered in Chapter 14 on art, music and creativity.

EU cases

HL v United Kingdom (Application no. 45508/99) Judgment, Strasbourg, 5 October 2004. Available at www.bailii.org/eu/cases/ECHR/2004/471.html (accessed 6 December 2014).

Storck v Germany (Application no. 61603/00) Judgment, Strasbourg, 16 June 2005. Available at www.worldlii.org/eu/cases/ECHR/2005/406.html (accessed 6 December 2014).

UK cases

YL (by her litigation friend the Official Solicitor) v Birmingham City Council and others [2007] UKHL. Available at www.publications.parliament.uk/pa/ld200607/ldjudgmt/jd070620/birm-1.htm (accessed 6 December 2014).

P (by his litigation friend the Official Solicitor) (Appellant) v Cheshire West and Chester Council and another (Respondents); P and Q (by their litigation friend the Official Solicitor) (Appellants) v Surrey County Council (Respondent) [2014] UKSC 19. On appeal from: [2011] EWCA Civ 1257; [2011] EWCA Civ 190. Available at www.supremecourt.uk/decided-cases/docs/UKSC_2012_0068_Judgment.pdf (accessed 6 December 2014).

Statute law

Care Act 2014. Available at www.legislation.gov.uk/ukpga/2014/23/contents/enacted (accessed 6 December 2014).

Equality Act 2010. Available at www.legislation.gov.uk/ukpga/2010/15/contents (accessed 6 December 2014).

Human Rights Act 1998. Available at www.legislation.gov.uk/ukpga/1998/42/pdfs/ukpga_1998 0042_en.pdf (accessed 18 May 2015).

European Convention on Human Rights, Article 5: The right to liberty and security. Available at www.equalityhumanrights.com/sites/default/files/documents/humanrights/hrr_article_5.pdf (accessed 6 December 2014).

Mental Capacity Act 2005, section 64. Available at www.legislation.gov.uk/ukpga/2005/9/section/64 (accessed 6 December 2014).

References

Alaszewski, H. and Manthorpe, J. (2000) Finding the balance: older people, nurses and risk. Education and Ageing, 15, 2, 195–209.

Alvaro, L.C. (2012) Competency: general principles and applicability in dementia [Article in Spanish]. Neurologia, 27, 5, 290–300.

Alzheimer Scotland (Scottish Government) (2010) Taking charge – a short guide to support for people with dementia and their carers. Available at www.alzscot.org/assets/0000/2160/taking-charge-self-directed-support.pdf (accessed 6 December 2014).

Audit Commission (2010) Financial Management of Personal Budgets: Challenges and Opportunities for Councils. London: Audit Commission.

Authors undisclosed (2012) Notes: after GINA, NINA? Neuroscience-based discrimination in the workplace. Vanderbilt Law Review, 65, 933–67.

BBC News (2014) Disabled people's access to High Street 'shocking', audit finds. Available at www.bbc.co.uk/news/uk-politics-30342957 (accessed 20 February 2015).

Beresford, P. (2012) What service users want from social workers. Community Care. Available at www.communitycare.co.uk/2012/04/27/what-service-users-want-from-social-workers/#.UpR46OIniiM (accessed 6 December 2014).

Beresford, P., Shamash, M., Forrest, V., Turner, M. and Branfield, F. (2005) Developing Social Care: Service Users' Vision for Adult Support. London: Social Care Institute for Excellence.

Bigby, C. and Frawley, P. (2010) Social Work Practice and Intellectual Disability. Basingstoke: Palgrave Macmillan.

Billings, P.R., Kohn, M.A., de Cuevas, M., Beckwith, J., Alper, J.S. and Natowicz, M.R. (1992) Discrimination as a consequence of genetic testing. The American Journal of Human Genetics, 50, 3, 476–82.

Bowman, C.E. (2001) Governance and autonomy in alternatives to hospital care. Age and Ageing, 30, Suppl. 3, 15–18.

Braak, H. and Braak, E. (1991) Neuropathological staging of Alzheimer-related changes. Acta Neuropathologica, 82, 239–59.

Brand, M., Labudda, K. and Markowitsch, H.J. (2006) Neuropsychological correlates of decision making in ambiguous and risky situations. Neural Networks, 19, 8, 1266–76.

Brearley, C. (1982) Risk and Social Work. London: Routledge and Kegan Paul.

Busemeyer, J.R. and Stout, J.C. (2002) A contribution of cognitive decision models to clinical assessment: decomposing performance on the Bechara gambling task. Psychological Assessment, 14, 253–62.

Carr, S. (2010) Enabling Risk, Ensuring Safety: Personal Budgets and Self Directed Support. SCIE Report 36. London: Social Care Institute for Excellence.

Carr, S. (2011) Enabling risk and ensuring safety: self-directed support and personal budgets. Journal of Adult Protection, 13, 3, 122–36.

Charter of Fundamental Rights of the European Union (2000/C 364/01). Available at www.europarl.europa.eu/charter/pdf/text_en.pdf (accessed 6 December 2014).

Chinthapalli, K. (2012) Personal health budgets: surplus of cash or deficit of ideas? British Medical Journal, 345, e8329.

Clare, L. (2003) Managing threats to self: awareness in early stage Alzheimer's disease. Social Science and Medicine, 57, 1017–29.

Clark, H. (2006) 'It's Meant That, Well, I'm Living a Life Now': Older People's Experience of Direct Payments. In J. Leece and J. Bornat (eds) Developments in Direct Payments. Bristol: Policy Press.

CLBC (2009) Belonging to One Another: Building Personal Support Networks. Victoria: CLBC.

De Boer, M.E., Hertogh, C.M., Dröes, R.M., Riphagen, I.I., Jonker, C. and Eefsting, J.A. (2007) Suffering from dementia – the patient's perspective: a review of the literature. International Psychogeriatrics, 19, 1021–39.

Delazer, M., Sinz, H., Zamarian, L. and Benke, T. (2007) Decision-making with explicit and stable rules in mild Alzheimer's disease. Neuropsychologia, 45, 8, 1632–41.

Department of Health (2007) Putting People First: A Shared Vision and Commitment to the Transformation of Social Care. Available at http://webarchive.nationalarchives.gov.uk/20130107105354/http:/www.dh.gov.uk/prod_consum_dh/groups/dh_digitalassets/@dh/@en/documents/digitalasset/dh_081119.pdf (accessed 6 December 2014).

Department of Health (2009) Personal Health Budgets: First Steps. London: Department of Health.

Department of Health (2010a) Nothing Ventured, Nothing Gained: Risk Guidance for Dementia. Available at www.gov.uk/government/uploads/system/uploads/attachment_data/file/215960/dh_121493.pdf (accessed 11 February 2015).

Department of Health (2010b) Equity and Excellence: Liberating the NHS. Available at www.gov.uk/government/uploads/system/uploads/attachment_data/file/213823/dh_117794.pdf (accessed 20 February 2015).

Department of Health (2012) Personal Health Budgets Guide: Integrating Personal Budgets – Myths and Misconceptions. Available at www.personalhealthbudgets.england.nhs.uk/_library/Resources/Personalhealthbudgets/Toolkit/MakingPHBHappen/Integration/IntegratingPersonalBudgetsMM.pdf (accessed 11 February 2015).

DNA Web Team (2014) Ahead of Alzheimer's Day, UN expert urges greater protections for people with dementia, Saturday, 20 September 2014. Available at www.dnaindia.com/health/report-ahead-of-alzheimer-s-day-un-expert-urges-greater-protections-for-people-with-dementia-2020164 (accessed 11 February 2014).

Dröes, R.-M., Boelens-Van der Knoop, E.C.C., Bos, J., Meihuizen, L. *et al.* (2006) Quality of life in dementia in perspective: an explorative study of variations in opinions among people with dementia and their professional caregivers, and in literature. Dementia, 5, 533–58.

Duffy, S. (2011) A Fair Society and the Limits of Personalisation: A Discussion Paper from The Centre for Welfare Reform, first presented at the Tizard Memorial Lecture, 4th March 2011. Available at www.centreforwelfarereform.org/uploads/attachment/261/a-fair-society-and-the-limits-of-personalisation.pdf (accessed 6 December 2014).

Ellis, K. (2007) Direct payments and social work practice: the significance of 'street-level bureaucracy' in determining eligibility. British Journal of Social Work, 37, 405–22.

Equality and Human Rights Commission (2014) Workplace adjustments. Available at www.equalityhumanrights.com/private-and-public-sector-guidance/employing-people/work-place-adjustments (accessed 6 December 2014).

Forder, J., Jones, K., Glendinning, C., Caiels, J. *et al.* (2012) Evaluation of the Personal Health Budget Pilot Programme (PSSRU Discussion Paper, Vol. 2840–2). Canterbury: PSSRU University of Kent, Canterbury.

Gastmans, C. (2013) Dignity-enhancing nursing care: a foundational ethical framework. Nursing Ethics, 20, 142–9.

Gilmour, H., Gibson, F. and Campbell, J. (2003) Living alone with dementia: a case study approach to understanding risk. Dementia, 2, 403–20.

Glasby, J. and Littlechild, R. (2009) Direct Payments and Personal Budgets: Putting Personalisation into Practice. Bristol: Policy Press.

Gleichgerrcht, E., Ibáñez, A., Roca, M., Torralva, T. and Manes, F. (2010) Decision-making cognition in neurodegenerative diseases. Nature Reviews Neurology, 6, 11, 611–23.

Glendinning, C., Challis, D., Fernandez, J., Jacobs, S. *et al.* (2008) Evaluation of the Individual Budgets Pilot Programme: Final Report. York: Social Policy Research Unit, University of York.

Goh, A.M., Chiu, E., Yastrubetskaya, O., Erwin, C. *et al.* Investigators of the Huntington Study Group (2013) Perception, experience, and response to genetic discrimination in Huntington's disease: the Australian results of the International RESPOND-HD Study. Genetic Testing and Molecular Biomarkers, 17, 2, 115–21.

Goodchild, C. (on behalf of the Mental Health Foundation) (2011) Personal budgets for people with dementia: a report on challenges and solutions to implementation based on interviews with eight local authorities in England. Available at www.mentalhealth.org.uk/content/assets/PDF/publications/Personal_budgets_for_people_living_with_dementia.pdf (accessed 6 December 2014).

Green, D. (2008) Risk and social work practice. Australian Social Work, 14, 3, 154–6.

Gridley, K., Brooks, J. and Glendinning, C. (2014) Good practice in social care: the views of people with severe and complex needs and those who support them. Health and Social Care in the Community, 22, 6, 588–97.

Griffith, R. (2014) Mental Capacity and Mental Health Acts part 3: deprivation of liberty. British Journal of Nursing, 23, 18, 998–9.

Ha, J., Kim, E.J., Lim, S., Shin, D.W. *et al.* (2012) Altered risk aversion and risk-taking behaviour in patients with Alzheimer's disease. Psychogeriatrics, 12, 3, 151–8.

Habell, M. (2013) Specialised design for dementia. Perspectives in Public Health, 133, 3, 151–7.

Hampton, A.N. and O'Doherty, J.P. (2007) Decoding the neural substrates of reward-related decision making with functional MRI. Proceedings of the National Academy of Sciences of the USA, 104, 4, 1377–82.

Hart, V. (2014) A View from Social Care Practice. In C. Needham and J. Glasby (eds) Debates in Personalisation. Bristol: Policy Press.

Health Foundation (2010) Report: personal health budgets – research scan. Available at www.health.org.uk/public/cms/75/76/313/2594/personal%20health%20budgets.pdf?realName=wiYPsk.pdf (accessed 6 December 2014).

Heggestad, A.K., Nortvedt, P. and Slettebø, A. (2013) Dignity and care for people with dementia living in nursing homes. Dementia (London), 2013 Dec 18 [Epub ahead of print].

Holland, A.C. and Kensinger, E.A. (2010) Emotion and autobiographical memory. Physics of Life Reviews, 7, 1, 88–131.

House of Lords (2014) Select Committee on the Mental Capacity Act 2005: Report of Session 2013–14 on Mental Capacity Act 2005: Post-Legislative Scrutiny. Available at www.publications.parliament.uk/pa/ld201314/ldselect/ldmentalcap/139/139.pdf (accessed 6 December 2014).

Hsu, M., Bhatt, M., Adolphs, R., Tranel, D. and Camerer, C.F. (2005) Neural systems responding to degrees of uncertainty in human decision-making. Science, 310, 1680–3.

Jacobs, S., Abell, J., Stevens, M., Wilberforce, M. *et al.* (2013) The personalization of care services and the early impact on staff activity patterns. Journal of Social Work, 13, 141–63.

Kemshall, H. and Pritchard, J. (eds) (1996) Good Practice in Risk Assessment and Risk Management. London: Jessica Kingsley Publishers.

Kendrick, M.J. and Sullivan, L. (2009) Appraising the leadership challenges of social inclusion. International Journal of Leadership in Public Services, 5, 67–75.

Kloeters, S., Bertoux, M., O'Callaghan, C., Hodges, J.R. and Hornberger, M. (2013) Money for nothing: atrophy correlates of gambling decision making in behavioural variant frontotemporal dementia and Alzheimer's disease. Neuroimage: Clinical, 2, 263–72.

Limb, M. (2012) Personal health budgets may be spent on 'laptops and travel passes'. British Medical Journal, 344, e2155.

Limb, M. (2014) Personal health budgets are good for the few but not for the many, conference hears. British Medical Journal, 27, 348. doi: 10.1136/bmj.g1149.

Macovei, M. (Council of Europe) (2002) The right to liberty and security of the person: a guide to the implementation of Article 5 of the European Convention on Human Rights. Available at www.supremecourt.ge/files/upload-file/pdf/article5eng.pdf (accessed 6 December 2014).

Mainsbridge, A. (2002) Employers and genetic information: a new frontier for discrimination. Macquarie Law Journal, 2, 61–85.

Manes, F., Torralva, T., Ibáñez, A., Roca, M., Bekinschtein, T. and Gleichgerrcht, E. (2011) Decision making in frontotemporal dementia: clinical, theoretical and legal implications. Dementia and Geriatric Cognitive Disorders, 32, 1, 11–17.

McDonald, A. (2010) The impact of the 2005 Mental Capacity Act on social workers' decision making and approaches to the assessment of risk. British Journal of Social Work, 40, 4, 1229–46.

McGettrick, G. (2014) The UN Disability Convention as an instrument for people with dementia and their carers. Presentation at the Alzheimer Europe Conference, Glasgow, October 2014.

McKee, M. (2013) Two key messages were overlooked in article on personal health budgets. British Medical Journal, 346, f34.

Mental Welfare Commission for Scotland (n.d.) Autonomy benefit and protection: How human rights can protect people with mental health conditions or learning disabilities from unlawful deprivation of liberty. Discussion paper prepared by Hilary Patrick, Mental Health Law and Practice. Available at www.mwcscot.org.uk/media/51750/Autonomy,_benefit_and_protection.pdf (accessed 6 December 2014).

Newbronner, L., Chamberlain, R., Bosanquet, K., Bartlett, C., Sass, B. and Glendinning, C. (2011) Keeping Personal Budgets Personal: Learning from the Experiences of Older People, People with Mental Health Problems and Their Carers, SCIE Report 40. London: Social Care Institute for Excellence.

NHS Confederation (2009) Shaping personal health budgets: a view from the top. Available at www.nhsconfed.org/~/media/Confederation/Files/Publications/Documents/ Shaping_personal_health_budgets-a_view_from_the_top.pdf (accessed 20 April 2015).

NHS Confederation (2011) Personal Health Budgets: The Views of Service Users and Carers. London: NHS Confederation.

Nordenfelt, L. (2004) The varieties of dignity. Health Care Analysis, 12, 69–81.
Nuffield Council on Bioethics (2009) Dementia: Ethical Issues. Nuffield Council Reports. London: Nuffield Council on Bioethics.
Nuffield Trust (2013) Personal health budgets: challenges for commissioners and policy makers. Research summary (authors: Vidhya Alakeson and Benedict Rumbold). Available at www.nuffieldtrust.org.uk/sites/files/nuffield/publication/130828_personal_health_budgets_summary_0.pdf (accessed 6 December 2014).
Perretta, J.G., Pari, G. and Beninger, R.J. (2005) Effects of Parkinson disease on two putative non-declarative learning tasks: probabilistic classification and gambling. Cognitive and Behavioural Neurology, 18, 185–92.
Policy Research Unit in Commissioning and the Healthcare System (2013) Personal budgets and health: a review of the evidence, February 2013 (author: Dr Erica Wirrmann Gadsby/PRU). Available at http://blogs.lshtm.ac.uk/prucomm/files/2013/04/Personal-Budgets-review-of-evidence_FINAL-REPORT.pdf (accessed 6 December 2014).
Power, A. (2013) Making space for belonging: critical reflections on the implementation of personalised adult social care under the veil of meaningful inclusion. Social Science and Medicine, 88, 68–75.
Rahman, S. (2014) Living Well with Dementia: The Importance of the Person and the Environment for Wellbeing. Oxford: Radcliffe Health.
Rahman, S., Sahakian, B.J., Hodges, J.R., Rogers, R.D. and Robbins, T.W. (1999) Specific cognitive deficits in mild frontal variant frontotemporal dementia. Brain, 122, 8, 1469–93.
Rahman, S., Sahakian, B.J., Cardinal, R.N., Rogers, R. and Robbins, T. (2001) Decision making and neuropsychiatry. Trends in Cognitive Sciences, 5, 6, 271–7.
Rapaport, J., Manthorpe, J., Moriarty, J., Hussein, S. and Collins, J. (2005) Advocacy and people with learning disabilities in the UK: how can local funders find value for money? Journal of Intellectual Disabilities, 9, 4, 299–319.
Rogers, J. (2011) Personal health budgets: a new way of accessing complementary therapies? Complementary Therapies in Clinical Practice, 17, 2, 76–80.
Rosenbloom, M.H., Schmahmann, J.D. and Price, B.H. (2012) The functional neuroanatomy of decision making. Journal of Neuropsychiatry and Clinical Neurosciences, 24, 3, 266–77.
Scottish Government (2009) Charter of Rights for People with Dementia and their Carers in Scotland. Available at www.alzscot.org/assets/0000/2678/Charter_of_Rights.pdf (accessed 6 December 2014).
Scottish Government (2011) Standards of Care for Dementia in Scotland: Action to Support the Change Programme, Scotland's National Dementia Strategy. Available at www.gov.scot/Resource/Doc/350188/0117212.pdf (accessed 20 February 2015).
Serino, S. and Riva, G. (2013) Getting lost in Alzheimer's disease: a break in the mental frame syncing. Medical Hypotheses, 80, 4, 416–21.
Shastry, B.S. and Giblin, F.J. (1999) Genes and susceptible loci of Alzheimer's disease. Brain Research Bulletin, 48, 2, 121–7.
Sinz, H., Zamarian, L., Benke, T., Wenning, G.K. and Delazer, M. (2008) Impact of ambiguity and risk on decision making in mild Alzheimer's disease. Neuropsychologia, 46, 7, 2043–55.
Slasberg, C., Beresford, P. and Schofield, P. (2012) How self directed support is failing to deliver personal budgets and personalization. Research, Policy and Planning, 29, 3, 161–77.
Social Care Institute for Excellence (SCIE) (2010) Dignity in Care, SCIE Guide 15. Available at www.scie.org.uk/publications/guides/guide15/index.asp (accessed 6 December 2014).
Swaffer, K. (2014) Reinvesting in life is the best prescription (1 December 2014). Australian Journal of Dementia Care. Available at http://journalofdementiacare.com/reinvesting-in-life-is-the-best-prescription (accessed 6 December 2014).
Taylor, N.S.D. (2008) Obstacles and dilemmas in the delivery of direct payments to service users with poor mental health. Practice: Social Work in Action, 20, 43–55.

The, A.-M. (2013) Motivatie is alles [Motivation is everything]. Nursing, 6, 49–51.
Tingle, J. (2012) Deprivation of liberty safeguards: a human rights issue. British Journal of Nursing, 21, 9, 554–5.
UNESCO (1997) Universal Declaration on the Human Genome and Human Rights. Available at http://portal.unesco.org/en/ev.php-URL_ID=13177&URL_DO=DO_TOPIC&URL_SECTION=201.html (accessed 20 February 2015).
United Nations General Assembly (2006) UN Convention on the Rights of Persons with Disabilities. Available at www.un.org/esa/socdev/enable/rights/convtexte.htm (accessed 6 December 2014).
Webber, M., Treacy, S., Carr, S., Clark, M. and Parker, G. (2014) The effectiveness of personal budgets for people with mental health problems: a systematic review. Journal of Mental Health, 23, 3, 146–55.
Weintraub, D., Siderowf, A.D., Potenza, M.N., Goveas, J. *et al.* (2006) Association of dopamine agonist use with impulse control disorders in Parkinson disease. Archives of Neurology, 63, 969–73.
White, C. (2011) Do personal health budgets lead to better care choices? British Medical Journal, 343, doi: http://dx.doi.org/10.1136/bmj.d6532.

Chapter 14

ART, MUSIC AND CREATIVITY FOR LIVING BETTER WITH DEMENTIA

'You can't use up creativity. The more you use, the more you have.'

Maya Angelou (1928–2014)

Introduction

Highly creative individuals weave together drive, skill and imagination to generate new ideas and actions. It is said that artists further employ the ability to link related sensory, conceptual and emotional images through a chosen medium (Seeley *et al.*, 2008). Sharing interests in art, music and creativity can break down perceived barriers in the community. But I couldn't agree more with the sentiment expressed in Killick and Craig (2012, p.17): '[C]reativity involves bringing something of the inside out, a letting go.' There are certain observations that are particularly noteworthy. The human species is the only animal that can draw a picture (Matsuzawa, 1991). Also, a topic that has long fascinated neuroscientists is whether the animal kingdom can 'enjoy' music (e.g. Fitch, 2013). It is also fast becoming clear that some people living with dementia can have quite staggering artistic talents unleashed.

Other jurisdictions will be able to share their own experiences of 'social prescribing'. In November 2007, the Scottish Development Centre for Mental

Health/Scottish Government published their well-received *Developing Social Prescribing and Community Referrals for Mental Health in Scotland.* It states:

> Social prescribing is a valuable complement to other recent and on-going developments within the NHS to promote access to psychological treatments and interventions. It is now widely understood that social, economic and environmental factors have a significant influence on the mental health and wellbeing of people in Scotland. (Scottish Development Centre for Mental Health/Scottish Government, 2007, p.5)

What is creativity?

There has been much discussion about what 'creativity' is. Many consider, for example, that the celebration of art and music is ultimately a triumph of individuality (e.g. Ramachandran and Hirstein, 1999). It is argued that the origins of creativity are, in fact, ancient and lie in Africa, suggesting that human anatomy and cognition might have been well developed by then (Morriss-Kay, 2010). Morriss-Kay (2010) argues, completely reasonably, that 3D art 'may have begun with human likeness recognition' (p.158), and emphasises the sophistication of the neural substrates of perception. However, she also refers to the creation of images from imagination or 'the mind's eye'; and the evolution of 'the mind's eye' is currently a fertile area of exploration (Caldwell, 2014). There is some sense in the literature of creativity being a 'unique achievement' judged by the quality of the 'finished products', such as Shakespeare's *The Tempest* or Charles Dickens' *Hard Times*, for example (Amabile, 1993). This is related, perhaps, to the property of 'novelty'; novelty has traditionally been closely linked to standard definitions of creativity (Kaufman, 2013). It has been argued further that 'originality is a required but insufficient condition; the work must also be of value' (El-Murad and West, 2004, p.189).

There has been some general discussion of the factors that are thought to promote creativity, as well as the factors that inhibit creativity. The notion of working in teams to promote creativity is also well known; benefits are thought to be mutual stimulation and the positive effect of feedback (e.g. King and Anderson, 1990). Fear might possibly be an inhibitor of creativity (e.g. Nickerson, 1999). These ideas are helpful for the general interpretation of the emergence of artistic talent which can happen in people living better with dementia.

Art and living better with dementia

Artistic talent and dementia

There are many aspects of the essence of art, and the perceptual qualia that underlie them, that are way beyond the scope of this chapter. For an excellent review of some of these phenomena – for example, 'a perceptual group', 'binding and reinforcing effects', 'contrast extraction' and 'symmetry' – the reader is encouraged to refer to the excellent article 'The science of art' by V.S. Ramachandran and William Hirstein (1999). This comprehensive review looks at the evidence behind various perceptual phenomena, even if we are far from understanding their neural substrates.

What happens to artistic ability for someone living with dementia?

The first thing to say is that each person living with dementia is an individual. But some interesting observations have been made.

Behaviourally, painting depends on various cognitive processes such as object recognition, visual representation, constructive ability, working memory and motor skills (Takahata *et al.*, 2014). Gordon (2005) opines that the development of exceptional and unexpected artistic skills at any age must be a matter of curiosity. This can occur among young children with severe learning difficulties, especially if they have autism. Some examples have previously been given in the literature, with descriptions of the way in which these children's brains may function (Snyder *et al.*, 2003). Kirk and Kertesz (1991) found that the 'drawings of patients with Alzheimer's disease displayed fewer angles, impaired perspective and spatial relations, simplification, and overall impairment compared with those of the control subjects' (p.73). These deficits appeared to be independent of memory and language and continued to deteriorate over the course of three years. Neglect was relatively uncommon. It has been shown that damage in this region can cause a symptom known as constructional apraxia (Piercy, Hecaen and de Ajuriaguerra, 1960), which refers to the inability to draw or copy figures despite spared motor ability.

One prominent example of a drastic change in artistic style following brain damage is the serial artworks created by the famous professional artist Willem de Kooning, who had continued to draw after progression of dementia of the Alzheimer type (Crutch and Rossor, 2006). Crutch, Isaacs and Rossor (2001) reported the case of a man with probable dementia of the Alzheimer type fulfilling the criteria of the DSM-IV (American Psychiatric Association, 2000). W.U. was a 66-year-old artist, born in south Philadelphia, who came to England in 1957. The authors felt that the rapidity and extent of change in artistic ability was indicative of a process above and beyond normal ageing, particularly given his relatively young age at onset. Over an interval of five years, there was an objective deterioration in the quality of artwork produced.

Studies of spontaneous drawing in people living well with dementia of the Alzheimer type have highlighted the presence of perceptual and executive visuospatial deficits. Neuropsychological measures of visuoperceptual and visuospatial function tend to show significant decline, as a component of the global cognitive impairment. Change in artistic styles as a consequence of focal brain damage has also been reported in patients with a cerebral stroke. The most cited region in relation to visual constructive ability is the right hemisphere (Magnus and Laeng, 2006). Cummings and Zarit (1987) also report the course of an artist with dementia of the Alzheimer type over a 30-month period. The patient's work became more simplified and primitive. His colour palette became increasingly restricted, and advanced techniques such as shading and perspective were lost.

The phenomenon of 'visual realism' is characterised by accurate and detailed representation of the scenes and objects in visual space. In primates, visual representation is constructed through hierarchical processing of lower-level perceptual information and higher-level visual representation (Marr, 1982). For realistic drawing, extraction of lower-level perceptual information – such as edge, contour, shape, colour, contrast, light and shadow – is necessary. This lower-level perceptual information corresponds to the so-called 'physical level' in Marr's classical computational model of visual representation (Marr, 1982). Magnus and Laeng (2006) included this perceptual information as the necessary components for expert drawing. Takahata and colleagues (2014) recently reported a case of left prefrontal stroke, where the patient showed enhancement of artistic skills of realistic painting after the onset of brain damage.

Rankin and colleagues (2007) did a 'head-to-head comparison' of artistic styles in dementia of the Alzheimer type and frontotemporal dementia (FTD). Despite equal performance on standard visuospatial tests, these groups of people living with dementia produced distinct patterns of artistic features. The visual art created by the semantic dementia (SD) group was characterised by significant facial distortion and overall bizarreness, compared with normal control drawings, regardless of whether they depicted people or objects. However, it is noteworthy that patients in this group did show trends towards more disorganised composition, which it is suggested may be due to frontal-executive dysfunction in the areas of visuospatial planning and organisation. Indeed, on neuropsychological testing, persons living with frontotemporal dementia performed the worst of all groups in almost all cognitive domains. Their drawings also demonstrated distortion of facial features, which may be due to damage to the fusiform face area, the posterior structure in the inferior temporal gyrus that is currently known to be implicated in the differentiation and characterisation of facial detail.

Ebersbach (2003) described an artist who depicted her visual hallucinations associated with Parkinson's disease. In this case, the artist was able to translate her symptoms into a beautiful artistic product. In another remarkable report, Sahlas described the accomplished artist, poet, novelist, illustrator and playwright Mervyn Peake (Sahlas, 2003). Diagnosed with dementia with Lewy bodies (DLB), in his fifth decade Peaks began to describe his visual hallucinations and paranoid delusions in sketches and poetry composed during his illness. Miller and colleagues (2000) reported on 12 patients with FTD who acquired, or sustained, new musical or visual abilities despite progression of their dementia. Intriguingly, they reported that artistic output shared many features. Talents were musical or visual, but never in the verbal sphere. Work lacked a symbolic or abstract component, and painters copied or remembered realistic landscapes and animals. Miller and colleagues (1998) also described, two years earlier, five persons with early FTD who became artists; their history, artistic process, neuropsychology and anatomy are described.

Chakravarty (2011) later described the case of an 82-year-old female with probable dementia of the Alzheimer type, who developed unusual artistic creativity after development of her disease. The person showed no inclination towards visual arts during her premorbid years. She had presented with progressive memory loss for mostly recent events, which was soon followed by getting lost inside her house and on the road, disorientation in time and place, and difficulty in naming and recognising her relatives. Her paintings were mostly of human figures, vibrant and rich in colour, and with attention to detail. There were many images of Hindu gods and goddesses (images and idols which she must have seen several times in the past). To explain behavioural improvement following brain injury, Kapur (1996) coined the term 'paradoxical functional facilitation', thought to be a compensatory augmentation occurring as a specific manifestation of central nervous system plasticity. This hypothesis has been verified to some extent through converging evidence elsewhere. For example, simulating such brain impairment in healthy people by directing low-frequency magnetic pulses into the left frontotemporal lobe has produced significant stylistic changes in drawing (Snyder *et al.*, 2003). (An alternative view has been proposed by Ambar Chakravarty (2010) called 'reverse diaschisis', the opposite of the situation in which reduced function of one brain area leads to reduced function of a remote brain area to which it is anatomically connected.)

Dementia does not always facilitate artistic creativity, however.

Budrys and colleagues (2007) reported the case of V.V., a professional artist from an artist family. After graduating from the Lithuanian Art Academy in 1988, she had produced paintings, engravings, poetry and performances. She was later found to have been living with neuronal intermediate filament inclusion disease (NIFID), a recently described new variant of early-onset frontotemporal dementia.

Arts and creativity in practice

Renée Beard (2012) completed a critique of the evidence base for arts therapies, including music, visual arts, drama and dance/movement therapies, between the years 1990 and 2010. Beard found that this evidence base is divided between studies focusing on the 'product' and those focusing on the 'process' of art.

A remarkable project on arts and creativity in Yorkshire has produced a photobook, '"We're not finished" – South Yorkshire Dementia Creative Arts Exhibitions 2009–2014', which celebrated the first six years of the South Yorkshire Dementia Creative Arts Exhibition, coordinated by the School of Nursing and Midwifery, University of Sheffield (University of Sheffield, 2014). The exhibition was successful in showcasing the talents of people living well with dementia, including families and care practitioners.

Music and living better with dementia

Why is music so important?

The ubiquity of music in human culture is indicative of its ability to produce pleasure and reward value. Music is a cultural universal of human societies, and the ability to appreciate music is widely prized. Many people experience a particularly intense, euphoric response to music which, because of its frequent accompaniment by an autonomic or psychophysiological component, is sometimes described as 'shivers-down-the-spine' or 'chills' (e.g. Panksepp, 1995). Chills comprise clear, discrete events.

Patients have few autobiographical memories (Rubin and Kozin, 1984), which are formed earlier in life (especially between 10 and 30 years), when the context of acquisition is particularly charged emotionally, and few flashbulb memories, which concern a public event when the context of acquisition is particularly unexpected, dramatic and charged emotionally (Brown and Kulik, 1977). A component of Brown and Kulik's argument about 'flashbulb memories' was that the emotional significance of the event – which they proposed included the arousal evoked by the event as well as the consequentiality of the event – would be a key determinant of whether the details of the event were retained.

Music and emotions

Blood and Zatorre (2001) found that subjective reports of chills were accompanied by changes in heart rate, electromyogram and respiration. As intensity of these chills increased, cerebral blood flow increased, and decreases were observed in brain regions thought to be involved in reward motivation, emotion and arousal, including ventral striatum, midbrain, amygdala, orbitofrontal cortex and ventral medial prefrontal cortex. Brain structures correlating with intensely pleasant emotion in the 2001 study differed considerably from those observed during unpleasant or pleasant responses to musical dissonance or consonance in Blood and colleagues' previous study (1999).

Music and the brain

Music–brain relationships can also be investigated by studying cases of musicians with cerebral lesions (Basso and Capitani, 1985; Signoret *et al.*, 1987). One of the most dramatic cases is that of the French composer of paternal Swiss and maternal Basque descent, Maurice Ravel (1875–1937), who is thought to have developed a progressive cerebral disease. Several historians and musicologists have reflected on Ravel's life, but most of these biographies say little about Ravel's last years (Amaducci, Grassi and Boller, 2002).

It is occasionally thought that language and music are two sides of the same intellectual coin, but research on brain-damaged patients has shown that the loss of verbal functions (aphasia) is not necessarily accompanied by a loss of musical abilities (amusia) (Basso, 1993). Amusia without aphasia has also been described. This double dissociation indicates functional autonomy in these mental processes (Amaducci *et al.*, 2002).

Music and memory

Music can affect and be affected by memory.

For example, participants who were induced into sad moods via music tended to recall negative (mood-congruent) autobiographical events first, followed by positive autobiographical events (Josephson, Singer and Salovey, 1996). However, while the perceptual and affective dimensions of music have received much attention, the cognitive organisation of music knowledge has been researched less widely. Omar and colleagues (2010) investigated these aspects of music knowledge in relation to musical perceptual abilities and extra-musical neuropsychological functions, and their results are indeed fascinating. The findings here perhaps suggest that music knowledge is fractionated, and superordinate musical knowledge is relatively more robust than knowledge of particular music. Under this hypothesis, it is reasonable to suggest, as indeed the authors did, that music constitutes a distinct domain of non-verbal knowledge but shares certain cognitive organisational features with other brain knowledge systems. Within the domain of music knowledge, dissociable cognitive mechanisms process knowledge derived from physical sources and the knowledge of abstract musical entities. Absolute pitch may be preserved after extensive left anterior temporal lobe damage (Zatorre, 1989), and the literature suggests perhaps that musical pitch may constitute a privileged route to naming in semantic dementia. Voxel-based morphometry of magnetic resonance brain images have showed that the recognition of famous tunes correlated with the degree of right anterior temporal lobe atrophy, particularly in the temporal pole, and the research background of this is interesting (e.g. Hsieh *et al.*, 2011).

Music may encourage not only autobiographical memory recall but also cognitive performance in category fluency (Thompson *et al.*, 2005). This study suggests that music improves both memory access and speech content and fluency. Listening to music, in particular popular songs, can stimulate memory by evoking autobiographical events. Musical semantic knowledge of a popular song seems to be relatively well preserved in patients with dementia of the Alzheimer type in the mild or moderate stages, and seems to be associated with a relatively well-preserved capacity of access to autobiographical memories. Results from Basaglia-Pappas and colleagues (2013) now suggest that music can enhance cognitive performance and can be used for reminiscence therapy. Emotional events often attain a privileged status in memory (LaBar and Cabeza, 2006).

There are several reasons to suspect that the medial prefrontal cortex (MPFC) might support the integration of memories, emotions and music. Meta-analyses of autobiographical memory retrieval tasks indicate MPFC involvement (Svoboda, McKinnon and Levine, 2006), and, more generally, the MPFC is engaged by judgments regarding self-relevance and affect (Ochsner *et al.*, 2004). The consistent finding is that musical memory is often surprisingly well-preserved in dementia of the Alzheimer type (Vanstone and Cuddy, 2010); this might be consistent with a crucial role for the caudal anterior cingulate and the ventral pre-supplementary motor area in the neural encoding of long-known as compared with recently known and unknown music (Jacobsen *et al.*, 2015).

Holland and Kensinger (2010) have recently discussed how findings from the clinical literature (e.g. regarding depression) and the social psychology literature (e.g. on emotion regulation) might inform future investigations of the interplay between the emotions experienced at the time of retrieval and the memories recalled, and they present ideas for future research in this domain. As beautifully explained by Salimpoor and colleagues (2009), the conundrum lies in the fact that there are no direct functional similarities between music and other pleasure-producing stimuli: it has no clearly established biological value (cf. food, love and sex), no tangible basis (cf. pharmacological drugs and monetary rewards) and no known addictive properties (cf. gambling and nicotine). It is reported that Freud and Nabokov seemed incapable of receiving any pleasure at all from music (see, for example, the brilliant *Musicophilia* by Oliver Sacks, 2011). Music reliably evokes strong physiological as well as cognitive emotional responses (Balteş *et al.*, 2011; Khalfa *et al.*, 2002), and these responses have been linked to a distributed cortico-subcortical brain network that mediates biological drives and rewards and the evaluation of emotional and social signals more generally (Peretz and Zatorre, 2005). However, the neurobiological role of music and the reasons these organised abstract sounds should hold such appeal for our species remain elusive (Mithen, 2005; Warren, 2008). One prominent theory is that music asserts its effects through influencing emotions (Meyer, 1956). It follows from this that music may evoke or enhance emotions, and that emotion in itself could be rewarding. The connection between emotional arousal and sympathetic nervous system activity has been well established (Ekman, Levenson and Friesen, 1983).

'Musicophilia'

As argued by Fletcher, Clark and Warren (2014), as an abstract stimulus, music is ideally suited to probe interactions between reward, affective and cortical information processing circuitry (Salimpoor *et al.*, 2013). Abnormally enhanced appreciation of music or 'musicophilia', reflected in increased listening to music, craving for music and/or willingness to listen to music even at the expense of other daily-life activities, may rarely signal brain disease: examples include neurodevelopmental disorders such as Williams syndrome (Martens, Reutens and Wilson, 2010), head trauma (Sacks, 2011), stroke (Jacome, 1984), temporal lobe epilepsy on anticonvulsant therapy (Rohrer, Smith and Warren, 2006) and focal degenerations, particularly involving the temporal lobes (Hailstone, Omar and Warren, 2009). Fletcher and colleagues (2013) found that musicophilia was more commonly associated with the syndrome of semantic dementia (SD; associated with focal anteromedial temporal lobe and inferior frontal lobe atrophy) than behavioural variant frontotemporal dementia (bvFTD).

Is there an evidence base for 'music therapy'?

Tanaka, Nogawa and Tanaka (2012) discussed the most effective music for Japanese persons living with dementia, using Japanese music. They proposed two hypotheses: (1) effective brain rehabilitation will be represented by increased activity throughout the prefrontal lobe after or during music therapy; and (2) music therapy with Japanese music will be more effective for Japanese patients than classical music. Recent clinical studies, namely in functional neuroimaging, have been able to evidence the favourable role of music therapy in the management of dementia of the Alzheimer type (Koger, Chapin and Brotons, 1999). Music-based therapy corresponds to two fundamental methods: a 'receptive' listening-based method and an 'active' method, based on playing musical instruments. Music therapy was defined by Munro and Mount (1978) as 'the controlled use of music, its elements and their influences on the human being to aid in the physiologic, psychologic and emotional integration of the individual during the treatment of an illness or disability' (p.1033).

Guétin and colleagues (2009) helpfully reported on a single-centre, comparative, controlled, randomised study, with blinded assessment of its results. The duration of follow-up was 24 weeks. Results from this study confirm the valuable effect of music therapy on anxiety and depression in patients with mild to moderate dementia of the Alzheimer type. One of the challenges in caring for people with dementia is organising stimulating activities. Zgola (1987) argues that the most successful programmes, both in adult day care and in residential care, have found that activities replacing skills that have been lost support positive roles and make success possible. A stimulating environment can help people with dementia by diverting attention from loss and illness. Over a decade ago Topo and colleagues (2004) found that multimedia products can be used in dementia care if support is available and the design of the product takes into account the user requirements of people with dementia.

In the 'Music therapy and dementia' workshop at the Alzheimer Europe conference in Malta (2013), Simone Willig presented 'A lot of things work better with music'. Willig trained at the University of Applied Sciences and has musically accompanied people with dementia for 15 years. With her colleague Silke Kammer, she is the author of the influential book *Mit Musik geht vieles besser: Der Königsweg in der Pflege bei Menschen mit Demenz* (2012; translated as 'A Lot of Things Work Better with Music: The Royal Road to People with Dementia'). The beginning of Willig's poster reads as follows:

> During recent years, music therapy has become an important part of the psycho-social services provided for people with dementia connecting to the encounters. Often serving as a different kind of language, music assists both in establishing contact with other people, and with one's own emotions and body. Music has the ability to build a bridge to a person's past and cultural origin and to promote a sense of belonging and a lasting feeling of security. (Willig, 2013, reproduced by kind permission)

Silke Kammer is a professional in music therapy from Bad Nauheim and Frankfurt am Main in Germany. She works with older people and people living well with dementia and other long-term neurological conditions. Kammer (2014) argues that in everyday life one can add quality to encounters with people with dementia by singing songs according to the situation. In her poster for the Alzheimer Europe conference held in Glasgow in 2014, Kammer argued that adding a 'simple catchy melody through a little song' can make events more meaningful. In terms of the bookcase analogy referred to in Chapter 15 on the reminiscence of sporting memories, it is as if Kammer is deliberating adding an emotional 'tag' to memories to give them more resilience in the memory databank of a person living well with dementia.

I previously introduced the concept of relationship-centred care in Chapter 7. Camic, Myferi Williams and Meeten (2011) conducted a useful study of ten people living with dementia and their family carers who participated in a Singing Together Group for ten weeks. It is argued by the authors that, in relation to Nolan's Senses Framework (see Chapter 7), it is clear from the interview responses that many of the 'senses' were met with the community singing group. The atmosphere of the group and personal characteristics of the music facilitator made people feel safe (sense of security) and 'valued'. Participants were immediately able to have a 'sense of purpose' and 'belonging', and the opportunity for new learning gave them a 'sense of fulfilment'. By connecting to old familiar songs, people were able to reminisce about their past working.

Conclusion

It is beginning to become clear that art, music and creativity can be 'unlocked' in some people living with dementia. This is an exciting phenomenon, and one that many people will find inspiring, especially as it contradicts all the negativity about dementia portrayed in the media. We should not be afraid of things even though we do not understand the cognitive neuroscience or cognitive neurology behind them. As a further example of people living with dementia having emotions unlocked, I now turn to sporting memories in Chapter 15. This award-winning initiative is fascinating.

References

Amabile, T.M. (1993) What does a theory of creativity require? Psychological Inquiry, 4, 2, 179–237.

Amaducci, L., Grassi, E. and Boller, F. (2002) Maurice Ravel and right-hemisphere musical creativity: influence of disease on his last musical works? European Journal of Neurology, 9, 1, 75–82.

American Psychiatric Association (2000) Diagnostic and Statistical Manual of Mental Disorders, 4th edition. Washington, DC: American Psychiatric Association.

Balteş, F.R., Avram, J., Miclea, M. and Miu, A.C. (2011) Emotions induced by operatic music: psychophysiological effects of music, plot, and acting: a scientist's tribute to Maria Callas. Brain and Cognition, 76, 1, 146–57.

Basaglia-Pappas, S., Laterza, M., Borg, C., Richard-Mornas, A., Favre, E. and Thomas-Antérion, C. (2013) Exploration of verbal and non-verbal semantic knowledge and autobiographical memories starting from popular songs in Alzheimer's disease. International Psychogeriatrics, 25, 5, 785–95.

Basso, A. (1993) Amusia. In F. Boller and J. Grafman (eds) Handbook of Neuropsychology, Vol. 8. Amsterdam: Elsevier.

Basso, A. and Capitani, E. (1985) Spared musical abilities in a conductor with global aphasia and ideomotor apraxia. Journal of Neurology, Neurosurgery and Psychiatry, 48, 407–12.

Beard, R. (2012) Art therapies and dementia care: a systematic review. Dementia: The International Journal of Social Research and Practice, 11, 5, 636–56.

Blood, A.J. and Zatorre, R.J. (2001) Intensely pleasurable responses to music correlate with activity in brain regions implicated in reward and emotion. Proceedings of the National Academy of Sciences of the USA, 98, 20, 11818–23.

Blood, A.J., Zatorre, R.J., Bermudez, P. and Evans, A.C. (1999) Emotional responses to pleasant and unpleasant music correlate with activity in paralimbic brain regions. Nature Neuroscience, 2, 4, 382–7.

Brown, R. and Kulik, J. (1977) Flashbulb memories. Cognition, 5, 73–99.

Budrys, V., Skullerud, K., Petroska, D., Lengveniene, J. and Kaubrys, G. (2007) Dementia and art: neuronal intermediate filament inclusion disease and dissolution of artistic creativity. European Neurology, 57, 3, 137–44.

Caldwell, C.E. (2014) The mind's eye. Journal of Neurology, Neurosurgery and Psychiatry, 85, 10, 1064.

Camic, P.M., Myferi Williams, C. and Meeten, F. (2013) Does a 'Singing Together Group' improve the quality of life of people with a dementia and their carers? A pilot evaluation study. Dementia, 12, 1, 157–76.

Chakravarty, A. (2010) The creative brain: revisiting concepts. Medical Hypotheses, 74, 606–12.

Chakravarty, A. (2011) De novo development of artistic creativity in Alzheimer's disease. Annals of Indian Academy of Neurology, 14, 4, 291–4.

Crutch, S.J. and Rossor, M.N. (2006) Artistic changes in Alzheimer's disease. International Review of Neurobiology, 74, 147–61.

Crutch, S.J., Isaacs, R. and Rossor, M.N. (2001) Some workmen can blame their tools: artistic change in an individual with Alzheimer's disease. Lancet, 357, 9274, 2129–33.

Cummings, J.L. and Zarit, J.M. (1987) Alzheimer's disease in an artist. Journal of the American Medical Association, 258, 19, 2731–4.

Ebersbach, G. (2003) An artist's view of drug-induced hallucinosis. Movement Disorders, 18, 833–4.
Ekman, P., Levenson, R. and Friesen, W.V. (1983) Autonomic nervous system activity distinguishes among emotions. Science, 221, 1208–10.
El-Murad, J. and West, D.G. (2004) The definition of creativity and measurement of creativity: what do we know? Journal of Advertising Research, June 2004, 188–201.
Fitch, W.T. (2013) Rhythmic cognition in humans and animals: distinguishing meter and pulse perception. Frontiers in Systems Neuroscience, 7, 68.
Fletcher, P.D., Clark, C.N. and Warren, J.D. (2014) Music, reward and frontotemporal dementia. Brain, 137, 10, e300.
Fletcher, P.D., Downey, L.E., Witoonpanich, P. and Warren, J.D. (2013) The brain basis of musicophilia: evidence from frontotemporal lobar degeneration. Frontiers in Psychology, 4, 347.
Gordon, N. (2005) Unexpected development of artistic talents. Postgraduate Medical Journal, 81, 962, 753–5.
Guétin, S., Portet, F., Picot, M.C., Pommié, C. *et al.* (2009) Effect of music therapy on anxiety and depression in patients with Alzheimer's type dementia: randomised, controlled study. Dementia and Geriatric Cognitive Disorders, 28, 1, 36–46.
Hailstone, J.C., Omar, R. and Warren, J.D. (2009) Relatively preserved knowledge of music in semantic dementia. Journal of Neurology, Neurosurgery and Psychiatry, 80, 808–9.
Holland, A.C. and Kensinger, E.A. (2010) Emotion and autobiographical memory. Physics of Life Reviews, 7, 1, 88–131.
Hsieh, S., Hornberger, M., Piguet, O. and Hodges, J.R. (2011) Neural basis of music knowledge: evidence from the dementias. Brain, 134, 9, 2523–34.
Jacobsen, J.H., Stelzer, J., Fritz, T.H., Chételat, G., La Joie, R. and Turner, R. (2015) Why musical memory can be preserved in advanced Alzheimer's disease. Brain. pii: awv135.
Jacome, D.E. (1984) Aphasia with elation, hypermusia, musicophilia and compulsive whistling. Journal of Neurology, Neurosurgery and Psychiatry, 47, 308–10.
Josephson, B.R., Singer, J.A. and Salovey, P. (1996) Mood regulation and memory: repairing sad moods with happy memories. Cognition and Emotion, 10, 437–44.
Kammer, S. (2014) PO36. Music is the key – it is? Programme of the 24th Alzheimer Europe Conference, 20–22 October, Glasgow. Available at www.alzheimer-europe.org/Conferences/Previous-conferences/2014-Glasgow/Detailed-Programme-abstracts-and-presentations/(language)/eng-GB (accessed 11 February 2015).
Kapur, N. (1996) Paradoxical functional facilitation in brain-behaviour research: a critical review. Brain, 119, 1775–90.
Kaufman, G. (2013) What to measure? A new look at the concept of creativity. Scandinavian Journal of Educational Research, 47, 3, 235–51.
Khalfa, S., Isabelle, P., Jean-Pierre, B. and Manon, R. (2002) Event-related skin conductance responses to musical emotions in humans. Neuroscience Letters, 328, 2, 145–9.
Killick, J. and Craig, C. (2012) Creativity and Communication in Persons with Dementia: A Practical Guide. London: Jessica Kingsley Publishers.
King, N. and Anderson, N. (1990) Innovation in Working Groups. In M.A. West and J.L. Farr (eds) Innovation and Creativity at Work. New York, NY: J. Wiley and Sons.
Kirk, A. and Kertesz, A. (1991) On drawing impairment in Alzheimer's disease. Archives of Neurology, 48, 73–7.
Koger, S.M., Chapin, K. and Brotons, M. (1999) Is music therapy an effective intervention for dementia? A meta-analytic review of literature. Journal of Music Therapy, 36, 2–15.
LaBar, K.S. and Cabeza, R. (2006) Cognitive neuroscience of emotional memory. Nature Reviews Neuroscience, 7, 1, 54–64.
Magnus, R. and Laeng, B. (2006) Drawing on either side of the brain. Laterality, 11, 71–89.

Marr, D. (1982) Vision. San Francisco, CA: Freeman.
Martens, M.A., Reutens, D.C. and Wilson, S.J. (2010) Auditory cortical volumes and musical ability in Williams syndrome. Neuropsychologia, 48, 9, 2602–9.
Matsuzawa, T. (1991) Chimpanzee Mind. Tokyo: Iwatani Shoten.
Meyer, L.B. (1956) Emotion and Meaning in Music. Chicago, IL: University of Chicago Press.
Miller, B.L., Boone, K., Cummings, J.L., Read, S.L. and Mishkin, F. (2000) Functional correlates of musical and visual ability in frontotemporal dementia. British Journal of Psychiatry, 176, 458–63.
Miller, B.L., Cummings, J., Mishkin, F., Boone, K. *et al.* (1998) Emergence of artistic talent in frontotemporal dementia. Neurology, 51, 4, 978–82.
Mithen, S.J. (2005) The Singing Neanderthals: The Origins of Music, Language, Mind and Body. Cambridge, MA: Harvard University Press.
Morriss-Kay, G.M. (2010) The evolution of human artistic creativity. Journal of Anatomy, 216, 158–76.
Munro, S. and Mount, B. (1978) Music therapy in palliative care. Canadian Medical Association Journal, 119, 1029–34.
Nickerson, R.S. (1999) Enhancing Creativity. In R. Sternberg (ed.) Handbook of Creativity. Cambridge: Cambridge University Press.
Ochsner, K.N., Knierim, K., Ludlow, D.H., Hanelin, J. *et al.* (2004) Reflecting upon feelings: an fMRI study of neural systems supporting the attribution of emotion to self and other. Journal of Cognitive Neuroscience, 16, 1746–72.
Omar, R., Hailstone, J.C., Warren, J.E., Crutch, S.J. and Warren, J.D. (2010) The cognitive organisation of music knowledge: a clinical analysis. Brain, 133, 4, 1200–13.
Panksepp, J. (1995) The emotional sources of 'chills' induced by music. Music Perception, 13, 171–207.
Peretz, I. and Zatorre, R.J. (2005) Brain organisation for music processing. Annual Review of Psychology, 56, 89–114.
Piercy, M., Hecaen, H. and de Ajuriaguerra, J. (1960) Constructional apraxia associated with unilateral cerebral lesions–left and right sided cases compared. Brain, 83, 225–42.
Ramachandran, V.S. and Hirstein, W. (1999) The science of art: a neurological theory of aesthetic experience. Journal of Consciousness Studies, 6, 6–7, 15–51.
Rankin, K.P., Liu, A.A., Howard, S., Slama, H. *et al.* (2007) A case-controlled study of altered visual art production in Alzheimer's and FTLD. Cognitive and Behavioral Neurology, 20, 1, 48–61.
Rohrer, J.D., Smith, S.J. and Warren, J.D. (2006) Craving for music after treatment for partial epilepsy. Epilepsia, 47, 5, 939–40.
Rubin, D.C. and Kozin, M. (1984) Vivid memories. Cognition, 16, 1, 81–95.
Sacks, O. (2011) Musicophilia: Tales of Music and the Brain. London: Picador.
Sahlas, D.J. (2003) Dementia with Lewy bodies and the neurobehavioural decline of Mervyn Peake. Archives of Neurology, 60, 889–92.
Salimpoor, V.N., Benovoy, M., Longo, G., Cooperstock, J.R. and Zatorre, R.J. (2009) The rewarding aspects of music listening are related to degree of emotional arousal. PLoS One, 4, 10, e7487.
Salimpoor, V.N., van den Bosch, I., Kovacevic, N., McIntosh, A.R., Dagher, A. and Zatorre, R.J. (2013) Interactions between the nucleus accumbens and auditory cortices predict music reward value. Science, 340, 216–19.
Scottish Development Centre for Mental Health/Scottish Government (2007) Developing Social Prescribing and Community Referrals for Mental Health in Scotland (November). Available at www.scotland.gov.uk/Resource/Doc/924/0054752.pdf (accessed 6 December 2014).
Seeley, W.W., Matthews, B.R., Crawford, R.K., Gorno-Tempini, M.L. *et al.* (2008) Unravelling Boléro: progressive aphasia, transmodal creativity and the right posterior neocortex. Brain, 131 (Pt 1), 39–49.

Signoret, J.L., Van Eeckhout, P., Poncet, M. and Castaigne, P. (1987) Aphasie sans amusie chez un organiste aveugle [Aphasia without amusia in a blind organist]. Revue Neurologique (Paris), 143, 172–81.

Snyder, A.W., Mulcahy, E., Taylor, J.L., Mitchell, D.J., Sachdev, P. and Gandevia, S.C. (2003) Savant-like skills exposed in normal people by suppressing the left fronto-temporal lobe. Journal of Integrative Neuroscience, 2, 149–58.

Svoboda, E., McKinnon, M.C. and Levine, B. (2006) The functional neuroanatomy of autobiographical memory: a meta-analysis. Neuropsychologia, 44, 2189–208.

Takahata, K., Saito, F., Muramatsu, T., Yamada, M. *et al.* (2014) Emergence of realism: enhanced visual artistry and high accuracy of visual numerosity representation after left prefrontal damage. Neuropsychologia, 57, 38–49.

Tanaka, Y., Nogawa, H. and Tanaka, H. (2012) Music therapy with ethnic music for dementia patients. International Journal of Gerontology, 6, 247–57.

Thompson, R.G., Moulin, C.J.A., Hayre, S. and Jones, R.W. (2005) Music enhances category fluency in healthy older adults and Alzheimer's disease patients. Experimental Aging Research, 31, 91–9.

Topo, P., Mäki, O., Saarinkalle, K., Clarke, N. *et al.* (2004) Assessment of a music-based multimedia program for people with dementia. Dementia, 3, 3, 33–50.

University of Sheffield (2014) 'We're not finished' – South Yorkshire Dementia Creative Arts Exhibitions 2009–2014. Collated by David Reid and Natasha Wilson, School of Nursing and Midwifery, University of Sheffield. Available at www.sheffield.ac.uk/polopoly_fs/1.402827!/file/Photobook_SYDCAE.pdf (accessed 23 February 2015).

Vanstone, A.D. and Cuddy, L.L. (2010) Musical memory in Alzheimer disease. Neuropsychological, Development and Cognition B: Aging, Neuropsychology and Cognition 17, 1, 108–28.

Warren, J. (2008) Book review: another musical mystery tour. Brain, 131, 890–4.

Willig, S. (2013) P1.4.1. A lot of things work better with music: Music therapy and dementia, Poster presented at the New Psychological Interventions for Alzheimer Europe Conference 2013, Malta. Available at www.alzheimer-europe.org/Media/Files/7.-Conferences/2013-Malta/P14.1-Simone-Willig (accessed 11 February 2015).

Willig, S. and Kammer, S. (2012) Mit Musik geht vieles besser: Der Königsweg in der Pflege bei Menschen mit Demenz [A Lot of Things Work Better with Music: The Royal Road to People with Dementia). Hannover: Vincentz Network.

Zatorre, R.J. (1989) Intact absolute pitch ability after left temporal lobectomy. Cortex, 25, 567–80.

Zgola, J.M. (1987) Doing Things: A Guide to Programming Activities for Persons with Alzheimer's Disease and Related Disorders. Baltimore, MD: Johns Hopkins University Press.

Chapter 15

EXPLAINING THE TRIGGERING OF SPORTING MEMORIES IN PEOPLE LIVING BETTER WITH DEMENTIA

'Without football, my life is worth nothing.'

Cristiano Ronaldo (b. 1985)

Introduction

A prominent message relating to the notion that it is possible to live well with dementia is that, with careful attention, a person living with dementia might be able to focus on what he or she can do, rather than what he or she has difficulty with. Of course, trying to persevere at anything that is difficult can be inherently demoralising for the best of us. That's why to put at ease a person living with dementia of the Alzheimer type, where very old memories can be very well preserved compared with a memory of what was done yesterday, it is easier to engage in conversation about things way in the past. Tony Jameson Allen of the

Sporting Memories Network often remarks that football is fully pervasive in English culture; Tony might possibly be right.

Types of memory

Declarative memory is recall of factual information such as dates, words, faces, events and concepts. Procedural memory is recall of how to do things such as riding a bike.

There are two types of declarative memory: semantic and episodic. Semantic memory is recall of general facts, while episodic memory is recall of personal facts. Remembering the capital of France and the rules for playing football uses semantic memory. Remembering what happened in each game of the World Series 2014 uses episodic memory. Declarative memory can be emotional or non-emotional.

This is shown schematically in Figure 15.1. See Tulving (1985) for a basic discussion of this construct.

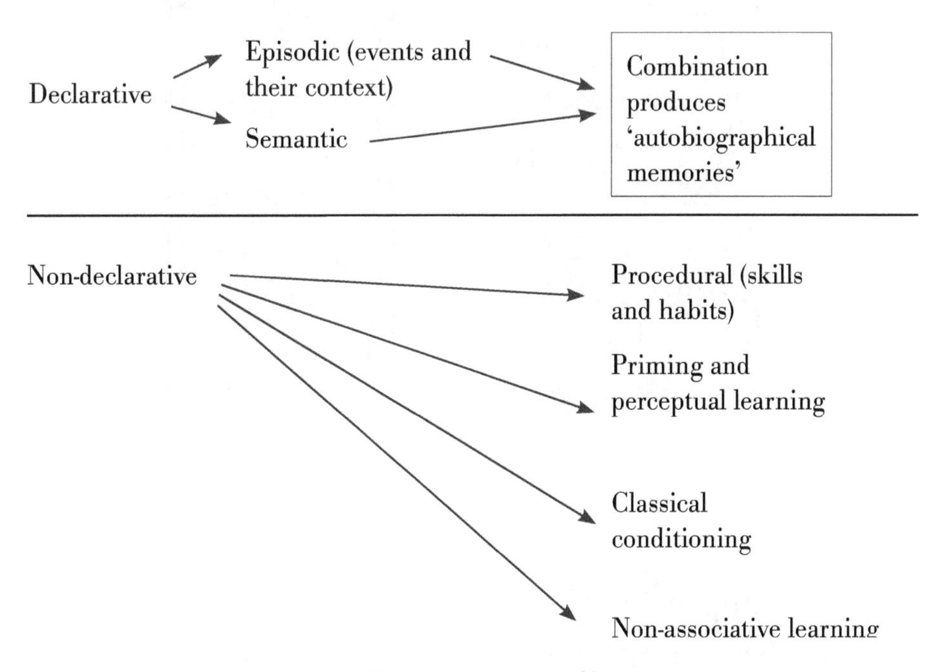

Figure 15.1 The neuroscience of long-term memory

This diagram is partly based on Figure 1 from Squire (2004) depicting a taxonomy of mammalian long-term memory systems. The taxonomy lists the brain structures thought to be especially important for each form of declarative and nondeclarative memory. This diagram, however, has been modified to reflect that there exists a complicated relationship emerging in cognitive neuroscience between episodic and autobiographical memory (Gilboa, 2004).

SOURCE: ADAPTED FROM GILBOA, 2004; SQUIRE, 2004

An illustration of the two bookcases for facts and emotional memories comprising the 'bookcase analogy' is shown in Figure 15.2. These pictures are intended to depict the analogy for when a person develops dementia of the Alzheimer type in its early stages. Whilst the bookcase made of balsa wood is unsteady, with books representing earliest memories liable to fall off the top shelf, the bookcase containing emotional memories, made of solid oak, is pretty sturdy. This is the analogy used in one of the activities of the Dementia Friends programme currently underway in England. For a fuller description of a comparable 'bookcase analogy' please refer to Jones (2004).

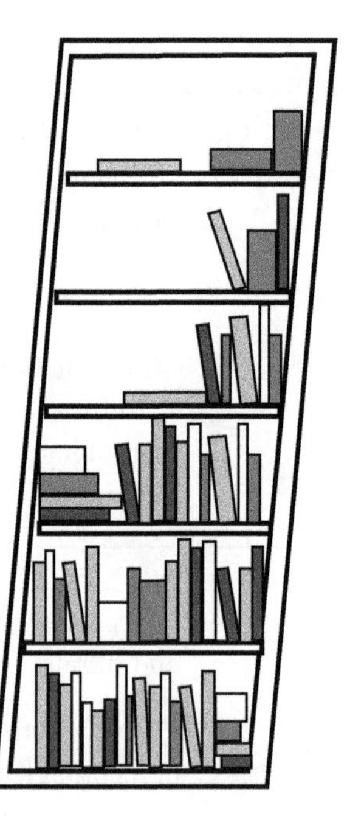

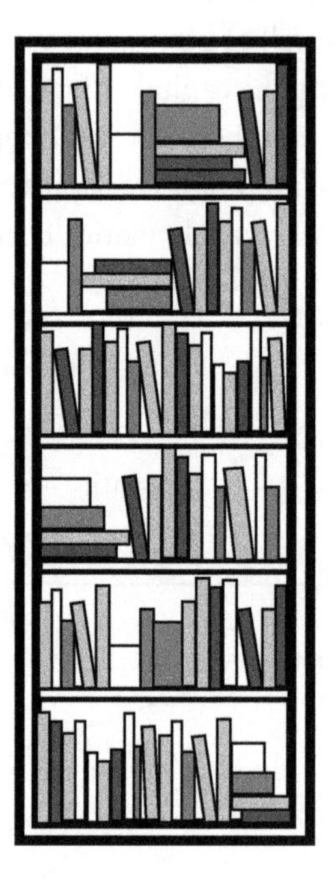

Figure 15.2 The bookcase analogy

'Picking off certain networks'

While there is more to a person living with dementia than the clinical diagnosis, the clinical diagnosis – if correct – does give very good clues normally as to which parts of a distributed neuronal network might be affected early on in disease. Whilst most attention has been given to pharmacological interventions, there is increasing recognition that psychosocial interventions may have comparable value, and may be preferable in some contexts – for example, where medication may be ineffective or have negative side effects (Woods *et al.*, 2009).

Anecdotal and empirical evidence suggests that emotionally important events hold a special place in memory, where they are bestowed with a unique subjective vivid character (Todd *et al.*, 2012). The successful retrieval of information from long-term memory requires the integrated activity of multiple brain regions. And the information does not only come from post-mortem studies. Current proposals, based primarily on findings from the human lesion literature, have focused on the role of the hippocampus and the temporofrontal region in long-term memory retrieval (Alvarez and Squire, 1994; Kroll *et al.*, 1997; Nadel and Moscovitch, 1997). The specific neural system engaged varies with the nature of the stimuli examined (verbal or non-verbal), the time frame of initial acquisition (recent or remote) and the type of information retrieved from long-term memory (personal or public). The amnesic syndrome has been the subject of much interest in neuropsychology because of what it might reveal about the organisation and neurological foundations of normal memory (Cohen and Squire, 1981).

Meanwhile, evidence from semantic dementia – and a converging range of sources – leads to a synthesis that the ventral and inferolateral parts of the anterior part of the temporal lobe are pivotal for the storage of semantic knowledge (e.g. Binney *et al.*, 2010).

In this chapter, I wish to discuss a curious phenomenon of how some football fans living with dementia appear to become very energised by 'sporting memories'. And the incredible thing is that this is all to be expected from an understanding of how the human brain and mind goes about its business.

Introduction to football memories

The Sporting Memories Network was established to promote and develop the use of sporting memories to improve the wellbeing of people through conversation and reminiscence.

'Bill's story' (Sporting Memories Network, n.d.) is a good introductory film to this unique initiative, only lasting a few minutes. Little was known about Bill Corbett's sporting prowess as a fine footballer playing for Celtic. It became known through participation in the memory group that his personal history included playing for Scotland. So he became 'unlocked' as a person. This group simply used photographs from his era of playing football. In a sporting memories group, the group leader might show an extensive range of memorabilia, including visual cues, such as photographs of players, advertisements from the grounds, cigarette and bubblegum cards, old boots and knitted woollen jerseys, and olfactory cues, such as the smells of liniment oil and pipe tobacco. The sessions can take place in care homes or in people's own homes. The recall is very detailed, specific to decades such as the 1930s and 1940s, including the names of the players and even the weather. The members of the group become happier and engage with each other socially.

The cognitive and behavioural processes involved in reactivating a football memory are especially interesting, given what we know about their putative neural substrates. Reactivating a 'football memory' is indeed a brilliant example of taking advantage of what a person living with dementia can do, rather than what he or she cannot do. Box 15.1 shows the framework for the types of questions the human brain will unwittingly consider in 'processing' a football memory.

Box 15.1 How will the brain approach a football memory?

1. Does the sports fan live with any type of dementia?
2. Is the picture triggering the memory recent or old?
3. Does the sports fan recognise any faces in the picture?
4. Does the picture trigger some memory relating to his or her own past?
5. Is the memory meaningful for that particular person?
6. Does the memory have any 'emotional gist', for example happiness or sorrow?
7. Are there any 'clues' to help, for example the smell of Bovril?

Neural substrates for visual football memories

Memories for the past

Some time last century, an amazing advance in understanding the cognitive neurology of memory was made. In 1957, William Scoville and Brenda Milner published the now-famous case of patient H.M. Scoville surgically removed large parts of the medial temporal lobe (including the bilateral hippocampi) in H.M., to relieve him from intractable epilepsy. This is the part of the brain quite close to the ear. The surgery was successful in controlling his epilepsy; however, it also elucidated that the hippocampus is essential for the formation of new memory traces (Scoville and Milner, 1957). The brain may handle this problem by temporarily storing as much information as possible, allowing associations that prove to be the most relevant to sort themselves out over time (Burnham, 1903, cited in Insel and Takehara-Nishiuchi, 2013).

Emotional arousal

Many of us have been spectators of football matches where emotions have run high. Although not quite a life-or-death experience, this emotional aspect can lead us to have a vivid recollection of what we were doing at the time. Emotions are associated with the mutually enhancing effects of sympathetic arousal (Anderson, Wais and Gabrieli, 2006) and altered attention (Schmitz, De Rosa and Anderson, 2009), which result in facilitated encoding of emotional events (De Martino *et al.*, 2009). It is well established that emotional events are more easily detected under impoverished conditions where attentional load is taxed (Soares and Ohman, 1993) or stimuli are presented at the threshold of awareness (Nielsen and Sarason, 1981). As reviewed in Phelps (2004), it has to be conceded that one of the primary advances in the study of memory over the past half-century is the growing recognition that there are multiple memory systems that are governed by distinct and interacting neural substrates. Investigations examining the influence of emotion on memory have primarily focused on two medial temporal lobe memory systems.

The first is linked to the amygdala and is more or less specialised for the processing of emotion. The hallmark of this memory system is that it is crucial for the acquisition and expression of fear conditioning, in which a neutral stimulus acquires aversive properties by virtue of being paired with an aversive event. The second is linked to the hippocampal complex and is necessary for declarative or episodic memory. This memory system can be thought of as a primary memory system in humans, in that it governs the function most often referred to as 'memory' – that is, the recollection of events at will.

Early theories that proposed to explain the neuropsychological basis of emotion perception (Cannon, 1929; James, 1884) emphasised the importance of feedback from bodily responses to an emotionally salient stimulus in determining the nature and extent of emotional feeling, but they did not distinguish between the identification of the emotive stimulus and the affective state produced in response to this. Various researchers (e.g. Clore and Ortony, 2000) have emphasised that appraisal or identification of stimulus salience, which may occur with or without conscious awareness, precedes the generation of emotional response.

Figure 15.3 shows a process map of how an emotion might be produced in response to a stimulus. This diagram is adapted from Phillips *et al.* (2003). The main processes important for emotion perception are: (1) appraisal and identification of the emotional significance of the stimulus; (2) production of a specific affective state and behaviour in response to the stimulus; and (3) regulation of the affective state and emotional behaviour, which may involve an inhibition or modulation of processes 1 and 2, so that the affective state, emotional experience and behaviours generated are contextually appropriate.

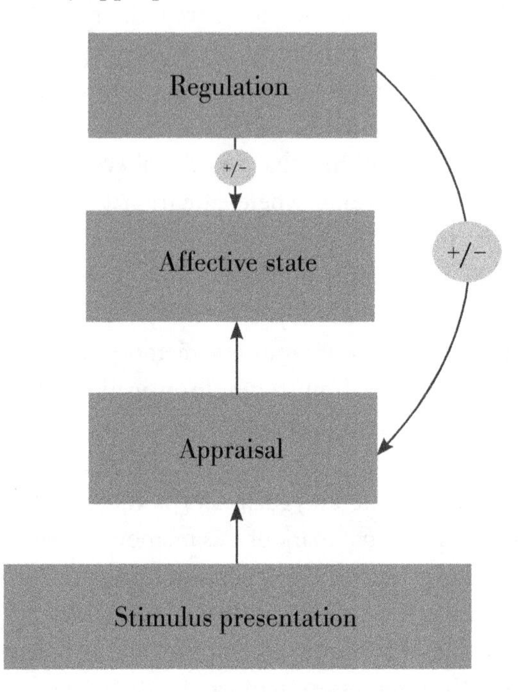

Figure 15.3 How an emotion might be produced in response to a stimulus
Source: Adapted from Phillips et al., 2003 (p.505)

A gradient for memories

But not all memories are the same. In dementia of the Alzheimer type, as I have already described, older memories can be quite well preserved compared with the memory from yesterday. In humans, damage limited to the hippocampus produces temporally graded retrograde amnesia, with relative sparing of remote memory compared with recent memory. This observation forms the cornerstone of the idea that as memories mature they are reorganised in a time-dependent manner. In the late part of the nineteenth century, the French psychologist Theodule Ribot

(1882) described how memory loss after brain insult was often related to the age of the memory: the effect on more recent memories was typically greater than that on older (or more remote) memories. The dissociation has become known as Ribot's law (or Ribot's gradient), and subsequent neuropsychological studies went on to establish a more precise relationship between the locus of brain damage and the gradient. Later studies of patients with more circumscribed lesions established that damage to the hippocampus, in particular, is responsible for this typical graded amnesia (Rempel-Clower *et al.*, 1996).

This observation forms the basis of the idea that memories are reorganised in a time-dependent manner. Within this general framework, the relative contributions of different brain regions may vary as a function of memory age. Accordingly, some regions may play important roles in the expression of newly formed (or recent) memory, but their contributions may fade over time. Conversely, other regions may play preferential roles in the expression of older (or remote) memories.

What happens when you get confronted by 'football memories'?

Memories of events evoking strong emotions, especially fear, selectively persist (Wagner *et al.*, 2006) because emotion enhances event-memory retention. The hippocampus is crucial in processing declarative and spatial long-term memory, whereas the amygdala drives emotion processing and emotional memory formation (LaBar and Cabeza, 2006). Whether or not emotion enhances event memory retention is controversial. By using photographs with affective valence as both encoding and recall stimuli, some authors have found that emotion accelerates episodic memory encoding (Bradley *et al.*, 1992). However, others speculate that emotion simply heightens the subjective sense of remembering, and that an increase in the subjective ratings of vividness, recollection and belief in accuracy does not indicate accurate memory (Sharot, Delgado and Phelps, 2004).

Overall, it appears that emotion can enhance memory accuracy, particularly for the fact that an event occurred, but emotion's impact on the sense of the vivid recollection of details exceeds its influence on memory for those details per se. In other words, emotion boosts memory accuracy to an extent, but it affects the subjective sense of recollection even more (Phelps and Sharot, 2008). Emotion's enhancement of the recollective experience – the subjective judgment of a memory's vividness and the rememberer's sense of confidence in it – is more robust and consistent than its enhancement of accuracy for objective details.

There is strong evidence in both humans and non-humans that the physiological changes that occur with arousal enhance the retention of events via the interaction of the amygdala and hippocampus. Such studies and others highlight the neural mechanisms by which emotion increases memory accuracy over time, at least for the occurrence of events (see Phelps, 2006, for a review).

There are currently few theories of retrograde amnesia, and a very detailed explanation of all of the current ones is far beyond the scope of the present chapter. Nevertheless, consolidation theory, which derives from nineteenth-century authors such as Ribot (1882), has more recently been popularised by Milner (1966) and Alvarez and Squire (1994). In its contemporary form, consolidation theory states that there is physiological consolidation of memories, associated with structural reallocation, such that the memories eventually become independent of the hippocampi and medial temporal lobes, and are thereby spared from the effects of medial temporal damage. Consolidation theory therefore predicts a temporal gradient (relative sparing of early memories) in retrograde amnesia, as has been found by Manns, Hopkins and Squire (2003). Furthermore, consolidation may be sensitive to 'runaway consolidation', a vicious circle in which one pattern becomes stronger through consolidation, becomes more likely to be consolidated in the next trial, and ends up monopolising all consolidation resources while crowding out other memories (Meeter, 2003).

The vital link to our past

The vital thing to note is that these memories are not divorced from us as people. They are intimately tagged in the timeline of our past. Autobiographical memories (ABM) of past experiences can often be elicited spontaneously; something we encounter in our environment or in our thoughts directly transports us back in time to mentally re-experience that one particular event (Berntsen and Hall, 2004). Other times, however, ABM retrieval requires much more effort: we have to actively search for a memory to answer some specific question about our past. ABM is undoubtedly a complex construct, generally taken to refer to memory for a personally experienced event that is imbued with a sense of recollection (Greenberg and Rubin, 2003). Episodic ABMs are typically emotionally laden (Piefke *et al.*, 2003), leaving durable and evocative memory traces (Berntsen and Rubin, 2002), often with a rich level of contextual sensory-perceptual details (Conway *et al.*, 2003).

Neuroimaging studies have pointed towards a large neural network subtending ABM retrieval including the hippocampus, parahippocampal gyrus, lateral temporal cortices, posterior parietal cortex, retrosplenial cortex, posterior cingulate cortex, precuneus, thalamus and the medial prefrontal cortex (Maguire, 2001). While, in most instances, the end goal of this generative retrieval process is the recovery of a specific ABM, the search process usually involves the retrieval of conceptual autobiographical knowledge and generic events prior to accessing the specific event that fulfils the search criteria (Graham *et al.*, 2003; Haque and Conway, 2001). Behavioural studies have revealed that general events are typically retrieved prior to the retrieval of specific episodic events (Haque and Conway, 2001). Thus, it has been predicted that brain regions supporting retrieval of generic ABMs, such as the lateral temporal cortex (Addis *et al.*, 2004; Graham *et al.*, 2003), would exhibit early activation.

'System-level memory consolidation theory' posits that the hippocampus initially links the neocortical representations, followed by a shift to a hippocampus-independent neocortical network. With consolidation, an increase in activity in the human subgenual ventromedial prefrontal cortex (vmPFC) has repeatedly been shown. Indeed, David Marr (1970) proposed that the hippocampus serves as a simple moment-by-moment capturing system, while the neocortex stores information in a structured way. The subgenual vmPFC is likely to be a critical brain region for the integration of information, and therefore could play quite an important role in the reactivation of sporting memories in various types of dementia.

A proposed critical role of the subgenual prefrontal cortex is shown in Figure 15.4. The subgenual vmPFC receives input from the separate areas of the limbic system – the amygdala, the hippocampus and the ventral striatum. The information is integrated and weighted, and it is subsequently stored. The integrated representation is used to suppress irrelevant information in the limbic structures. Autobiographical memory encompasses our recollections of specific, personal events, and is related to the general memory for events. This is what makes understanding the neural substrates of reactivation of sporting memories fascinating. The emotional content of an experience can influence the way in which the event is remembered, and emotions and emotional goals experienced at the time of autobiographical retrieval can influence the information recalled (Holland and Kensinger, 2010). The subgenual part of the ventromedial prefrontal cortex is hypothesised to integrate separate representations of value in the ventral striatum and also from the hippocampus and amygdala (Nieuwenhuis and Takashima, 2011). This network involving reward-sensitive areas would explain the emotional and motivational effects on 'sporting memories'.

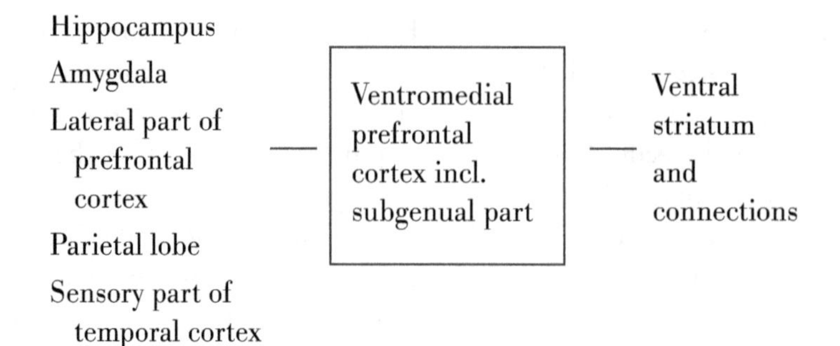

Figure 15.4 A critical role for the subgenual part of the prefrontal cortex in reactivating 'sporting memories'?

Source: Based on observations from Nieuwenhuis and Takashima, 2011; Holland and Kensinger, 2010

Only a few controlled studies have been carried out on autobiographical memory in the temporal or frontal variants of frontotemporal dementia (Hodges *et al.*, 1999; Neary *et al.*, 1998). Patients with behavioural variant frontotemporal dementia (bvFTD) were significantly impaired across all categories of contextual details, whereas patients with dementia of the Alzheimer type showed deficits for event and emotion/thoughts details only (Irish *et al.*, 2011). Curiously, since the anterior temporal lobe plays a well-known role in semantic memory, this may imply that remote ABM acquires a semantic nature, whereas recent memories remain episodic (Cermak, 1984).

A crucial aspect of the recollection of episodic memories is the concurrent retrieval of incidental 'contextual' information that is not task-relevant. For instance, the 'remember/know' procedure (Mandler, 1980; Tulving, 1985; Yonelinas *et al.*, 2001) operationalises episodic recollection ('remembering') in terms of the ability to retrieve incidental information concerning the external (time, place, etc.) or internal (current thoughts, feelings, etc.) context of the event in question. More generally, events are often embedded within a rich context of incidental associations to other autobiographical and semantic knowledge (e.g. Burgess and Shallice, 1996; Conway and Pleydell-Pearce, 2000; Levine *et al.*, 2004).

The importance of 'emotional gist'

Gist is an interesting concept. 'Gist' can be defined as global (overall) emotionality, whereby the scene can be rapidly identified as positive, negative or neutral without having to explore the individual (local) features of the scene. To take an example, a picture of the aftermath of the Twin Towers scene would hold a negative gist, whereby every scene feature would be negative and related to the overall 'story' – for example, buildings being demolished or aeroplanes crashing; there is not just one negative feature but an overall negative emotional valence (Humphrey, Underwood and Lambert, 2012). It is also possible that aversive, and potentially dangerous, stimuli are processed as more immediately salient for survival than positive stimuli that usually signal feeding, procreative or social opportunities (Liberzon *et al.*, 2003).

The special nature of faces

Cognitive psychologists have been interested in the special nature of faces because there is evidence that faces are somehow perceived differently to other patterned objects, and thus may represent a 'special' class of stimuli (Gauthier and Nelson, 2001). Farah (1996), among others, has suggested that face recognition differs from object recognition in that the former involves representing a face as a single, complex whole, whereas the latter typically involves decomposition into constituent elements. Faces represent the stimuli we rely on the most for social interaction. They inform us, amongst other things, about the identity, mood, gender, age, attractiveness, race and likely social friendliness of a person.

In the human lesion literature, the recognition and identification of famous faces has commonly been used to study the neural regions critical for retrieval of information from long-term memory (Greene and Hodges, 1996; Marslen-Wilson and Teuber, 1975; Warrington and James, 1967; Warrington and McCarthy, 1988). It is generally acknowledged that famous faces produce automatic retrieval of person-identity information from long-term memory (Bruce and Young, 1986; Burton, Bruce and Johnston, 1990). Thus, the comparison of famous and unfamiliar faces provides an opportunity to examine the neural systems activated when pre-existing semantic and biographical information is available for retrieval. Neuroimaging studies of memory for unfamiliar faces have demonstrated right hippocampal activation during encoding, but no hippocampal activity during subsequent recognition (e.g. Clark, Maisog and Haxby, 1998). Memory for unfamiliar faces has also produced frontal activation, although the side of activation has differed across studies. Haxby and colleagues (1996) found left frontal activation during encoding, whereas Kelley and colleagues (1998) observed increased right frontal activation.

But just because you recognise someone it does not necessarily mean you know who the person is. As Yovel and Paller (2004, p.789) inquire: 'Have you ever seen someone who looks familiar, while at the same time been unable to remember the circumstances of any previous meeting or anything else about the person?' This, as they describe, is a common example of a memory failure known as experiencing familiarity in the absence of recollection. It can occur when seeing someone in an atypical setting, as in George Mandler's (1980) classic example of seeing the butcher on the bus. The context of the bus provides none of the clues concerning the butcher's identity that are typically present when the butcher is encountered in the butcher's shop.

'The smell of Bovril' in aiding football memories

Visual memories do not operate in isolation.

One of the most profound questions for neuroscientists of all interests is why the human brain has exploded relatively in size, compared with its counterparts in the animal kingdom. Professor Horace Barlow, a previous chair in physiology at Cambridge, thought this was fundamental: for example, why the visual part of our brain – the visual cortex – was so substantially different to the film of the eye recording images in the fly's retina.

As described in an article entitled 'Perfumes aid dementia research' (Challis, 2014), smells can trigger powerful emotional memories from the past more effectively than other senses such as sight and sound, and smells – cut grass, baked bread or perfumes, for instance – can therefore be powerful memory stimulants for someone with dementia. These examples also point to brain regions which, early in phylogeny, were mainly engaged in odour (Brodal, 1947), but later on were necessary for processing emotions and memory. Even in human beings, it has been found that our first memories are strongly related to odour: Willander and Larsson (2006) presented odour, word and picture cues to elicit past memories from adults and found that the odour cues elicited mainly memories from the first decade of life, whereas the word and picture cues elicited mainly past events from the second decade of life.

The brain regions, initially (in phylogeny) relevant for odour processing, are subsumed under the heading 'limbic system' (Markowitsch, 1999) and are discussed as mediating between the phylogenetically old structures of the brain stem and the advanced structures of the neocortex (MacLean, 1970). Among them, the amygdala is necessary for a proper interpretation of the social and biological environment (LeDoux, 1998) and the hippocampal formation for the transfer of memory from short-term to long-term storage and possibly also for retrieval. Other limbic and paralimbic (Nauta, 1979) structures such as the septal nuclei and the medial and anterior thalamic nuclei support the emotional colourisation of memories and are nowadays seen as overlapping with the so-called default mode network, a system of structures active when the brain is at wakeful rest and not focused towards stimuli in the outer world (reviewed in Markowitsch, 2013).

Conclusion

In this chapter and in Chapter 14, I have provided examples of innovative approaches from art, music and 'football memories' which comprise an alternative to pharmacological treatments for dementia. This is an important thrust of my thesis. Enhancing wellbeing through such priorities must be a legitimate aim of dementia-friendly communities, and we are in desperate need of high-quality research with the aspiration of living better with dementia. I have also already described in detail one large systemic innovation to promote wellbeing – that is, whole-person care (Chapter 10). I now go back to components of large-scale transformation in the next two chapters of my book to promote living better with dementia. Chapter 16 is mainly about the use of antipsychotics in care homes, and Chapter 17 looks at 'radical' leadership challenges by people living well with dementia themselves.

References

Addis, D.R., Moscovitch, M., Crawley, A.P. and McAndrews, M.P. (2004) Recollective qualities modulate hippocampal activation during autobiographical memory retrieval. Hippocampus, 14, 752–62.

Alvarez, P. and Squire, L.R. (1994) Memory consolidation and the medial temporal lobe: a simple network model. Proceedings of the National Academy of Sciences of the USA, 91, 7041–5.

Anderson, A.K., Wais, P.E. and Gabrieli, J.D. (2006) Emotion enhances remembrance of neutral events past. Proceedings of the National Academy of Sciences of the USA, 103, 1599–604.

Berntsen, D. and Hall, N.M. (2004) The episodic nature of involuntary autobiographical memories. Memory and Cognition, 32, 789–803.

Berntsen, D. and Rubin, D.C. (2002) Emotionally charged autobiographical memories across the life span: the recall of happy, sad, traumatic and involuntary memories. Psychology and Aging, 17, 636–55.

Binney, R.J., Embleton, K.V., Jefferies, E., Parker, G.J. and Ralph, M.A. (2010) The ventral and inferolateral aspects of the anterior temporal lobe are crucial in semantic memory: evidence from a novel direct comparison of distortion-corrected fMRI, rTMS, and semantic dementia. Cerebral Cortex, 20, 11, 2728–38.

Bradley, M.M., Greenwald, M.K., Petry, M.C. and Lang, P.J. (1992) Remembering pictures: pleasure and arousal in memory. Journal of Experimental Psychology: Learning, Memory, and Cognition, 18, 379–90.

Brodal, A. (1947) The hippocampus and the sense of smell: a review. Brain, 70, 2, 179–222.

Bruce, V. and Young, A. (1986) Understanding face recognition. British Journal of Psychology, 77, 305–27.

Burgess, P.W. and Shallice, T. (1996) Confabulation and the control of recollection. Memory, 4, 359–411.
Burnham, W.H. (1903) Retroactive amnesia: illustrative cases and a tentative explanation. American Journal of Psychology, 14, 3–4, 382–96.
Burton, A.M., Bruce, V. and Johnston, R.A. (1990) Understanding face recognition with an interactive activation model. British Journal of Psychology, 81, 361–80.
Cannon, W.B. (1929) Bodily Changes in Pain, Hunger, Fear and Rage, Vol. 2. New York, NY: Appleton.
Cermak, L.S. (1984) The Episodic-Semantic Distinction in Amnesia. In L.R. Squire and N. Butters (eds) Neuropsychology of Memory. New York, NY: Guilford Press.
Challis, C. (2014) Perfumes aid dementia research. Available at http://home.bt.com/lifestyle/fashionbeauty/fashionbeautynews/perfumes-aid-dementia-research-11363903520277 (accessed 6 December 2014).
Clark, V.P., Maisog, J.M. and Haxby, J.V. (1998) fMRI study of face perception and memory using random stimulus sequences. Journal of Neurophysiology, 79, 3257–65.
Clore, G.L. and Ortony, A. (2000) Cognition in Emotion: Always, Sometimes or Never? In R. Lane, L. Nadel, G. Ahern, J. Allen *et al.* (eds) Cognitive Neuroscience of Emotion. New York, NY: Oxford University Press.
Cohen, N.J. and Squire, L.R. (1981) Retrograde amnesia and remote memory impairment. Neuropsychologia, 19, 3, 337–56.
Conway, M.A. and Pleydell-Pearce, C.W. (2000) The construction of autobiographical memories in the self-memory system. Psychology Review, 107, 261–88.
Conway, M.A., Pleydell-Pearce, C.W., Whitecross, S.E. and Sharpe, H. (2003) Neurophysiological correlates of memory for experienced and imagined events. Neuropsychologia, 41, 334–40.
De Martino, B., Kalisch, R., Rees, G. and Dolan, R.J. (2009) Enhanced processing of threat stimuli under limited attentional resources. Cerebral Cortex, 19, 127–33.
Farah, M.J. (1996) Is face recognition 'special'? Evidence from neuropsychology. Behavioural Brain Research, 76, 181–9.
Gauthier, I. and Nelson, C.A. (2001) The development of face expertise. Current Opinion in Neurobiology, 11, 2, 219–24.
Gilboa, A. (2004) Autobiographical and episodic memory: one and the same? Evidence from prefrontal activation in neuroimaging studies. Neuropsychologia, 42, 10, 1336–49.
Graham, K.S., Lee, A.C., Brett, M. and Patterson, K. (2003) The neural basis of autobiographical and semantic memory: new evidence from three PET studies. Cognitive, Affective, and Behavioral Neuroscience, 3, 234–54.
Greenberg, D.L. and Rubin, D.C. (2003) The neuropsychology of autobiographical memory. Cortex, 39, 687–728.
Greene, J.D. and Hodges, J.R. (1996) Identification of famous faces and famous names in early Alzheimer's disease: relationship to anterograde episodic and general semantic memory. Brain, 119, 111–28.
Haque, S. and Conway, M.A. (2001) Sampling the process of autobiographical memory construction. European Journal of Cognitive Psychology, 13, 529–47.
Haxby, J.V., Ungerleider, L.G., Horwitz, B., Maisog, J.M., Rapoport, S.I. and Grady, C.L. (1996) Face encoding and recognition in the human brain. Proceedings of the National Academy of Sciences of the USA, 93, 922–7.
Hodges, J.R., Patterson, K., Ward, R., Garrard, P. *et al.* (1999) The differentiation of semantic dementia and frontal lobe dementia (temporal and frontal variants of fronto-temporal dementia) from early Alzheimer's disease: a comparative neuropsychological study. Neuropsychology, 13, 31–40.
Holland, A.C. and Kensinger, E.A. (2010) Emotion and autobiographical memory. Physics of Life Reviews, 7, 1, 88–131.

Humphrey, K., Underwood, G. and Lambert, A. (2012) Salience of the lambs: a test of the saliency map hypothesis with pictures of emotive objects. Journal of Vision, 12, 1, 1–15.

Insel, N. and Takehara-Nishiuchi, K. (2013) The cortical structure of consolidated memory: a hypothesis on the role of the cingulate-entorhinal cortical connection. Neurobiology of Learning and Memory, 106, 343–50.

Irish, M., Hornberger, M., Lah, S., Miller, L. *et al.* (2011) Profiles of recent autobiographical memory retrieval in semantic dementia, behavioural-variant frontotemporal dementia, and Alzheimer's disease. Neuropsychologia, 49, 9, 2694–702.

James, W. (1884) What is an emotion? Mind, 9, 188–205.

Jones, G.M.M. (2004) Metaphors for teaching about changing memory and cognition in Alzheimer's disease. Bookcases in a library. In G.M.M. Jones and B.M.L. Mielsen (eds) Care-giving in Dementia: Research and Applications (Vol. 3). Hove: Brunner-Routledge.

Kelley, W.M., Miezin, F.M., McDermott, K.B., Buckner, R.L. *et al.* (1998) Hemispheric specialization in human dorsal frontal cortex and medial temporal lobe for verbal and nonverbal memory encoding. Neuron, 20, 927–36.

Kroll, N.E., Markowitsch, H.J., Knight, R.T. and Von Cramon, D.Y. (1997) Retrieval of old memories: the temporofrontal hypothesis. Brain, 120, 1377–99.

LaBar, K.S. and Cabeza, R. (2006) Cognitive neuroscience of emotional memory. Nature Reviews Neuroscience, 7, 1, 54–64.

LeDoux, J.E. (1998) The Emotional Brain. New York, NY: Touchstone.

Levine, B., Turner, G.R., Tisserand, D., Hevenor, S.J. and McIntosh, A.R. (2004) The functional neuroanatomy of episodic and semantic autobiographical remembering: a prospective functional MRI study. Journal of Cognitive Neuroscience, 16, 1633–46.

Liberzon, I., Phan, K.L., Decker, L.R. and Taylor, S.F. (2003) Extended amygdala and emotional salience: a PET activation study of positive and negative affect. Neuropsychopharmacology, 28, 4, 726–33.

MacLean, P.D. (1970) The Triune Brain, Emotion, and the Scientific Bias. In F.O. Schmitt (ed.) The Neurosciences: Second Study Program. New York, NY: Rockefeller University Press.

Maguire, E.A. (2001) Neuroimaging studies of autobiographical event memory. Philosophical Transactions of the Royal Society of London, Series B: Biological Sciences, 356, 1441–51.

Mandler, G. (1980) Recognizing: the judgment of previous occurrence. Psychological Review, 87, 252–71.

Manns, J.R., Hopkins, R.O. and Squire, L.R. (2003) Semantic memory and the human hippocampus. Neuron, 38, 127–33.

Markowitsch, H.J. (1999) Limbic System. In R. Wilson and F. Keil (eds) The MIT Encyclopedia of the Cognitive Sciences. Cambridge, MA: MIT Press.

Markowitsch, H.J. (2013) Memory and self-neuroscientific landscapes. ISRN Neuroscience, 176027.

Marr, D. (1970) A theory for cerebral neocortex. Proceedings of the Royal Society of London, Series B: Biological Sciences, 176, 1043, 161.

Marslen-Wilson, W.D. and Teuber, H.L. (1975) Memory for remote events in anterograde amnesia: recognition of public figures from news photographs. Neuropsychologia, 13, 353–64.

Meeter, M. (2003) Control of consolidation in neural networks: avoiding runaway effects. Connection Science, 15, 45–61.

Milner, B. (1966) Amnesia Following Operation on the Temporal Lobes. In C.W.M. Whitty and O.L. Zangwill (eds) Amnesia. London: Butterworth.

Nadel, L. and Moscovitch, M. (1997) Memory consolidation, retrograde amnesia and the hippocampal complex. Current Opinion in Neurobiology, 7, 217–27.

Nauta, W.J.H. (1979) Expanding Borders of the Limbic System Concept. In T. Rasmussen and R. Marino (eds) Functional Neurosurgery. New York: Raven Press.

Neary, D., Snowden, J.S., Gustafson, L., Passant, U. *et al.* (1998) Frontotemporal lobar degeneration: a consensus on clinical diagnostic criteria. Neurology, 51, 1546–54.

Nielsen, S.L. and Sarason, I.G. (1981) Emotion, personality, and selective attention. Journal of Personality and Social Psychology, 41, 945–60.
Nieuwenhuis, I.L. and Takashima, A. (2011) The role of the ventromedial prefrontal cortex in memory consolidation. Behavioural Brain Research, 218, 2, 325–34.
Phelps, E.A. (2004) Human emotion and memory: interactions of the amygdala and hippocampal complex. Current Opinion in Neurobiology, 14, 2, 198–202.
Phelps, E.A. (2006) Emotion and cognition: insights from studies of the human amygdala. Annual Review of Psychology, 57, 27–53.
Phelps, E.A. and Sharot, T. (2008) How (and why) emotion enhances the subjective sense of recollection. Current Directions in Psychological Science, 17, 2, 147–52.
Phillips, M.L., Drevets, W.C., Rauch, S.L. and Lane, R. (2003) Neurobiology of emotion perception I: the neural basis of normal emotion perception. Biological Psychiatry, 54, 5, 504–14.
Piefke, M., Weiss, P.H., Zilles, K., Markowitsch, H.J. and Fink, G.R. (2003) Differential remoteness and emotional tone modulate the neural correlates of autobiographical memory. Brain, 126, 650–68.
Rempel-Clower, N.L., Zola, S.M., Squire, L.R. and Amaral, D.G. (1996) Three cases of enduring memory impairment after bilateral damage limited to the hippocampal formation. Journal of Neuroscience, 16, 16, 5233–55.
Ribot, T. (1882) Diseases of Memory. New York, NY: Appleton-Century-Crofts.
Schmitz, T.W., De Rosa, E. and Anderson, A.K. (2009) Opposing influences of affective state valence on visual cortical encoding. Journal of Neuroscience, 29, 7199–207.
Scoville, W.B. and Milner, B. (1957) Loss of recent memory after bilateral hippocampal lesions. Journal of Neurochemistry, 20, 1, 11–21.
Sharot, T., Delgado, M.R. and Phelps, E.A. (2004) How emotion enhances the feeling of remembering. Nature Neuroscience, 7, 1376–80.
Soares, J.J. and Ohman, A. (1993) Backward masking and skin conductance responses after conditioning to non-feared but fear-relevant stimuli in fearful subjects. Psychophysiology, 30, 5, 460–6.
Sporting Memories Network (n.d.) Home page. Available at www.sportingmemoriesnetwork.com/smn (accessed 6 December 2014).
Squire, L.R. (2004) Memory systems of the brain: a brief history and current perspective. Neurobiology of Learning and Memory, 82, 3 171–7.
Todd, R.M., Talmi, D., Schmitz, T.W., Susskind, J. and Anderson, A.K. (2012) Psychophysical and neural evidence for emotion-enhanced perceptual vividness. Journal of Neuroscience, 32, 33, 11201–12.
Tulving, E. (1985) Memory and consciousness. Canadian Psychologist, 26, 1–12.
Wagner, U., Hallschmid, M., Rasch, B. and Born, J. (2006) Brief sleep after learning keeps emotional memories alive for years. Biological Psychiatry, 60, 788–90.
Warrington, E.K. and James, M. (1967) An investigation of facial recognition in patients with unilateral cerebral lesions. Cortex, 3, 317–26.
Warrington, E.K. and McCarthy, R.A. (1988) The fractionation of retrograde amnesia. Brain and Cognition, 7, 184–200.
Willander, J. and Larsson, M. (2006) Smell your way back to childhood: autobiographical odour memory. Psychonomic Bulletin and Review, 13, 2, 240–4.
Woods, R.T., Bruce, E., Edwards, R.T., Hounsome, B. *et al.* (2009) Reminiscence groups for people with dementia and their family carers: pragmatic eight-centre randomised trial of joint reminiscence and maintenance versus usual treatment: a protocol. Trials, 10, 64.
Yonelinas, A.P., Hopfinger, J.B., Buonocore, M.H., Kroll, N.E. and Baynes, K. (2001) Hippocampal, parahippocampal and occipital-temporal contributions to associative and item recognition memory: an fMRI study. Neuroreport, 12, 359–63.
Yovel, G. and Paller, K.A. (2004) The neural basis of the butcher-on-the-bus phenomenon: when a face seems familiar but is not remembered. Neuroimage, 21, 2, 789–800.

Chapter 16

INNOVATION, ANTIPSYCHOTICS AND LIVING BETTER WITH DEMENTIA

'To achieve and sustain this we also need to extend research on the clinical and cost effectiveness of non-pharmacological methods of treating behavioural problems in dementia and of other pharmacological approaches as an alternative to antipsychotic medication. Training and building skills are at the heart of the sustainability of this plan, and recommendations are made concerning improving the curriculum and skills in primary care and in care home settings, where a national vocational qualification in dementia is proposed.'

Professor Sube Banerjee, 'The use of antipsychotic medication for people with dementia: time for action' (2009)

Introduction

The G8 Summit Declaration (2013, p.1) made a 'Call for greater innovation to improve the quality of life for people with dementia and their carers while reducing emotional and financial burden'. This group then stated that it therefore welcomed the UK's decision to appoint a global Dementia Innovation Envoy 'to draw together international expertise to stimulate innovation and to co-ordinate international efforts to attract new sources of finance, including exploring the possibility of developing a private and philanthropic fund to support global dementia innovation' (G8 Summit Declaration, 2013, p.1). Thus far, however, this group has been slow to appoint a person living well with dementia on to its board membership.

The NHS has aspirations to be a 'learning organisation' (Timpson, 1998). There are some clues about which factors and issues need to be considered in order to ensure effective adoption and implementation of innovation (Koch and Iliffe, 2011). Greenhalgh and colleagues (2004) have reviewed the diffusion of innovations in service organisations. One of the key initial considerations is whether the intended innovation means the same thing for the adopter as the innovator, the so-called 'innovation-system fit' (see, for example, Koch and Iliffe, 2011). Professor Clayton Christensen has had a massive impact in his revolutionary work on disruptive innovations (e.g. Christensen *et al.*, 2006). As Christensen and colleagues (2006) suggest in the *Harvard Business Review*, innovation is often achieved by a move away from expense and complexity.

For example, the role of the specialist clinical nurse might be to provide for people with dementia and their families the appropriate end-of-life support services that are currently available to others with long-term illnesses and to ensure that coordinated care is delivered (Robinson and Sampson, 2009). Such an innovative approach could reduce inappropriate hospital and respite admissions, reduce carer stress and ensure that the person with dementia is ultimately cared for in his or her preferred place of care. The concept of collaborative working in the assessment and coordination of care for individuals is not new and is considered an opportunity for more effective, efficient, timely interventions for service users, carers and practitioners alike (Cameron and O'Neill, 2005). I will return to collaboration in my conclusion (Chapter 18).

Traditionally, supports and services for people diagnosed with dementia of the Alzheimer type have focused on the carers. Circle of Care, a community-based home support agency in Toronto, has developed a support group for individuals with early-stage dementia (Goldsilver and Gruneir, 2001). Positive themes emerged to reveal feelings of affirmation, camaraderie and improved confidence, while feelings of helplessness and frustration were also raised. In the alternative, Carbonneau, Caron and Desrosiers (2010) propose a conceptual framework of the positive aspects of caregiving based on an integrative literature review. This conceptual framework provides a comprehensive model that should improve understanding of the positive aspects of caregiving. It could also contribute to the development of innovative support programmes based on the positive aspects of caregiving instead of the negative aspects.

Innovations are new creations of economic and/or societal significance, mainly carried out by firms (private or public). They may be new products or new processes. The firms produce (and sell) products that may be material goods or intangible services (new products are product innovations) by means of technological or organisational processes (new processes are process innovations). For these reasons, public organisations do not normally influence the innovation processes directly but influence (change, reinforce, improve) the context in which the innovating firms operate (Edquist, 2011). At national and local levels, a number of concerns have been raised regarding inter-agency working, particularly between health and social work services in supporting older people and the quality of the services they receive (Cameron and O'Neill, 2005). The authors identified that the issues raised included lack of coordination of local services from a patient's perspective, involving poor information sharing between agencies, barriers between organisations, lack of clarification of respective roles and responsibilities, multiple points of contact, lack of shared care management with common operational standards and lack of community rehabilitation with few opportunities to carry out maintenance or restorative treatments.

Partanen, Chetty and Arto Rajala (2014) offer helpful advice on the likely success of 'systemic innovations'. Systemic innovation has major technological implications that offer new opportunities, which need a major adaptation to other parts of the system, building on core competences within the system (Teece, 1996). The opportunities that systemic innovations create can only be exploited when adjustments are well integrated and coordinated in the whole system.

There have also been interesting product innovations. Anthony Pak-Hin Kong (2014) has outlined a preliminary study to explore the implementation of apps on iPads to conduct cognitive exercises in a clinical setting for clients with early-stage dementia. Joseph Martin Alisky (2006) proposes the hypothesis that mobile phones, internet communication and global positioning satellite (GPS) receivers could be integrated into computer-based caregiving systems to provide orientation and safety cues, daily reminders of activities, protection against wandering and direct links to medical assistance in case of incapacitation. The broad gist of this is that home computers, mobile phones, GPS receivers and personal data assistant (PDA) devices could be integrated into ambulatory and home-based systems to compensate for deficits in memory and judgment.

Antipsychotics

Antipsychotics are medications that affect the action of a number of brain chemicals (neurotransmitters) and were initially developed to manage psychosis. Antipsychotics fall into two classes: typical and atypical. Typical antipsychotics were first developed in the 1950s to treat psychosis. Sometimes called psychotropic or psychotherapeutic medications, they were intended to change the lives of people with mental disorders for the better (National Institute for Mental Health, revised 2008). In 2012, the Australian Government provided all residential and community care services with two new decision-making guidelines: 'Responding to Issues of Restraint in Aged Care in Residential Care' and 'Responding to Issues of Restraint in Aged Care in Community Care' (Pieisah and Skladzien, 2014). There are few topics that arouse such strong emotions as the use of antipsychotics. The general perception is that they can be useful and necessary, but they are not without their problems; for example, while they might quieten a person living with dementia who is agitated, they can also cause confusion, and some of the side effects are much more serious (Pulsford and Thompson, 2013).

The use of antipsychotics in care homes tends to underplay some major pre-existent difficulties. One is the extent to which healthcare professionals actually listen to patients – the 'users' or 'survivors' of the service. Themes of 'depersonalisation' and 'objectification' are, for example, evident in accounts of relations with doctors: 'Doctors are described as ignoring patients in the apparent belief that they are not fully human' (Crossley and Crossley, 2001, p.1481). Indeed, Crossley and Crossley undertake a very elegant analysis of 'patient voices' and their relationship to professional authority in mental health services.

Care home research can be problematic. A review of research in UK care homes concluded that information on dementia prevalence and impact was becoming increasingly outdated (Bisla *et al.*, 2011). It has been estimated that in England 376,250 older people reside in 10,331 care homes, costing approximately £16 billion in direct government funding alone (e.g. Care Quality Commission, 2010). The multitude of different companies, organisations and individuals owning care homes makes them a very disparate group. Negative media representations, the stigma of antipsychotic use and its assumed association with suboptimal care could make care home managers reluctant participants in a research survey (Backhouse *et al.*, 2014). In line with the work of Kitwood (1997) on the concept of person-centred care, Cohen-Mansfield (2001) proposed the highly influential model of unmet needs to explain the challenging behaviour of people with dementia. When there are too many environmental stimuli, the stress threshold is exceeded and symptoms of 'challenging behaviour' may appear.

I have previously discussed widely held concerns about terms such as 'challenging behaviour' and 'wandering' (e.g. Chapter 12). To prevent so-called 'challenging behaviour', it is argued, for example, that the amount of environmental stimulus should be adjusted to the processing capabilities of the person with dementia (Hall and Buckwalter, 1987). The National Service Framework for Older People (Department of Health, 2001), the National Institute for Health and Care Excellence dementia guidelines (2006) and a market analysis also highlight the importance of training for care staff and the need to improve access to effective non-pharmacological therapies.

The Department of Health has also conducted a review of antipsychotic prescribing for people with dementia (Department of Health, 2011; see also Banerjee, 2009), which recommends a substantial reduction in unnecessary prescribing. The National Dementia Strategy vision of enabling people with dementia in care homes to live well with dementia needs to be underpinned by effective, evidence-based interventions that are standardised, consistent, practical and can be delivered as part of the NHS. Whitaker and colleagues (2013) describe a protocol for a feasibility study of an optimised person-centred intervention to improve mental health and reduce antipsychotics amongst people with dementia in care homes.

Antipsychotic medications are often prescribed to manage the behavioural and psychological symptoms of dementia (BPSD). Several large studies have demonstrated a clear association between treatment with antipsychotic drugs and increased morbidity and mortality in people with dementia (Ballard, Creese and Aarsland, 2011; Schneider, Dagerman and Insel, 2005). Treatment guidelines recommend that the first-line management of BPSD should be detailed assessment to identify any treatable cause of symptoms (e.g. hunger, thirst, pain, infection, loneliness). Furthermore, underlying causes should be treated and alternative non-pharmacological interventions explored before the initiation of antipsychotics. Risperidone is the only antipsychotic licensed in the United Kingdom for this indication, and then only for short-term use. Nevertheless, other antipsychotic agents are often prescribed and used on a long-term basis with infrequent medication review (Azermai *et al.*, 2012).

The debate on the use of antipsychotics is not as clear-cut as it might first appear. Cornegé-Blokland and colleagues (2012) conducted a survey in 23 nursing homes in the Netherlands, and, on each dementia ward, the physician selected one or two patients who had recently started antipsychotics. Physicians, nurses and family carers generally considered the possible benefits of antipsychotics to outweigh the risk of side effects. The interviewed nursing home physicians and nurses expected almost half of their patients with dementia and behavioural disturbances to benefit from antipsychotic therapy. Serious side effects were expected to occur only sporadically.

The widespread use of antipsychotic drugs in nursing homes has been a concern for many years. US data indicate that as many as 40% of residents with dementia receive antipsychotics, many at doses above the recommended level (Mitka, 2012). Also, despite safety warnings from the US Food and Drug Administration (FDA), there has been little change in the rate of antipsychotic prescription in US nursing homes over the past decade (Liperoti *et al.*, 2003). Evidence regarding the use of antipsychotics in European long-term care facilities is modest, but studies from the Netherlands, Austria and Germany describe rates of antipsychotic prescription as high as 50% to 70% in nursing home residents, whereas Belgian and earlier Finnish studies report rates between 30% and 40% (Foebel *et al.*, 2014). Data from European nursing homes suggest that, once initiated, prescription of these drugs continues (Richter *et al.*, 2012). Initiatives aimed at reducing the use of antipsychotics in nursing homes through facility staff training, high-quality care promotion and abuse prevention have been promoted, and there is evidence to suggest that withdrawal of antipsychotic drugs may reduce mortality (Ballard *et al.*, 2011).

Behavioural and psychological symptoms of dementia

BPSD are an integral part of dementia syndrome. They are considered to be major contributors to the burden of dementia for both patients and carers, affecting 50% to 80% of patients (Finkel, 2000). The prevalence in nursing homes even rises above 80% (Brodaty *et al.*, 2001; Cornegé-Blokland *et al.*, 2012).

BPSD increase morbidity and burden, affect quality of life and impact cost of care. Available literature suggests that BPSD can manifest in multiple ways; the most common components are behavioural, affective, psychotic and somatic in nature (Kar, 2009). The NICE guideline CG42 'Dementia: supporting people with dementia and their carers in health and social care' (NICE, 2006), gives recommendations on the care of people with all types of dementia; this includes managing behavioural and psychological symptoms of dementia (NICE, 2013). Furthermore, non-cognitive symptoms and behaviour that challenges are included in the NICE quality standard on dementia (NICE, 2013). 'Challenging behaviour' is a term that has been adapted from the field of learning disability, and incorporates various other terms to do with behaviour (Krishnamoorthy and Anderson, 2011) and the 'behavioural and psychological symptoms of dementia' are the most commonly used in this field, but all have their limitations and critics as well as their supporters (British Psychological Society, 2013). It is important to remember that many of the behaviours identified as challenging are not symptoms of dementia; rather, they are symptoms of human distress, disorientation and misperception. As such, it seems counterproductive to frequently treat such behaviours through tranquillisation and sedation without first attempting to deal with the distress and cognitive confusion (British Psychological Society, 2013).

'Challenging behaviour' is very common in nursing homes; more than 80% of nursing home residents with dementia show one or more forms of challenging behaviour (Zuidema *et al.*, 2007). The presence of challenging behaviour in nursing homes diminishes the quality of life of residents, is associated with the use of physical restraints and results in higher costs (Murman *et al.*, 2002). Even though prescribing psychoactive drugs or using restraints to control challenging behaviour is a relatively straightforward treatment, many current models emphasise that the management of challenging behaviour requires an analysis of the meaning of behaviour. The Grip on Challenging Behavior care programme was developed using the current guidelines and models on managing challenging behaviour in dementia in nursing homes (Zwijsen *et al.*, 2014). It had been hypothesised that the use of the care programme would lead to a decrease in challenging behaviour and in the prescription of psychoactive drugs without increase in use of restraints. Zwijsen and colleagues (2014) found that the Grip on Challenging Behavior programme was able to diminish some forms of challenging behaviour and the use of psychoactive drugs.

BPSD can cause significant carer stress to family members and care home staff, which, without intervention, may rapidly lead to acute hospital admission and/or transfer to a more intensive care setting (de Vugt *et al.*, 2005). Antipsychotic medication may be viewed as an easier option than non-pharmacological alternatives, and the risks are rarely discussed or documented. Thompson Coon and colleagues (2014) found that interventions to reduce inappropriate prescribing of antipsychotic medications to people with dementia who were resident in care homes may be effective in the short term, but longer, more robust studies are needed.

The use of antipsychotics in care homes

Backhouse and colleagues (2014) sent a postal survey to all care homes registered as specialising in the care of older people or older people with dementia within four counties in the East of England. This survey was a first attempt to estimate the use of antipsychotics in care homes. Despite measures to reduce antipsychotic use for all people with dementia in England, they found that 12% of care home residents were still prescribed antipsychotic medication. Around half of all care home managers reported they had experienced behaviours they found difficult. Antipsychotic medications and a variety of non-pharmacological interventions appear to be used concurrently in many care homes. Barnes and colleagues (2012) provided an estimate of the prevalence of antipsychotic use for dementia in secondary mental health services in the UK and collected data relevant to quality improvement initiatives for such prescribing practice. Of the 1001 (62%) patients prescribed treatment for more than six months, only three-quarters had a documented review of therapeutic response in the previous six months.

The potential misuse of antipsychotic medications (APMs) is an ongoing quality concern in nursing homes, especially given recent black box warnings and other evidence regarding the risk of APMs when used in nursing home populations. Lucas and colleagues (2014) found that predictors of inappropriate use are found to be consistent with other measures of nursing home quality, supporting the validity of the proposed measure. There is general concern about their general contribution to clinical care. Indeed, in a cost–benefit analysis of second-generation antipsychotics and placebo in a randomised trial of the treatment of psychosis and aggression in dementia of the Alzheimer type, Rosenheck and colleagues (2007) found that there were no differences in measures of effectiveness between initiation of active treatments or placebo (which represented watchful waiting), but the placebo group had significantly lower healthcare costs. At the time of their introduction in clinical practice, atypical antipsychotics have been reported to be characterised by a better safety profile compared with conventional medications, especially with respect to extrapyramidal symptoms (EPS) such as Parkinsonism and tardive dyskinesia (Liperoti, Pedone and Corsonello, 2008). Atypical antipsychotics have been licensed since the 1990s and approved by the US Food and Drug Administration (FDA) exclusively for the treatment of schizophrenia. Rapidly after their introduction in clinical practice, these medications became the new standard of care for BPSD due to their reported advantages over conventional agents, particularly with respect to EPS and tardive dyskinesia (Liperoti *et al.*, 2008).

It is reported that treatment with atypical antipsychotics among patients with dementia has been linked to some risk of lengthening of interval in electrocardiogram (Hennessy *et al.*, 2002; Straus *et al.*, 2004). However, the current data available have suggested that atypical antipsychotics may not increase the risk of clinical outcomes related to QTc prolongation, including ventricular arrhythmias and sudden death, and with respect to cardiac toxicity they may be safer than conventional medications (Liperoti *et al.*, 2003; Ray *et al.*, 2001).

Atypical antipsychotics are, further, known to cause a spectrum of metabolic adverse effects such as diabetes, hyperlipidaemia and weight gain among young and adult patients with schizophrenia.

But the situation is by no means clear.

Van de Ven-Vakhteeva and colleagues (2013) assessed 290 patients with dementia living in nine nursing homes throughout the Netherlands in a longitudinal study. The measurements were repeated every six months over two years. They studied the change in neuropsychiatric symptoms (NPS) and antipsychotic drugs use and their effect on quality of life over time in two separate, generalised estimating equations. They found that antipsychotic use does not necessarily have detrimental effects on the quality of life of patients with dementia; rather, NPS consistently and negatively affects quality of life. The use of antipsychotics to treat NPS is justified when used carefully (i.e. their benefits and side effects should be monitored). Despite serious safety concerns, antipsychotic medications continue to be used widely in US nursing homes. Huybrechts and colleagues (2012) studied the variation in antipsychotic treatment choice across US nursing homes. They found that antipsychotic treatment choice is to some extent influenced by an individual nursing home's underlying prescribing culture. Indeed, the tendency of a facility to prescribe one antipsychotic class over another may reflect underlying values, experiences and exposure to pharmaceutical detailing shared by healthcare providers within that nursing home (Gruneir and Lapane, 2008).

All-Party Parliamentary Group: 'Always a last resort: inquiry into the prescription of antipsychotic drugs to people with dementia living in care homes' (April 2008)

In November 2007, the All-Party Parliamentary Group (APPG) on Dementia announced that it would be undertaking an inquiry into the prescription of antipsychotic drugs to people with dementia in a care home setting. The APPG conducted this inquiry because of concerns expressed by carers, patient organisations and academics about the appropriateness and safety of prescribing antipsychotic drugs to people with dementia. The inquiry requested evidence from a variety of stakeholder groups including people with dementia, carers, health and social care professionals, care home providers, academics, regulators and trade bodies.

These organisations and individuals were invited to submit views on the following issues (APPG on Dementia, 2008, p.vi):

» How widespread is the use of antipsychotic drugs for people with dementia in care homes?

» Why are people with dementia in care homes being prescribed antipsychotic drugs?

» To what extent is the use of these drugs appropriate?

» What alternatives are there to the use of antipsychotics?

» What steps should be taken to ensure the appropriate prescription of antipsychotic drugs for people with dementia?

The APPG made recommendations to ensure the appropriate prescription of antipsychotic drugs to people with dementia in care homes and to ensure that alternatives to the drugs are available and implemented. The overall recommendation is that the National Dementia Strategy for England must include an action plan to reduce the number of prescriptions. Specific recommendations are as follows (APPG on Dementia, 2008, p.x):

» Dementia training should be mandatory for all care home staff.

» Care homes must receive effective support from external services including GPs, community psychiatric nurses, psychologists and psychiatrists, which should involve regular, proactive visits to the care home.

» The use of antipsychotics for people with dementia must be included in Mental Capacity Act training for all care home staff.

» Protocols for the prescribing, monitoring and review of antipsychotic medication for people with dementia must be introduced.

» There should be compulsory regulation and audit of antipsychotic drugs for people with dementia.

The case for behavioural interventions

The case for behavioural interventions as an alternative to prescribing antipsychotic medication is strong (Cohen-Mansfield, 2001). It is estimated that behavioural interventions cost £27.6 million more per year than antipsychotic drugs for the cohort of 133,713 individuals with dementia requiring antipsychotic drugs in England (NHS Institute for Innovation and Improvement/Matrix Evidence, 2011). However, the behavioural interventions will generate nearly £70.4 million in healthcare cost savings due to reduced incidence of stroke and falls. In addition to the healthcare cost savings, behavioural interventions generate quality-of-life improvements. If these quality-of-life improvements are valued monetarily at the lower end of the NICE threshold, behavioural interventions would generate an additional £12 million in benefits per annum. It has previously been suggested that, combining healthcare cost savings and quality-of-life improvements, behavioural interventions generate a net benefit of nearly £54.9 million per year. This net benefit ranges from nearly £2.8 million per year in North East SHA to £7.3 million per year in North West SHA (NHS Institute for Innovation and Improvement/Matrix Evidence, 2011). Recently, Richter and colleagues (2012) reported on a systematic review of evidence to support the effectiveness of psychosocial interventions for reducing antipsychotic medication in care home residents. A number of empirical studies have examined whether non-pharmacological approaches can be used as alternatives to medication. Despite some mixed reviews (e.g. Forsetlund *et al.*, 2011), those studies with the best control have shown that regular input from a trained clinician can lead to a significant reduction in the use of antipsychotics (Fossey *et al.*, 2006).

The 'stepped care model'

An individual with dementia may present with particular behaviours that require a higher intensity of intervention, in which case the person can be 'stepped up'. The 'stepped care model' provides signposts to interventions that meet individual needs with the aim of preventing a further increase in distress for the individual and the carer. However, there is the opportunity for movement from one step to another if the behaviour continues to be unresolved.

The 'stepped care model' from the British Psychological Society's briefing paper 'Alternatives to antipsychotic medication: psychological approaches in managing psychological and behavioural distress in people with dementia' (2013) identifies the appropriate interventions that meet the presenting need, reinforcing the message that antipsychotic medication can be implemented as a secondary alternative. The model reinforces the need to ask: 'Why is the behaviour occurring?'

The steps describe the level of assessment and treatment input, identifying the person/professional who can perform the task. They are shown in Figure 16.1.

Step 4: Specialist intervention (individualised formulation-led interventions)
Individualised assessment, formulation and interventions
(specialist practitioners and carers/care staff)

Step 3: High-intensity interventions (protocol-led interventions)
Interventions tailored to specific presentations and needs
(experienced practitioners and carers/care staff)

Step 2: Low-intensity interventions (management of contextual issues)
Thorough assessment and general good practice in the care environment (GP and carers/care staff) – four weeks

Step 1: Recognition
Identification of difficulties, physical health and initial monitoring (GP and carers/care staff) – four weeks

Figure 16.1 The 'stepped care model'
Source: British Psychological Society, 2013 (p.5) (reproduced by kind permission of the British Psychological Society)

The 'call to action'

Mobilising communities is thought to be a very important aspect of creating change. The capacity of an organising campaign to produce such outcomes depends on systematic mobilisation as well as deployment of constituency resources – time, money and skill (Ganz, 2012). Social movement scholars interested in framing processes begin by taking as problematic what, until the mid-1980s, the literature had largely ignored: meaning work, the struggle over the production of mobilising and countermobilising ideas and meanings (Benford and Snow, 2000).

A resource pack from the Royal Pharmaceutical Society, Dementia Action Alliance and NHS Institute for Innovation and Improvement (2009) entitled 'The Right Prescription: A Call to Action. Reducing the inappropriate use of antipsychotic drugs for people with dementia' was published to help pharmacists to take action. The Dementia Action Alliance and NHS Institute for Improvement and Experiment identified eight groups of people to achieve their aim of reviewing antipsychotic prescriptions by 31 March 2012. These groups are listed in Box 16.1.

Box 16.1 Groups chosen for 'The Right Prescription: a call to action on the life of antipsychotic drugs for people with dementia'

* People with dementia, their carers and families
* Commissioners in health, social care and GP commissioning
* General practitioners and primary care teams
* Hospital doctors and multidisciplinary teams
* Leaders of care homes
* Pharmacists
* Psychiatrists and mental health teams
* Medical and nursing directors

Source: Adapted from Dementia Action Alliance/NHS Institute for Innovation and Experiment, 2012

Although antipsychotic treatment for dementia is most commonly initiated in secondary care, prescribing responsibility is commonly transferred subsequently to primary care, with the risk of undefined responsibility for continued medication review (Barnes *et al.*, 2012). This may be further compounded by poor communication between general practitioners and psychiatrists (Soyinka and Lawley, 2007).

It is indeed correctly argued in the NHS Improving Quality document 'Mobilising and organising for large scale change in healthcare. "The Right Prescription: A Call to Action on the use of antipsychotic drugs for people with dementia"' (Boyd *et al.*, 2013) that 'Strategy involves identifying resources through relationships and through identifying political, economic and cultural opportunities to create a structure for action' (p.23). There has been much interest in the potential innovative use of e-prescriptions in England (O'Hanlon, 2014). When patients are admitted to hospital, doctors should be able to view their current drugs and allergies in the GP core record. This allows for safer, more accurate and complete care from day one, thus avoiding the risk of critical medications being interrupted or delayed, which can lead to complications and longer hospital stays.

Tasked with bringing down prescriptions by 66%, the Dementia and Prescribing Antipsychotic Project in London was set up by NHS London in 2011 to support 31 London primary care organisations. It found that GPs and pharmacists were successful in effecting a reduction in antipsychotic prescribing for behavioural and psychological symptoms in dementia when they worked together (Oboh, 2014). Ensuring appropriate use of antipsychotics is currently mandated and is consistent with high-quality, person-centred care; simple yet individualised educational innovation comprising intervention and assessment can serve as a model for use in other long-term care facilities (Watson-Wolfe *et al.*, 2014).

The overall importance of innovation

Hospitals and other health systems increasingly must rely on innovation as they seek creative approaches for improving patient outcomes while simultaneously dealing with regulatory and cost constraints (Duarte, Goodson and Dougherty, 2014). The concept of open innovation, launched by Chesbrough (2007) and others, has gained interest and acceptance among researchers and practitioners in recent years. It argues that companies should not just rely on internally developed ideas and knowledge, but increasingly also look to ideas and knowledge developed externally; and that they can commercialise internal ideas through channels outside of their current businesses in order to generate value (Chesbrough, Vanhaverbeke and West, 2006). Creation and sharing of knowledge in networks is essential to make open innovation strategies work.

We are social animals. It is therefore unsurprising that digital collaboration is fundamental to happiness at work. Workers are apparently percentage points higher in their stated satisfaction with their workplace culture when they have access to digital collaboration tools (Deloitte, 2013). Michelfelder and Kratzer (2013) draw on social network theory, suggesting that the contradictory theories of the strength of weak ties and weak network structures on the one hand and the theory of strong ties and closed network structures on the other have a mutually reinforcing effect on innovation outcomes if combined rather than considered separately. And yet the innovation process varies markedly in different countries and regions (Nelson, 1993), and scholars and policy makers want to understand why. It is clear that the innovation culture of a whole country can be critical.

Along with the widespread interest that collaboration has received, there is a particular recognition of the significance collaboration has for innovation

(Gupta, Raj and Wilemon, 1985). Schleimer and Sculman (2011) question why innovation research remains dominated by research that focuses on products and processes rather than on services. Intriguingly, they further remark that, where firms engage simultaneously in intra-firm and inter-firm collaboration for the development of a new service, only inter-firm trust and commitment have a direct and positive impact on new service development success.

Conclusion

This chapter has looked at the 'innovation culture' with a strong thrust towards reducing inappropriate antipsychotic prescription numbers in care homes. I believe that the health and social care sectors for people living better with dementia will benefit massively from innovative changes, and this is not at all simply driven by cost. I feel strongly that the goals of people living well with dementia will be advanced if they work collectively, as an independent force, and retain ownership over projects and programmes. Whilst traditional leaders are to be applauded for putting dementia on the world stage, it is striking that in policy documents now it is urged that 'national leaders' should spearhead national policies for dementia. I critiqued the approach of national policies in Chapter 4. In the penultimate chapter of this book, I argue that world leaders could and should come from the citizens who are currently living well with dementia. Like leaders on the ward who are 'champions', these are global 'champions' – and they are championing a dementia-friendly community where their legal rights establishing autonomy and dignity are pivotal.

Leadership will therefore be the subject of my penultimate chapter, before concluding in Chapter 18.

References

Alisky, J.M. (2006) Integrated electronic monitoring systems could revolutionize care for patients with cognitive impairment. Medical Hypotheses, 66, 6, 1161–4.

All-Party Parliamentary Group (APPG) on Dementia (2008) Always a last resort: inquiry into the prescription of antipsychotic drugs to people with dementia living in care homes. Available at www.alzheimers.org.uk/site/scripts/download.php?fileID=322 (accessed 24 February 2015).

Azermai, M., Petrovic, M., Elseviers, M.M., Bourgeois, J., Van Bortel, L.M. and Vander Stichele, R.H. (2012) Systematic appraisal of dementia guidelines for the management of behavioural and psychological symptoms. Ageing Research Reviews, 11, 1, 78–86.

Backhouse, T., Killett, A., Penhale, B., Burns, D. and Gray, R. (2014) Behavioural and psychological symptoms of dementia and their management in care homes within the East of England: a postal survey. Aging and Mental Health, 18, 2, 187–93.

Ballard, C., Creese, B. and Aarsland, D. (2011) Atypical antipsychotics for the treatment of behavioural and psychological symptoms of dementia with a particular focus on longer term outcomes and mortality. Expert Opinion on Drug Safety, 10, 35–43.

Banerjee, S. (2009) The use of antipsychotic medication for people with dementia: a report for the Minister of State for Care Services. Available at www.rcpsych.ac.uk/pdf/Antipsychotic%20 Bannerjee%20Report.pdf (accessed 12 February 2015).

Barnes, T.R., Banerjee, S., Collins, N., Treloar, A., McIntyre, S.M. and Paton, C. (2012) Antipsychotics in dementia: prevalence and quality of antipsychotic drug prescribing in UK mental health services. British Journal of Psychiatry, 201, 3, 221–6.

Benford, R.D. and Snow, D.A. (2000) Framing processes and social movements: overview and assessment. Annual Review of Sociology, 26, 611–39.

Bisla, J., Calem, M., Begum, A. and Stewart, R. (2011) Have we forgotten about dementia in care homes? The importance of maintaining survey research in this sector. Age and Ageing, 40, 5–6.

Boyd, A., Burnes, B., Clark, E. and Nelson, A./University of Manchester/NHS Improving Quality (2013) Mobilising and organising for large scale change in healthcare. The Right Prescription: A Call to Action on the use of antipsychotic drugs for people with dementia. Available at www.nhsiq.nhs.uk/media/2414209/dementia_report_nov_2013.pdf (accessed 6 December 2014).

British Psychological Society (Division of Clinical Psychology) (2013) Briefing paper. Alternatives to antipsychotic medication: psychological approaches in managing psychological and behavioural distress in people with dementia. Available at www.psige.org/public/files/BPS%20 FPoP%20-%20Alternatives%20to%20Anti-Psychotic%20Medication%20-%20report%20 -%20March%202013.pdf (accessed 6 December 2014).

Brodaty, H., Draper, B., Saab, D., Low, L.F. *et al.* (2001) Psychosis, depression and behavioural disturbances in Sydney nursing home residents: prevalence and predictors. International Journal of Geriatric Psychiatry, 16, 5, 504–12.

Cameron, K. and O'Neill, K. (2005) Carenap (Care Needs Assessment Package): a practical example of innovation in joint working and single shared assessment. Dementia, 4, 1, 149–55.

Carbonneau, H., Caron, C. and Desrosiers, J. (2010) Development of a conceptual framework of positive aspects of caregiving in dementia. Dementia, 9, 327–53.

Care Quality Commission (2010) The Adult Social Care Market and the Quality of Services. London: Care Quality Commission.

Chesbrough, H. (2007) The market for innovation: implications for corporate strategy. California Management Review, 49, 3, 45–66.

Chesbrough, H., Vanhaverbeke, W. and West, J. (2006) Open Innovation: Researching a New Paradigm. Oxford: Oxford University Press.

Christensen, C., Baumann, H., Ruggles, R. and Sadtler, T.M. (2006) Disruptive innovation for social change. Harvard Business Review, December, 94–101.

Cohen-Mansfield, J. (2001) Nonpharmacologic interventions for inappropriate behaviors in dementia: a review, summary, and critique. American Journal of Geriatric Psychiatry, 9, 361–81.

Cornegé-Blokland, E., Kleijer, B.C., Hertogh, C.M. and van Marum, R.J. (2012) Reasons to prescribe antipsychotics for the behavioural symptoms of dementia: a survey in Dutch nursing homes among physicians, nurses, and family caregivers. Journal of the American Medical Directors Association, 13, 1, 80.e1–6.

Crossley, M.L. and Crossley, N. (2001) 'Patient' voices, social movements and the habitus: how psychiatric survivors 'speak out'. Social Science and Medicine, 52, 10, 1477–89.

Deloitte (2013) Digital collaboration: delivering innovation, productivity and happiness. Available at www2.deloitte.com/content/dam/Deloitte/se/Documents/technology-media-telecommunications/deloitte-digital-collaboration.pdf (accessed 20 April 2015).

Dementia Action Alliance/NHS Institute for Innovation and Experiment (2012) The Right Prescription: a call to action on the use of antipsychotic drugs for people with dementia. Available at www.institute.nhs.uk/images/Call_to_Action/DementiaC2Acommitmentstatements finalcopy.pdf (accessed 27 May 2015).

Department of Health (2001) National Service Framework for Older People (DH publication number 23633). London: Department of Health.

Department of Health (2011) National Dementia Strategy: Equalities Action Plan. Available at www.gov.uk/government/uploads/system/uploads/attachment_data/file/215522/dh_128525. pdf (accessed 6 December 2014).

de Vugt, M.E., Stevens, F., Aalten, P., Lousberg, R., Jaspers, N. and Verhey, F.R. (2005) A prospective study of the effects of behavioural symptoms on the institutionalization of patients with dementia. International Psychogeriatrics, 17, 4, 577–89.

Duarte, N.T., Goodson, J.R. and Dougherty, T.-M.P. (2014) Managing innovation in hospitals and health systems: lessons from the Malcolm Baldrige National Quality Award Winners. International Journal of Healthcare Management, 7, 1, 21–34.

Edquist, C. (2011) Design of innovation policy through diagnostic analysis: identification of systemic problems (or failures). Industrial and Corporate Change, 20, 6, 1725–53.

Finkel, S. (2000) Introduction to behavioural and psychological symptoms of dementia (BPSD). International Journal of Geriatric Psychiatry, 15, S2–4.

Foebel, A.D., Liperoti, R., Onder, G., Finne-Soveri, H. *et al.* SHELTER Study Investigators (2014) Use of antipsychotic drugs among residents with dementia in European long-term care facilities: results from the SHELTER Study. Journal of the American Medical Directors Association, 15, 12, 911–17.

Forsetlund, L., Eike, M.C., Gjerberg, E. and Vist, G.E. (2011) Effect of interventions to reduce potentially inappropriate use of drugs in nursing homes: a systematic review of randomised controlled trials. BMC Geriatrics, 11, 16.

Fossey, J., Ballard, C., Juszczak, E., James, I. *et al.* (2006) Effect of enhanced psychosocial care on antipsychotic use in nursing home residents with severe dementia: cluster randomised trial. British Medical Journal, 332, 7544, 756–61.

G8 Summit Declaration (2013) Available at www.gov.uk/government/uploads/system/uploads/ attachment_data/file/265869/2901668_G8_DementiaSummitDeclaration_acc.pdf (accessed 6 December 2014).

Ganz, M. (2012) Actors, not spectators. New Statesman, July 2012, 52–4.

Goldsilver, P.M. and Gruneir, M.R. (2001) Early stage dementia group: an innovative model of support for individuals in the early stages of dementia. American Journal of Alzheimer's Disease and Other Dementias, 16, 2, 109–14.

Greenhalgh, T., Robert, G., Macfarlane, F., Bate, P. and Kyriiakidou, O. (2004) Diffusion of innovations in service organisations: systematic review and recommendations. Milbank Quarterly, 82, 4, 581–629.

Gruneir, A. and Lapane, K.L. (2008) It is time to assess the role of organisational culture in nursing home prescribing patterns. Archives of Internal Medicine, 168, 238–9.

Gupta, A.K., Raj, S.P. and Wilemon, D. (1985) The R&D-marketing interface in high-technology firms. Journal of Product Innovation Management, 2, 1, 12–24.

Hall, G.R. and Buckwalter, K.C. (1987) Progressively lowered stress threshold: a conceptual model for care of adults with Alzheimer's disease. Archives of Psychiatric Nursing, 1, 399–406.

Hennessy, S., Bilker, W.B., Knauss, J.S., Margolis, D.J. *et al.* (2002) Cardiac arrest and ventricular arrhythmia in patients taking antipsychotic drugs: cohort study using administrative data. British Medical Journal, 325, 1070–4.

Huybrechts, K.F., Rothman, K.J., Brookhart, M.A., Silliman, R.A. *et al.* (2012) Variation in antipsychotic treatment choice across US nursing homes. Journal of Clinical Psychopharmacology, 32, 1, 11–17.

Kar, N. (2009) Behavioural and psychological symptoms of dementia and their management. Indian Journal of Psychiatry, 51, Suppl. 1, S77–86.
Kitwood, T. (1997) Dementia Reconsidered: The Person Comes First. Buckingham: Open University Press.
Koch, T. and Iliffe, S. (2011) Implementing the National Dementia Strategy in England: evaluating innovative practices using a case study methodology. Dementia, 10, 487–98.
Krishnamoorthy, A. and Anderson, D. (2011) Managing challenging behaviour in older adults with dementia. Progress in Neurology and Psychiatry 15, 3, 20–6.
Liperoti, R., Mor, V., Lapane, K.L., Pedone, C., Gambassi, G. and Bernabei, R. (2003) The use of atypical antipsychotics in nursing homes. Journal of Clinical Psychiatry, 64, 9, 1106–12.
Liperoti, R., Pedone, C. and Corsonello, A. (2008) Antipsychotics for the treatment of behavioural and psychological symptoms of dementia (BPSD). Current Neuropharmacology, 6, 2, 117–24.
Lucas, J.A., Chakravarty, S., Bowblis, J.R., Gerhard, T. *et al.* (2014) Antipsychotic medication use in nursing homes: a proposed measure of quality. International Journal of Geriatric Psychiatry, 29, 10, 1049–61.
Michelfelder, I. and Kratzer, J. (2013) Why and how combining strong and weak ties within a single interorganisational R&D collaboration outperforms other collaboration structures. Journal of Product Innovation Management, 30, 6, 1159–77.
Mitka, M. (2012) CMS seeks to reduce antipsychotic use in nursing home residents with dementia. Journal of the American Medical Association, 308, 119–21.
Murman, D.L., Chen, Q., Powell, M.C., Kuo, S.B., Bradley, C.J. and Colenda, C.C. (2002) The incremental direct costs associated with behavioural symptoms in AD. Neurology, 59, 11, 1721–9.
National Institute for Health and Care Excellence (NICE) (2006) Dementia: supporting people with dementia and their carers in health and social care. NICE guidelines CG42. Available at www.nice.org.uk/guidance/cg42 (accessed 6 December 2014).
National Institute for Health and Care Excellence (NICE) (2013) Key therapeutic topics: low-dose antipsychotics in people with dementia. Available at www.nice.org.uk/advice/ktt7/resources/non-guidance-lowdose-antipsychotics-in-people-with-dementia-pdf (accessed 6 December 2014).
National Institute for Mental Health (2008) Introduction: Mental Health Medications, NIH Publication No. 08-3929. Available at www.nimh.nih.gov/health/publications/mental-health-medications/index.shtml (accessed 6 December 2014).
Nelson, R.R. (ed.) (1993) National Innovation Systems. New York, NY: Oxford University Press.
NHS Institute for Innovation and Improvement/Matrix Evidence (2011) An economic evaluation of alternatives to antipsychotic drugs for individuals living with dementia. Available at www.institute.nhs.uk/images//Call_to_Action/20%2010%202011%20An%20economic%20evaluation%20of%20alternatives%20to%20antipsychotic%20drugs%20for%20individuals%20living%20with%20dementia%20%20Final%20Report.pdf (accessed 2 March 2015).
Oboh, L. (2014) Reduce antipsychotic prescriptions to save dementia patients. Health Services Journal, 15 September 2014. Available at www.hsj.co.uk/home/innovation-and-efficiency/reduce-antipsychotic-prescriptions-to-save-dementia-patients/5074502.article#.VHtC-4vA4_U (accessed 6 December 2014).
O'Hanlon, S. (2014) E-prescriptions change the game for acute trusts. Health Service Journal, 18 February 2014. Available at www.hsj.co.uk/home/innovation-and-efficiency/e-prescriptions-change-the-game-for-acute-trusts/5067830.article (accessed 6 December 2014).
Pak-Hin Kong, A. (2014) Conducting cognitive exercises for early dementia with the use of apps on iPads. Communication Disorders Quarterly, doi: 10.1177/1525740114544026.
Partanen, J., Chetty, S.K. and Arto Rajala, A. (2014) Innovation types and network relationships. Entrepreneurship Theory and Practice, 38, 5, 1027–55.

Pieisah, C. and Skladzien, E. (Alzheimer's Australia) (2014) The use of restraints and psychotic medications in people with dementia. Paper 38. Available at www.agedcarevic.org.au/resources/Alzheimers%20Australia%20Use%20of%20Restraints%20and%20Psychotropic%20Medications.pdf (accessed 6 December 2014).

Pulsford, D. and Thompson, R. (2013) Dementia: Support for Family and Friends. London: Jessica Kingsley Publishers.

Ray, W.A., Meredith, S., Thapa, P.B., Meador, K.G., Hall, K. and Murray, K.T. (2001) Antipsychotics and the risk of sudden cardiac death. Archives of General Psychiatry, 58, 1161–7.

Richter, T., Meyer, G., Möhler, R. and Köpke, S. (2012) Psychosocial interventions for reducing antipsychotic medication in care home residents. Cochrane Database of Systematic Reviews, 12, CD008634.

Robinson, L. and Sampson, E.L. (2009) Editorial. End of life care in dementia: research needed urgently to determine the acceptability and effectiveness of innovative approaches. Dementia, 8, 417–19.

Rosenheck, R.A., Leslie, D.L., Sindelar, J.L., Miller, E.A. *et al.* Clinical Antipsychotic Trial of Intervention Effectiveness-Alzheimer's Disease (CATIE-AD) investigators (2007) Cost-benefit analysis of second-generation antipsychotics and placebo in a randomized trial of the treatment of psychosis and aggression in Alzheimer disease. Archives of General Psychiatry, 64, 11, 1259–68.

Royal Pharmaceutical Society, Dementia Action Alliance and NHS Institute for Innovation and Improvement (2009) The Right Prescription: A Call to Action. Reducing the inappropriate use of antipsychotic drugs for people with dementia. Available at www.rpharms.com/support-pdfs/the-right-prescription.pdf (accessed 6 December 2014).

Schleimer, S.C. and Sculman, A.D. (2011) When intra-firm and inter-firm collaborations co-occur: comparing their impact across new services versus new product innovations. International Journal of Innovation Management, 15, 5, 869–98.

Schneider, L., Dagerman, K. and Insel, P. (2005) Risk of death with atypical antipsychotic drug treatment for dementia: meta-analysis of randomised placebo-controlled trials. Journal of the American Medical Association, 294, 1934–43.

Soyinka, A. and Lawley, D. (2007) Antipsychotic prescribing for behavioural and psychological symptoms of dementia. Psychiatric Bulletin, 31, 176–8.

Straus, S.M., Bleumink, G.S., Dieleman, J.P., van der Lei, J. *et al.* (2004) Antipsychotics and the risk of sudden cardiac death. Archives of Internal Medicine, 164, 1293–7.

Teece, D.J. (1996) Firm organisation, industrial structure, and technological innovation. Journal of Economic Behavior and Organization, 31, 193–224.

Thompson Coon, J., Abbott, R., Rogers, M., Whear, R. *et al.* (2014) Interventions to reduce inappropriate prescribing of antipsychotic medications in people with dementia resident in care homes: a systematic review. Journal of the American Medical Directors Association, 15, 10, 706–18.

Timpson, T. (1998) The NHS as a learning organisation: aspirations beyond the rainbow? Journal of Nursing Management, 6, 261–74.

van de Ven-Vakhteeva, J., Bor, H., Wetzels, R.B., Koopmans, R.T. and Zuidema, S.U. (2013) The impact of antipsychotics and neuropsychiatric symptoms on the quality of life of people with dementia living in nursing homes. International Journal of Geriatric Psychiatry, 28, 5, 530–8.

Watson-Wolfe, K., Galik, E., Klinedinst, J. and Brandt, N. (2014) Application of the Antipsychotic Use in Dementia Assessment audit tool to facilitate appropriate antipsychotic use in long term care residents with dementia. Geriatric Nursing, 35, 1, 71–6.

Whitaker, R., Ballard, C., Stafford, J., Orrell, M. *et al.* (2013) Feasibility study of an optimised person-centred intervention to improve mental health and reduce antipsychotics amongst people with dementia in care homes: study protocol for a randomised controlled trial. Trials, 14, 13.

Zuidema, S.U., Derksen, E., Verhey, F.R. and Koopmans, R.T. (2007) Prevalence of neuropsychiatric symptoms in a large sample of Dutch nursing home patients with dementia. International Journal of Geriatric Psychiatry, 22, 632–8.

Zwijsen, S.A., Smalbrugge, M., Eefsting, J.A., Twisk, J.W. *et al.* (2014) Coming to grips with challenging behavior: a cluster randomized controlled trial on the effects of a multidisciplinary care program for challenging behavior in dementia. Journal of the American Medical Directors Association, 15, 7, 531.e1–10.

Chapter 17

PROMOTING LEADERSHIP FOR LIVING BETTER WITH DEMENTIA

> 'All Russia is our orchard. The earth is so wide, so beautiful, so full of wonderful places. [Pause.] Just think, Anya. Your grandfather, your great-grandfather and all your ancestors owned serfs, they owned human souls. Don't you see that from every cherry-tree in the orchard, from every leaf and every trunk, men and women are gazing at you? If we're to start living in the present isn't it abundantly clear that we've first got to redeem our past and make a clean break with it? And we can only redeem it by suffering and getting down to real work for a change.'
>
> Anton Chekhov, *The Cherry Orchard* (1904)

Introduction

The #G7dementia leaders imposed some degree of finality by promising a dementia treatment or cure by 2025. But they are not real leaders in this context as there is no guarantee that they will physically be there in 2025, in which case it will be impossible to attribute blame or success to them. And they did appear rather oblivious to much of the world around them. 'Living well with dementia' is exactly the sort of arena that will not benefit from a hierarchy of power, mandating people how to live well: a request not to think of elephants will quite often elicit the opposite result. In contrast, an approach that promotes leadership from the community of people living well with dementia would do a lot to dispel the taboos, stereotypes and prejudices. For example, in *Leadership for Person-Centred Dementia Care* (2013), Buz Loveday talks about fostering a learning culture. One of the most powerful myths is that someone who has been diagnosed with a dementia is totally incapable of new learning, so it is utterly appropriate that people living well with dementia as leaders should be included in this learning culture.

That there are books on leadership for staff in person-centred care in dementia but none for leadership for people living well with dementia is a sad indictment. Professor Dawn Brooker (2007) talks about the need to include people living with dementia in conversations, against the backdrop of the 'Dementia Care Mapping' construct, with core themes of enabling, attachment and empathy. Empathy is relatively unaffected in most people in the early stages of dementia, although there is good evidence that empathy – measured as one's ability to read other people's minds – may be affected in early behavioural variant dementia (Gregory *et al.*, 2002). It is consistently argued that successful leadership for staff in person-centred care necessitates working out other people's strengths and weaknesses. It would therefore be very demeaning to deny recognition of a person with dementia having leadership skills in 'reading' the wishes of others.

This chapter on leadership for living well with dementia is organised around four heads:

1. The NHS policy background
2. Background
3. Who leads 'change', where and when for living well with dementia?
4. A critical role for 'Dementia Champions'.

#G7dementia has in fact provided a perfect opportunity for proponents of living well with dementia to set out and implement the case for radical change, but not in the way that Big Pharma intended perhaps.

In this chapter, I argue that people living better with dementia should be primarily leading on dementia policy with caregivers; but clearly others are involved including experienced professionals and practitioners.

The NHS policy background

Leadership has to be authentic

In June 2013, the NHS Leadership Academy published a document entitled 'Towards a new model of leadership for the NHS' by John Storey and Richard Holti from the Open University Business School. This paper was commissioned by the NHS Leadership Academy as a contribution to thinking about the future development of leadership in and around the NHS.

There are three main areas of leadership discussed in this document, and they are very relevant to promoting living well with dementia.

1. Provide and justify a clear sense of purpose and contribution

This focuses on the needs and experiences of 'service users', and calls for an interpretation of the wider environment.

2. Motivate teams and individuals to work effectively

Consideration is a leadership behaviour showing a concern and respect for followers; initiating structure are those behaviours accentuating goal attainment. A meta-analysis of the relationship of the Ohio State leadership behaviours – consideration and initiating structure – with leadership, conducted by Judge and colleagues, found that both consideration and initiating structure had moderately strong relations with leadership outcomes (Judge, Piccolo and Ilies, 2004).

3. Focus on improving system performance

Large-scale, whole-systems interventions in health care require imaginative approaches to evaluation that go beyond assessing progress against predefined goals and milestones.

A 'sustaining innovation' does typically not create new markets or value networks, but rather only evolves existing ones with better value, allowing the firms within to compete against each other's sustaining improvements. A 'disruptive innovation' is an innovation that helps create a new market and value network, and eventually disrupts an existing market and value network (over a few years or decades), displacing an earlier technology.

Christensen and colleagues (2000) propose that the benefits of disruptive innovations in health care are immense. Nurse specialists, general practitioners and even patients, arguably, can do things in less expensive, decentralised settings that could once be performed only by expensive specialists in centralised, inconvenient locations. Service innovations were more likely to progress if grounded in good established relationships between clinicians and managers (Greenhalgh *et al.*, 2009). There is a discussion to be had about the extent to which service disruptive innovations can be outsourced or remain in house, which could be a matter for shared decision making.

Background

A political framework

Leadership in the NHS inevitably has to take account of current political approaches, as well as the views of patients, perhaps represented by patient leaders, or professionals, perhaps represented by professional organised groups. Leaders in the NHS are ever constrained by the political, professional and public acceptability of unpopular but often pragmatic decisions to change the delivery of healthcare services (Leech, 2008).

This is, of course, a very difficult 'juggling act' for leaders in the NHS, who will be less concerned about the financial constraints of the service unless such constraints jeopardise safety within the service, but will wish to produce the best possible 'outcomes' for a person living with dementia. The question is, of course, what outcomes, where and when. The macroeconomic decisions about dementia provision, such as the ongoing debate about competition, fragmentation, integration and collaboration, are there in the background in the English jurisdiction (Iliffe and Manthorpe, 2014).

A competency framework

Smythe and colleagues (2014) used and included focus groups, questionnaires and interviews to develop a 'competency framework' with eight main clusters. These were: skills for working effectively with people with dementia and their families; advanced assessment skills; enhancing psychological wellbeing; understanding behaviours; enhancing physical wellbeing; clinical leadership; understanding ethical and legal issues; and demonstrating skills in personal and professional development.

This research was conducted within an NHS Trust serving a large, urban multicultural population, in collaboration with a local university. The Trust was seeking to identify the training needs and competencies required to ensure that staff are equipped with the necessary knowledge and skills to ensure people with dementia receive high-quality care. Two NHS-focused competency frameworks had previously identified generic competencies required across the whole of the healthcare workforce (Department of Health, 2004) and the mental health workforce (National Institute for Mental Health in England, 2004), respectively. But working out what strategy to pursue to ensure people receive high-quality care is not as easy as it sounds.

Who leads 'change', where and when for living well with dementia?

Who sets the agenda?

A 'culture' is 'a set of shared, taken-for-granted implicit assumptions that members of an organisation hold and that determines how they perceive, think about and react to things' (Schein, 1992, cited in West *et al.*, 2014, p.5).

The culture of the NHS is bound to be biased, one could argue, to a biomedical model, but holding out for a 'cure' may be an unfeasible path to follow. However, forces could be unleashed such that people living well with dementia *are* the change agents. They might *insist* on change more in keeping with the powerful disability rights model.

Bushe and Coetzer (2007) recently encouraged a re-think on group formation in terms of membership (when people want to join the group and wish to be identified with the group) and competence (when members of the group think of themselves as 'we'). People are searching for at least one other person with whom they can pair up and form interpersonal bonds (Beck, 1974), and members are searching for others who will confirm their role identity in the group (Srivastva, Obert and Neilsen, 1977). There are a number of candidates for 'leaders' to promote living well with dementia, including physicians, psychiatrists, social care workers, nurses, people living well with dementia and other members of the public. The recent literature has driven in the overall direction that leadership comes from both the leaders themselves and the relationships among them.

West and colleagues (2014) correctly observe that organisational performance does not rest simply on the number or quality of individual leaders. They instead discuss how formal and informal leaders work collectively in support of the organisation's goals and in embodying the values that underpin the desired culture. In this context, the organisation does not act in isolation. Pooling the energy from a wide range of leaders allows an energy of itself to drive the cultural change, avoiding a paralysis from the sheer prospect of planning a change (see Isern and Pung, 2007).

The reason it would be dangerous to write off people who have been diagnosed with dementia from participating in the debate about policy is that there is a strong history of community activism bringing about change. There is no doubt that there is a sense of 'control' from the registered medical profession, who can prescribe medications for dementia, and the notion that people fundamentally oppose change has come under scrutiny (Jansen, 2000). Van Dijk and Van Dick (2009) introduced the notion of a 'person-oriented resistance to change... including the feelings of loss experienced by people as a result of departures from the status quo' (p.144).

As Marshall Ganz, currently a senior lecturer in public policy at Harvard, points out in the *New Statesman* magazine (2012), organising and storytelling might be key components.

People living well with dementia might be the leaders, and other members of the general public might be followers. Or, in the alternative, clinical leaders might be leaders, and members of the public might be followers. Or even, perhaps, people living well with dementia might be the leaders, and clinical leaders the followers. The permutations are, in fact, endless. As Follett (1996) remarked in 1933, her contemporaries had the view that one was 'either a leader or nothing of much importance' (p.170).

One particularly interesting aspect is the cultural change within a person with dementia going from a pharmacological-based approach to a living well one. One paradigm that has informed this research is Prochaska and DiClemente's (1982) transtheoretical model (TTM), which asserts that people use different processes during different stages of lifestyle change. The TTM posits that people progress through five stages when making any lifestyle change: precontemplation (unawareness or denial of the problem), contemplation (considering change), preparation (increasing commitment and taking initial steps), action (changing behaviour) and maintenance (sustaining the new behaviour). In smoking cessation, cognitive processes were used more in the earlier stages than were behavioural processes. In exercise adoption and diet change, use of behavioural and cognitive processes increased together. For a person living well with dementia, the decision to put more emphasis on approaches that optimise living well, rather than medications which might temporarily improve mini-mental score but do not change the underlying disease process, might be more behavioural than cognitive, and this would be an interesting area of further research.

But there are problems with change being driven entirely by followers: a large number of followers can lead to a lot of disagreement about which strategic path to follow, and also the pace of change, instead of taking on energy, takes on an air of indecision and lethargy.

Leading change from the 'edge'

There is currently an interesting debate as to where change might come from within the NHS, and this is elegantly described by Helen Bevan and Steve Fairman (2014) in a white paper entitled 'The new era of thinking and practice in change and transformation'. This is not without its corpus of critics who are stakeholders on the front line within the health and social care systems.

Indeed, people living well with dementia who feel things are going 'their way' – with less emphasis on medications and more emphasis on living well – often report this on the basis of language and day-to-day conversations that they are having in real life. This chimes with the organisational development literature (e.g. Bushe and Marshak, 2014), where such conversations are represented as empowering, democratic and a reality with authenticity. This is somewhat in contrast to how drug companies can often look contrived in fronting their rush for a pharmacological cure for dementia with people currently living with dementia.

Escaping the 'silos'

There has long been a notion that not everybody has the capability to be a 'great leader'. In finding 'great leaders', there should be an effort to form dialogues and exchanges with people lower down in organisations, for all tensions and conflicts to be aired constructively, and to develop people 'outside their silos' (Ready, 2004). For leadership in dementia, this might mean, for example, spending time talking to staff who are caring for or supporting a person with dementia, particularly if these staff are from diverse disciplinary backgrounds. This has potential repercussions for recruitment. Douglas Ready's article in the *Harvard Business Review* in 2004 (Ready, 2004) offers generic advice on leadership but could be very usefully applied in the dementia leadership ecosystem; this includes the articulation of clear policy, a pro-active of outreach of 'high calibre candidates' from across the organisation, active search for managing conflicts, encouraging employees outside their 'comfort zones'.

From 'tempered radicals' to building connections

It might be very difficult for people to bring about radical change, and Debra Meyerson (2001) contributed the seminal piece of work on 'tempered radicals' to tackle this in a noteworthy article entitled 'Radical change, the quiet way'. This is a triumphant piece of work which was begun when Meyerson was working with Professor Maureen Scully at the Simmons Graduate School of Management in Boston. Meyerson famously says that they want to rock the boat, but they also do not want to fall out. The whole perspective Meyerson offers is brilliant for channelling energy from tolerating mediocrity to following one's aspirations for improved value. Meyerson herself observes that change can occur primarily in one of two ways: through drastic action or through evolutionary adaptation. Radical change, Meyerson observes, is 'discontinuous' and often forced upon an organisation in a sudden way, due to a technological advance, scarcity or abundance of critical resources, or by sudden changes in the regulatory, legal or political landscape. However, evolutionary change is usually gentle and incremental, and produces long-lasting change with less upheaval.

With the huge amount of money that Big Pharma can put into lobbying senior politicians and large charities, as well as media coverage of its efforts, it sometimes feels as if promoting living well with dementia is a 'David v Goliath' scenario. But we've been here before. Marshall Ganz (2009, p.251) sets out to answer three questions, the first two of which are: 'How can the powerless sometimes challenge the powerful successfully? How can strategic resourcefulness compensate for lack of resources?' We sometimes see some of the more refreshing elements in policy and research coming from the smaller charities. For example, BRACE is a smaller registered charity for Alzheimer's research based in Bristol, which hosted a very successful 'Hope for the future' day on 4 November 2014 (BRACE, 2014). I asked a question on the new forthcoming English dementia strategy at this event.

Ganz's third question was: 'And how can we exercise leadership to turn what we have into what we need to get what we want?' (Ganz, 2009, p.251). The David referred to in the title is the biblical David, with only a mere sling shot. As John Kotter (2012, p.46) says in his highly influential article in the *Harvard Business Review*, 'The hierarchical structures and organisational processes we have used for decades to run and improve our enterprises are no longer up to the task of winning in this faster-moving world.'

Helpfully, though, Kotter does qualify this statement. Traditional hierarchies and management processes might be quite good at running their organisations, but Kotter argues that they are not so good at navigating themselves through 'risks and opportunities', where nimblenesss might be considered a virtue. Kotter feels that many change agents are required, but it is not 'paid appointees' but volunteers who can spread the message. Kotter feels this is a question of leadership, not management, and appealing to people's emotions.

Kotter (2012) identifies a number of 'accelerators of change', which build around identifying 'a single big opportunity', creating 'short time wins' and the need to 'build and maintain a guiding coalition'.

In terms of language and narrative, the relationship between society and dementia has often been framed in the popular media as 'a war against dementia'.

So how will we know when the 'war against dementia' is over? For those of us who wish to change the parameters of the debate from a neuropsychopharmacological cure solely to a strategy that also recognises living well with dementia, Kotter (2012, p.56) offers some very useful advice: 'A new direction or method must sink into the very culture of the enterprise – and it will do so if the initiative produces visible results and sends your organization into a strategically better future.'

Medicine and nursing are two examples of professions that are intensely hierarchical. The NHS itself is enormous and prone to be very bureaucratic. This fact in itself is a trigger for concern that change in such professions is difficult; it is the policy equivalent of changing the direction of a 'supertanker'.

Some leaders, however, are surprisingly successful at changing their organisations. In a thought-provoking article entitled 'The network secrets of great change agents' by Julie Battilana and Tiziana Casciaro in the *Harvard Business Review* (2013), the authors found that 'Change agents who were central in the organisation's informal network had a clear advantage, regardless of their position in the formal hierarchy' (p.64). On the other hand, 'People who bridged disconnected groups and individuals were more effective at implementing dramatic reforms, while those with cohesive networks were better at instituting minor changes' (p.64).

But all this tends to assume that change initiatives come primarily from the top leader or leaders of an organisation. Indeed, the success or failure of the change initiative is solely dependent upon the actions or attributes of the leader. Charismatic leaders who initiate changes based on their personal characteristics and inspire others to follow their vision would fall into this category of change leadership. A change in approach from one that relies on pharmacological interventions to one that consists of thinking about living well with dementia, such as advocacy, design and information, is an example of a 'divergent change'. In a cohesive network, the people in your network are closely connected to one another. According to Battilana and Casciaro, the nature of this network builds trust and mutual support, facilitating communication and coordination.

Most people in the change agent's network will trust his or her intentions. Those who are harder to convince will be pressured by others in the network to cooperate and will probably give in because the change is not too disruptive. For more dramatic transformations, however, a bridging network works better – first, because 'unconnected resisters', in Battilana and Casciaro's terminology, are less likely to form a coalition; and, second, because the change agent can vary the timing and framing of messages for different contacts, highlighting issues that speak to individuals' needs and goals. The difference between a 'cohesive' and a 'bridging' network is potentially highly significant for change agents wishing to bring about a change from an approach based on neuropsychopharmacology to living well with dementia. Therefore, one can see that organisations are intrinsically volatile, and while entropy possibly provides that organisations aim towards chaos, the aim is to create a coherent narrative through the appropriate mobilisation of 'social capital'. Agents in such networks are shown in Figure 17.1.

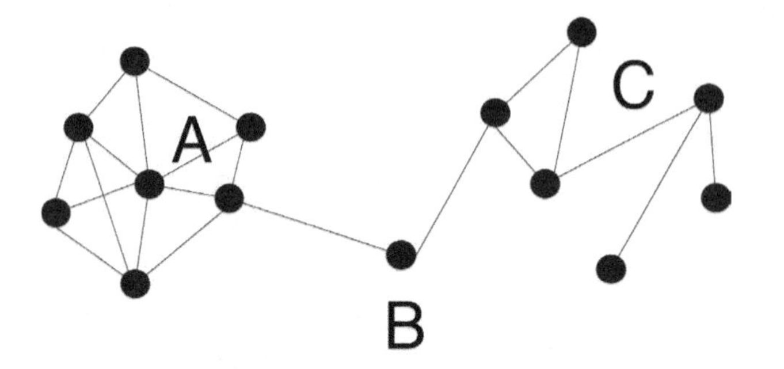

Figure 17.1 Creating a coherent network through 'social capital'

Social capital is typically defined as 'resources embedded in a social structure that are accessed and/or mobilized in purposive action' (Lin, 2001, p.29). In a 'cohesive' (close) network such as **A**, members in the network are connected in close proximity. This builds trust and mutual support, discourages opportunistic flow of information, facilitating communication but minimising interpersonal conflicts. A 'sparse' network (**C**) is effectively opposite to cohesive networks. In bridging networks, the 'bridge' (**B**) acts between disparate individuals and groups, giving control over the quality and volume of information exchange.

A critical role for 'Dementia Champions'

As Billie Jean King said, 'Champions keep playing until they get it right' (Conner, 2014, p.19).

Mayrhofer and colleagues see the role 'Dementia Champions' as being to influence and develop dementia care and service development. The authors argue that a 'community of practice needs robust and multi-pronged support during its first few years, until it reaches a critical mass that is resilient enough to cope with key changes in composition of membership and/or changing policy agendas' (Mayrhofer, Goodman and Holman, 2015, p.265). They remark how 'most [Dementia Champion] roles have developed organically rather than strategically. It is the context in which a [community of practice] is located that determines the mechanisms that need to be employed to support its functioning' (p.260). Knowledge sharing, transfer or dissemination is clearly critical for the highest quality of current communities of practice, as indeed dementia knowledge networks demonstrate. For example, in Scotland, dementia knowledge networks offer up-to-date knowledge, resources and points of discussion to improve practice (Scottish Dementia Champions Managed Knowledge Network, 2014). But, as Graeme Currie, Professor of Public Services Management at Nottingham Business School, points out, it is very hard to ignore that often the most substantial barriers to knowledge sharing are not only organisational, but professional (Currie, 2006).

The background to the paper by Mayrhofer and colleagues is important. Health Education England commissioned a project that had as its aims to 'develop and maintain a system wide initiative to support dementia champions across Hertfordshire'. The project was conceptualised as developing a 'Virtual Dementia Champion Community of Practice' through which Dementia Champions' inter-professional and inter-disciplinary sharing and transfer of knowledge could be facilitated. In this construct, communities of practice are useful multi-professional and multi-disciplinary constructs for healthcare professionals to engage in. They are seen as providing the means for shared staff and organisational learning and development that operate beyond boundaries (Aveling *et al.*, 2012). In any case, the whole issue of whether 'organisations' have boundaries has rightly come under scrutiny, not least because of technological advances and increased 'flexibility' in employer–employee relations (Starbuck, 2007).

Emma-Louise Aveling and colleagues (2012) noted that key lessons include 'the need for co-ordination and leadership alongside the lateral influence of peers' (p.158). Communities of practice commonly function in the existence of 'knowledge brokers' (Conklin *et al.*, 2013). Conklin and colleagues refer to these agents as having a shared purpose 'to develop and operate, facilitate exchanges among people with similar concerns and interests, and help groups and individuals to create, explore, and apply knowledge in their practice' (p.1). Clearly, Dementia Champions in the clinical community can serve this function. This chimes very well with the culture of collective leadership which is characterised by all staff focusing on continual learning and, through this, on the improvement of patient care; such an approach to leadership requires high levels of dialogue, debate and discussion to achieve shared understanding about quality problems and solutions (West *et al.*, 2014).

The role of nurses is seen as central to the future care of people with dementia (Bridges and Wilkinson, 2011; Hoe and Thompson, 2010). However, Draper and colleagues (2009), working in Australia, drew attention to the challenges involved in communicating the findings of the growing body of research focusing on dementia to the mix of individuals required to facilitate change – for example, policy makers, service providers, educators and members of the public. The importance of interpersonal contact in the transfer of knowledge and implementation of change has been emphasised, including:

- Opinion leaders: source of advice
- Facilitators: formal role in implementing change
- Champions: advocates of ideas or projects with enthusiasm and strong connections
- Linking agents: problem solvers
- Change agents: work with people to change behavior.

(Waugh *et al.*, 2014, p.721)

The findings of a range of initiatives have stressed the benefits of key individuals championing change (e.g. Cherry, Hahn and Vickrey, 2009; McCrae and Banerjee, 2011; Ploeg *et al.*, 2010). Despite disparity between the titles used to describe these individuals and their exact remit, there appears to be some consensus that interpersonal contact increases the probability of behavioural change in health care (Beer *et al.*, 2010; Thompson, Estabrook and Degner, 2006).

But it is noteworthy that people living with dementia can act as 'knowledge brokers' too. So it can be seen that people at the 'edge' of organisations, as proposed by Bevan and Fairman (2014), are able to work closely with people living with dementia, with values in common that allow the possibility of synergy in outcome.

Conclusion

Arguably, then, people living better with dementia and caregivers should be encouraged to lead change in keeping with a 'whole systems' approach, 'Start with a coalition of the willing, build an evidence base, build outwards' (Timmins, 2015) might appear therefore to be suitable advice for thought leaders including people living better with dementia and carers. If the person living with dementia is David, and Big Pharma is Goliath, David can aim his sling shot to tell Goliath that there is a role for anti-dementia drugs. But David and close to a million others in the UK deserve a chance to live well with dementia, with dignity, with information about their conditions, with information about what to do if they get unfairly dismissed from work, and with help about any aspects of their health and care. The impetus for a cultural change has been the underwhelming gamut of medications on offer, though admittedly some are good for some people in some circumstances. Leaders of living well with dementia do not exclusively need to be clinicians, but the NHS needs to foster an environment where such leaders can be identified and nurtured safely. In fact, there is considerable evidence that hierarchies will not lead to the very best knowledge sharing or creativity in producing solutions to the challenges of living well with dementia.

Whilst the NHS in England has clear guidance on what leadership is, in the form of reams and reams of paperwork, leadership for living well with dementia is pretty obvious when you see it. And the principles apply all over the world. Putting dementia on the world stage has inevitably raised expectations, but it has demanded that the NHS and social care systems in every jurisdiction take a long hard look at what sort of care they are leading. Above all, leaders in dementia should never make promises they cannot keep. Future leaders in dementia, one suspects, will not come from traditional training routes, but they all will have one thing in common: an ability to build bridges, convincing others that wellbeing in dementia matters.

I believe that people living well with dementia and all carers are the real champions for the future.

References

Aveling, E.L., Martin, G., Armstrong, N., Banerjee, J. and Dixon-Woods, M. (2012) Quality improvement through clinical communities: eight lessons for practice. Journal of Health Organisation and Management, 26, 158–74.

Battilana, J. and Casciaro, T. (2013) The network secrets of great change agents. Harvard Business Review, 91, 7–8, 62–8.

Beck, A.P. (1974) Phases in the Development of Sructure in Therapy and Encounter Groups. In D.A. Wexler and L.N. Rice (eds) Innovations in Client-Centered Therapy. New York, NY: John Wiley.

Beer, C., Lowry, R., Horner, B., Almeida, O.P. *et al.* (2010) Development and evaluation of an educational intervention for general practitioners and staff caring for people with dementia living in residential facilities. International Psychogeriatrics, 23, 221–9.

Bevan, H. and Fairman, S. (2014) White paper. The new era of thinking and practice in change and transformation. NHS Improving Quality. Available at www.nhsiq.nhs.uk/resource-search/publications/white-paper.aspx (accessed 6 December 2014).

BRACE (2014) Information on the event 'Dementia: Hope for the Future' held at Bristol, 4 November 2014. Available at www.alzheimers-brace.org/events/dementia-hope-future (accessed 6 December 2014).

Bridges, J. and Wilkinson, C. (2011) Achieving dignity for older people with dementia in hospital. Nursing Standard, 25, 42–7.

Brooker, D. (2007) Person-Centred Dementia Care: Making Services Better. London: Jessica Kingsley Publishers.

Bushe, G.R. and Coetzer, G.H. (2007) Group development and team effectiveness: using cognitive representations to measure group development and predict task performance and group viability. Journal of Applied Behavioural Science, 43, 184–212.

Bushe, G.R. and Marshak, R.J. (2014) The dialogic mindset in organisation development. Research in Organisational Change and Development, 22, 55–97.

Cherry, D.L., Hahn, C. and Vickrey, B.G. (2009) Educating primary care physicians in the management of Alzheimer's disease: using practice guidelines to set quality benchmarks. International Psychogeriatrics/IPA, 21, 1, 44–52.

Christensen, C.M., Verlinder, M. and Westerman, G. (2002) Disruption, disintegration and the dissipation of differentiability. Industrial and Corporate Change, 11, 5, 955–93.

Conklin, J., Lusk, E., Harris, M. and Stolee, P. (2013) Knowledge brokers in a knowledge network: the case of Seniors Health Research Transfer Network knowledge brokers. Implementation Science, 8, 1–10. Available at www.implementationscience.com/content/pdf/1748-5908-8-7.pdf (accessed 6 December 2014).

Conner, M. (2014) The Hill Worth Climbing. In Change Agents Worldwide, Changing the World of Work: One Human at a Time. Available at www.changeagentsworldwide.com/assets/doc/caww_ebook_11.pdf (accessed 25 February 2015).

Currie, G. (2006) Managing knowledge across organisational and professional boundaries within public services. Public Money and Management, April, 83–4.

Department of Health (2004) NHS Knowledge and Skills Framework (NHS KSF) and the Development and Review Process. London: The Stationery Office.

Draper, B., Low, L., Withall, A., Vickland, V. and Ward, T. (2009) Translating dementia research into practice. International Psychogeriatrics, 21, 72–80.

Follett, M.P. (1996) The Essentials of Leadership. In P. Graham (ed.) Mary Parker Follett: Prophet of Management. Boston: Harvard Business School Publishing.

Ganz, M. (2009) Why David Sometimes Wins. Oxford: Oxford University Press.

Ganz, M. (2012) Actors not spectators. New Statesman, 16 July, 52–4.

Greenhalgh, T., Humphrey, C., Hughes, J., Macfarlane, F., Butler, C. and Pawson, R. (2009) How do you modernize a health service? A realist evaluation of whole-scale transformation in London. Milbank Quarterly, 87, 2, 391–416.

Gregory, C., Lough, S., Stone, V., Erzinclioglu, S. *et al.* (2002) Theory of mind in patients with frontal variant frontotemporal dementia and Alzheimer's disease: theoretical and practical implications. Brain, 125, 4, 752–6.

Hoe, J. and Thompson, R. (2010) Promoting positive approaches to dementia care in nursing. Nursing Standard, 25, 47–56.

Iliffe, S. and Manthorpe, J. (2014) A new settlement for health and social care? British Medical Journal, 349, g4818.

Isern, J. and Pung, C. (2007) Driving radical change. McKinsey Quarterly, November, McKinsey and Co. Available at www.mckinsey.com/insights/organization/driving_radical_change (accessed 6 December 2014).

Jansen, K.J. (2000) The emerging dynamics of change: resistance, readiness, and momentum. Human Resource Planning, 23, 53–5.

Judge, T.A., Piccolo, R.F. and Ilies, R. (2004) The forgotten ones? The validity of consideration and initiating structure in leadership research. Applied Psychology, 89, 1, 36–51.

Kotter, J.P. (2012) Accelerate! Harvard Business Review, 90, 11, 43–58.

Leech, D. (2008) Interpreting the new language of leadership. British Journal of Healthcare Management, 20, 7, 310.

Lin, N. (2001) Social capital: A theory of social structure and action. Cambridge: Cambridge University Press.

Loveday, B. (2013) Leadership for Person-Centred Dementia Care. Bradford Dementia Group (Good Practice Guide). London: Jessica Kingsley Publishers.

Mayrhofer, A., Goodman, C. and Holman, C. (2015) Establishing a community of practice for dementia champions (innovative practice). Dementia (London), 14, 2, 259–266.
McCrae, N. and Banerjee, S. (2011) Modernizing mental health services for older people: a case study. International Psychogeriatrics/IPA, 23, 10–19.
Meyerson, D.E. (2001) Radical change, the quiet way. Harvard Business Review, October, 92–100.
National Institute for Mental Health in England (NIMHE) (2004) The Ten Essential Shared Capabilities: A Framework for the Whole of the Mental Health Workforce. London: NIMHE.
NHS Leadership Academy (authors: J. Storey and R. Holti) (2013) Towards a new model of leadership for the NHS. Available at www.leadershipacademy.nhs.uk/wp-content/uploads/2013/05/Towards-a-New-Model-of-Leadership-2013.pdf (accessed 6 December 2014).
Ploeg, J., Skelly, J., Rowan, M., Edwards, N. *et al.* (2010) The role of nursing best practice champions in diffusing practice guidelines: a mixed methods study. Worldviews on Evidence-Based Nursing, 7, 4, 238–51.
Prochaska, J.O. and DiClemente, C.C. (1982) Transtheoretical therapy: toward a more integrative model of change. Psychotherapy: Theory, Research and Practice, 19, 276–88.
Ready, D.A. (2004) How to grow great leaders. Harvard Business Review, 82, 12, 93–100.
Schein, E. (1992) Organisational Culture and Leadership. San Francisco, CA: Jossey Bass.
Scottish Dementia Champions Managed Knowledge Network (MKN) (2014) Home page. Available at www.knowledge.scot.nhs.uk/dementia.aspx (accessed 6 December 2014).
Smythe, A., Jenkins, C., Bentham, P. and Oyebode, J. (2014) Development of a competency framework for a specialist dementia service. Journal of Mental Health Training, Education and Practice, 9, 1, 59–68.
Srivastva, S., Obert, S. and Neilsen, E. (1977) Organizational Analysis through Group Processes: A Theoretical Perspective for Organization Development. In C. Cooper (ed.) Organizational Development in the UK and USA: A Joint Evaluation. New York: Petrocello Books.
Starbuck, W.H. (2007) Living in mythical places. Organisation Studies, 28, 21–5.
Thompson, G.N., Estabrook, C.A. and Degner, L.F. (2006) Clarifying the concepts in knowledge transfer: a literature review. Journal of Advanced Nursing, 53, 691–701.
Timmins, N. (2015) The practice of system leadership: Being comfortable with chaos. London: The King's Fund. Available at www.kingsfund.org.uk/sites/files/kf/field/field_publication_file/System-leadership-Kings-Fund-May-2015.pdf (accessed 23 May 2015).
Van Dijk, R. and Van Dick, R. (2009) Navigating organisational change: change leaders, employee resistance and work-based identities. Journal of Change Management, 9, 2, 143–63.
Waugh, A., Henderson, J., Sharp, B., Brown, M., Oliver, J. and Marland, G. (2014) Enriching the care of patients with dementia in acute settings? The Dementia Champions Programme in Scotland. Dementia (London), 13, 6, 717–36.
West, M., Eckert, R., Stewart, K. and Pasmore, W. (2014) Developing Collective Leadership for Health Care. London: King's Fund. Available at www.kingsfund.org.uk/sites/files/kf/field/field_publication_file/developing-collective-leadership-kingsfund-may14.pdf (accessed 6 December 2014).

Chapter 18

CONCLUSION

The World Health Organization (2014) defines mental health as:

> a state of wellbeing in which every individual realizes his or her own potential, can cope with the normal stresses of life, can work productively and fruitfully, and is able to make a contribution to her or his community.

Introduction

It turns out we are not all 'patients' – in that we can live well with a long-term condition and never have any contact with health or social care sectors (in theory). It turns out we are not all 'consumers' – unless we have a real choice and an ability to pay. But we are all persons. As I have mooted several times in this book, language matters.

It is sometimes hard to see the big picture in the policy regarding dementia in England. There are three dementia challenge champion groups, each focusing on one of the main areas for action: driving improvements in health and social care, creating dementia-friendly communities and improving dementia research. Essential to this is to encourage a pro-social approach, not a fragmented one. The terminology of 'dementia friendly communities' does matter a lot though; it might be more accurate to call these communities 'dementia inclusive communities', reflecting the dimension of equality under the law.

On the one hand, some people feel that we are under-diagnosing dementia, and that there are people languishing in England as they wait weeks or months for a diagnosis. Chris Roberts, himself living with dementia, and a leading advocate for people living with dementia, often warns that it is essential that, despite the wait, the diagnosis is correct. On the other hand, there are concerns, particularly if teams in primary care are financially incentivised for doing so, that there might be a plethora of over-diagnosed cases. The concern here is that there might be alternative interests determining why such people might be diagnosed, such as being recipients of compounds from drug companies which attach to proteins in the brain, and which might be useful in diagnosing dementia. Or are we building a 'new model army' of people who are ageing but are being shoehorned into the illness model because of their memory problems?

Another issue is potential 'competition' between dementia charities. Essentially, all dementia charities in England want the same thing and will need to attract an audience through various 'unique selling points', to use that awful marketing terminology. But in the next few years we may see commissioning arrangements change where the NHS may involve the third sector performing different complementary roles, such as advising and providing specialist nursing, in the same contractual arrangement. The law might shortly, in England, force people to work together here.

Another problem is the potential 'cure versus care' schism in international policy. This debate has accelerated in the last few years, with the perception – rightly or wrongly – that cure – in other words, the drive to find a magic bullet for dementia – is vying for attention with care. This narrative has a complicated history, in fact, in parallel with moves in the US which likewise have seen an overall trend towards desire for a 'smaller state'. But claims about finding a cure for dementia have to be realistic, and, while comparisons can be made with HIV and cancer about the impact that a cure may have for potentially removing stigma, such a debate has been done there incredibly carefully. For example, attention for cures and collaboration between Big Pharma and 'better regulation' potentially constitute a diversion of resources away from care. In the NHS strategy for England, with social care on its knees, a drive towards personalised medicine on the back of advances from the Human Genome Project can end up looking vulgar.

Medicalisation

The biomedical model needs to give in gracefully. However, it fits in with many narratives, and one philosophy in particular: 'the magic bullet'. The model of 'successful ageing' is now established as the counterpoint to those accounts of 'burdensome and vulnerable old age' that underpin gloomy predictions of the economic and emotional 'costs' to the State, to communities and to families of an ageing population (Dolan, 2013). To 'sell' the case for dementia, people are keen to tell you how much it costs, rather than the value brought to you by people living with dementia. Everything has to be seen through 'the productivity lens'.

But the State has an ability to implement strategies 'of force' in a coercive manner, as elegantly articulated by Szasz (2001). 'Leading physicians fuel the propaganda for therapeutic coercions as remedies for social problems' (Szasz, 2001, p.500).

The experience from other jurisdictions is rather ominous too. This is provided by Salem and colleagues (2012). Over-registration of dementia has been observed in young patients with a register-based dementia diagnosis for whom there was no mention of dementia in their medical records and no rater-based diagnosis of dementia. The authors suggest that an over-diagnosis may be explained by the wide range of conditions (e.g. depression, hepatic encephalopathy in alcohol abusers and chronic psychiatric diseases). A constellation of subjective cognitive symptoms as well as functional impairment are misinterpreted as dementia (Salem *et al.*, 2012). The evidence from Roses and Saunders (1997) points at a wider concern, about the accuracy of working dementia diagnoses, including post-mortem observations.

There are many unanswered questions as to who actually benefits from the clinical over-diagnosis of dementia. And indeed there are powerful forces at play. According to Heath (2013): 'They have permeated and polluted the drug and medical technology industries, medical research and regulatory bodies, clinical practice, payment systems, guideline production, and national healthcare systems. They are the cause of an astonishing amount of waste and harm' (p.1).

Recovery

That there has to be a 'cure' for everything is an ideological stranglehold of the medical approach. This is subconsciously framed in any argument from a physician that dementia takes second place because 'there is no cure for it'. Part of the struggle in changing this attitude to dementia is getting clinicians to proactively promote living better with dementia. To assist, there has been a dramatic expansion in the scientific study of wellbeing and the positive aspects of mental health in recent years. However, the financial investment put into dementia compared with other symptomatic clusters such as cancer is historically small. And the amount of money being put into high-quality research on living better with dementia, compared with cure, care or prevention, is embarrassingly tiny, in no small part reflecting the priorities of the large dementia charities worldwide. Conversely, mental health recovery is a worldwide vision and a goal in social policy, in mental health research and in psychosocial rehabilitation (Wilken and Hollander, 2008).

There has, instead, been some concern about whether people living with dementia symptoms have become 'consumers' because of their presentation.

There is, however, an encouraging possibility for recovery to become a dominant policy-directed model of many mental health care organisations. A boundary to this – for example, in older-adult acute mental health inpatient settings – is a training issue: some nurses, for instance, do not have a clear description of how to be recovery-oriented (McKenna *et al.*, 2014). In mental health organisations, 'recovery-oriented care' evolves naturally out of person-centred care. A focus of living better with dementia could be to orient the person with dementia in the community, and seek timely diagnosis and post-diagnostic support (Adams, 2010). Recovery-oriented care is gaining traction in mental health care provision in many countries in the developed world (e.g. Drennan, Law and Alred, 2012). The WHO definition at the beginning of this chapter emphasises that mental health is more than the absence of mental illness. Over 25 years ago, a model of psychological wellbeing was put forth by Ryff (1989) to address omissions in formulations of positive human functioning that prevailed in the 1980s.

Living better with dementia could be 'flourishing', which relates to the experience of life going well. It is a combination of feeling good and functioning effectively. Flourishing is synonymous with a high level of mental wellbeing; it epitomises mental health being related to the prototypical concept of 'eudaimonia' (Keyes, 2002; Ryff, 2014; Ryff and Singer, 1998). For too long, it is argued, the focus of mental health research and practice has been on the treatment of pathologies such as depression and anxiety, and to some extent on their prevention (Huppert and So, 2013). 'Recovery-oriented mental health rehabilitation' is described as the guiding principle in system reforms and should be available to everyone with a mental illness (Lancet Global Mental Health Group, 2007). Ways of surviving, recovering from and experiencing mental distress have become a significant social movement (Chassot and Mendes, 2014). Park and Peterson (2009, p.422) have argued: 'What does it mean to live well? How can people achieve a good life and sustain it? We can think of no more important questions about the human condition and thus for psychology as the quintessential human science.' Negative affect may have direct pertinence to interventions to promote resilience or help older adults adapt to adversity (Meeks *et al.*, 2012).

A study by Casadi Marino (2015) throws useful light on this as part of the first stage of development of a social recovery measure. Marino found that 'social recovery' involved developing a sense of being a worthy person with something to offer others. Individuals needed environments in which they could be both vulnerable and competent. Participants in Marino's study further emphasised the importance of 'a felt sense of belonging to a community in which they were valued' (Marino, 2015, p.70). They needed acceptance, safety and encouragement to take on challenges and continue to grow. Policy has clearly come a long way, rather fast. Deinstitutionalisation (the process of closing the asylums and developing community-based services) gathered pace from the 1950s onwards, fuelled by the development of phenothiazine medications (the first antipsychotic drugs) and a general increasing awareness of the negative effects of transfer into residential settings (Killaspy, 2014). In mental health services research, the strong focus on illness, symptoms and deficits as the target for change has begun to shift towards strengths and resources only in recent decades. Psychiatry, as acknowledged by the World Psychiatric Association, has often failed to promote wellbeing, and the contemporary shift in the mental health field argues for a focus on wellbeing regardless of the presence of mental illness (Schrank *et al.*, 2014).

Clearly, there is still much to do. For example, it will be interesting to examine precisely the capacity of some to experience and sustain their wellbeing, perhaps even deepen it, despite the challenges that life presents to them (Shmotkin, 2005). Tackling this issue will produce a fundamental sea change in the service delivering a philosophy of 'living better with dementia'.

Chapter 2 comprised a preliminary analysis of stigma, citizenship and the notion of 'living better with dementia'. Stigmatisation means that people are not truly socially accepted (Goffman, 1963). Reducing stigma has, of course, been a critical policy drive of dementia-friendly communities at an international level. But even here there is an intensely strong need for caution – as Kate Swaffer (2014, p.713), living well with dementia, notes, 'I have been uncertain that "dementia-friendly communities" is the right phrase as I am worried it encourages division rather than includes people.'

Strengthening the dignity and autonomy of people with dementia as individuals is likely to lead to stronger communities, even though the whole is not just the sum of its constituent parts. Throughout this book there have been different examples of how the sense of wellbeing of persons living with dementia might be improved. Chapter 13 considered a number of important contemporary issues, with a main emphasis on human rights and 'rights-based approaches'. Chapter 14 was primarily concerned with art and creativity, focusing on how living with dementia could in fact lead to enhanced art and creativity, and how the cultural needs of people living with dementia could best be furnished through laughter, poetry and art galleries or museums within communities. Chapter 17 looked at how leadership could be promoted by people living with dementia themselves.

Families

Chapter 5 considered the impact of the diagnosis of young-onset dementia on the partner of the person with dementia as well.

Unfortunately, the quality of family life has been a previously neglected area of health care. This research blind spot therefore needs to be addressed in order to provide appropriate support for the patient and the family unit (Golics *et al.*, 2013). Many people feel that they are fighting in a situation for which they have received little preparation and warning. 'Coping responses and behaviors (coping responses) involve efforts used by or resources available to persons to manage intrinsic and extrinsic stimuli that are perceived as stressful' (Clark, 2004, p.551). Ducharme and colleagues (2014) note 'booster sessions' as a means of maintaining the benefits of psycho-educational programmes, with a significant positive effect of the booster session being the emergence of preparedness to provide care.

A recent study was published by Reinhardt and colleagues (2014). This consisted of a six-month, prospective, randomised trial, and tested the effect of an intervention consisting of a face-to-face, structured conversation about end-of-life care options with family members of nursing home residents with advanced dementia (Reinhardt *et al.*, 2014). A comparison group received only social contact via telephone. Their results showed that intervention families had higher satisfaction with care than comparison families at the six-month time point, and they were more likely to have decided on medical options listed in residents' advance directives (Do Not Resuscitate, Intubate, Hospitalise) over time. It had been difficult, previously, to define what constitutes high-quality end-of-life care for people with dementia from the perspective of family carers (Davies *et al.*, 2014). Sampson and colleagues (2011) designed an intervention to improve end-of-life care through advance care planning (ACP), but they struggled to engage carers in ACP.

Sullivan and colleagues (2014) recently provided some preliminary data on a tool for assessing the negative thoughts that family carers of people with dementia may experience. Given that these thoughts are implicated in depression but may be modified, the capacity to identify dysfunctional thoughts early on may prove useful in carer support programmes. It has also been questioned whether a family meetings intervention was superior to usual care in postponing the nursing home placement of patients with dementia. Joling and colleagues (2013), however, found that this family meetings intervention for primary carers of patients with dementia did not postpone patient transfer into residential settings more than usual care. The way in which families can interact might arise from anomalies in the general brain processing of social and emotion processing. These can occur in types of dementia, particularly frontotemporal dementia. In particular, a loss of empathy – the ability to understand the feelings and take the perspective of others – has been reported as an early symptom by carers of patients with behavioural variant frontotemporal dementia and semantic dementia (Perry *et al.*, 2001). Providing care for a person with dementia can be associated with both positive and negative carer outcomes (Brodaty and Donkin, 2009), although the research language invariably tends to revolve around 'burden'. Various carer outcomes can co-occur. They may have different triggers and impacts, and they may be pertinent at different time points. They might be explained by the progression of atrophy in regions that are known to be critical for empathy and social behaviour; this has implications for the delivery and planning of services in dementia (Hsieh *et al.*, 2013).

According to recent evidence, the annual costs of caring for a person with dementia are substantial, with informal care being by far the largest contributor to the total societal costs (Joling *et al.*, 2013). Providing care to a person with dementia of the Alzheimer type is associated with emotional, physical and financial considerations, because of the diverse impact on the carer's lifestyle, professional career and financial status (Adams, 2006). It is stating the obvious to say that dementia is a prime public health issue. With its characteristic symptoms and signs, dementia influences not only a person's life but also the lives of family members who provide care and support for him or her. It is critical that all parties 'come out of the shadows' (the name given to a plank of German dementia policy). Jayne Goodrick, Rachel Niblock and Louise Langham have done outstanding work in the Dementia Action Alliance Carers' 'Call to Action' (see www.dementiaaction.org.uk/carers). As their physical and intellectual impairment increases, persons with dementia can lose the ability to function on their own and have to be helped by others, usually their close relatives, in daily life activities (Warchol-Biedermann *et al.*, 2014).

Furthermore, dementia can run in families: 25% of all people aged 55 years and older have a family history of dementia (Slooter *et al.*, 1998). For most, the family history is due to a genetically complex make-up, where many genetic variations of small effect interact to increase the risk of dementia.

Genetics forms the cusp of care and raw medicine and cure. For example, the AlzGene database (www.alzgene.org) provides a collection of meta-analysis results of genetic association studies using risk of dementia of the Alzheimer type as the primary phenotype in either population-based or family-based cohorts (Bertram *et al.*, 2007). This first, pioneering 'big data' project for Alzheimer's disease has been launched to enable scientists to analyse the entire genome sequence of more than 800 individuals. I discussed the significance of the 'big data' drive in global policy in Chapter 5. It is hoped that this ADNI whole genome sequencing project, coupled with very rich multimodal ADNI phenotypes, will provide important new insights into the genetic mechanisms of dementia of the Alzheimer type, which in turn will impact the development of new diagnostic, therapeutic and preventive approaches (Shen *et al.*, 2014). But the key point is not to witness a further 'Alzheimerisation' of all dementia policy considerations (Iliffe and Manthorpe, 2007).

The genetics of all the dementias are complicated and ever-changing, and counselling can be challenging professionally. But they do need to find their rightful place in a properly funded health service. Members of families where dementias run in families may be psychologically fragile, and those at risk facing the decision to be tested may face family pressure to not pursue testing. The whole issue of the pre-diagnosis examination for all dementias merits attention, and this is a frequent criticism of people currently living with a dementia diagnosis. In general, uptake of pre-symptomatic genetic testing is likely to be low in future. Experience has shown that, thus far, genetic testing for frontotemporal dementias can be offered safely following protocols similar to those developed for Huntington's disease (Quaid, 2011).

The field is progressing fast. A lot of attention has been focused on the formulation of high-quality guidelines such as the Joint Practice Guidelines of the American College of Medical Genetics and the National Society of Genetic Counselors (Goldman *et al.*, 2011). Motives and considerations for pursuing genetic testing always need to be explored. It is generally felt that counselling should be an exploration of personal experiences, values and beliefs, and personal and family needs. Genetic testing should be discussed within the context of adapting to familial risk and when clients feel keen to learn a more refined estimate of their risks to enhance their quality of life. It is finally being realised that policy strands can impact on various stakeholders in different ways. What is best for the 'peace of mind' of the carer is not necessarily the same as what is best for the peace of mind of the person living better with dementia. In Chapter 12, I considered whether 'wandering' is an appropriate term. The main emphasis of this chapter was the legal and ethical considerations in the use of 'global positioning systems' in enhancing the quality of life of persons with dementia and their closest ones.

Relationships and collaboration

In addition to families, general relationships are pivotal. In Chapter 3, I looked at the various issues facing the timely diagnosis and post-diagnostic support of people living with dementia from diverse cultural backgrounds, including people from black, Asian and ethnic minority backgrounds, people who are lesbian, bisexual, gay or transsexual, and people with prior learning difficulties.

Relationships between persons clearly matter from the history of policy of personhood too. Relationships between people living with dementia and those around them matter, as observed elegantly by Kitwood (1997). However, increasingly, we are understanding now that relationships matter between persons living with dementia and bodies 'corporate', such as the third sector or health and social care sectors. My exploration of 'living better with dementia' began with Chapter 1, which provided an introduction to policy in England as it currently stands, including a review of the need for a timely diagnosis as well as the right to timely post-diagnostic care. We all agree that much has to be done to up our game in England on the standards and expectations of post-diagnostic care, particularly if we are to close the 'diagnosis gap' through various initiatives. Whatever happens in policy, peer support is vital for the whole timeline for a person receiving a diagnosis of dementia. Peer support is well established in fields such as the disability movement and mental health, and is increasingly recognised as one way of enabling support by and for people with a diagnosis of dementia and their immediate carers (Keyes *et al.*, 2014).

Members of the highly influential Dementia Alliance International group, which consists of people living well with dementia but does not contain carers, have given a presentation at the Alzheimer's Disease International conference held in Puerto Rico in 2014 on successful internet peer support groups. Increasingly, people with dementia had been turning to social media to connect. Furthermore, people with dementia were finding each other at 'webinars' and connecting to create a sustainable community. A few messages came from this experience. There were frequent references to the positive impact and quality of relationships that emerged within peer support groups. People were able to both give and receive information, in 'pooling shared resources'. In the literature, there have been clear examples of peer support as an enabling mechanism, challenging the traditional medical deficit understanding of dementia.

It is inevitable that relationships do change over time, as do people (Mahieu, Anckaert and Gastmans, 2014). Ablitt, Jones and Muers (2009) found that different forms of relationship evolve as the dementia evolves. A neglect of direct evidence from the person with dementia is identified, and possible ways of combating this are considered.

Greenwood and colleagues (2013) published a thematic analysis of 13 in-depth interviews with nine carers and four peer volunteers which revealed that peer support helped both carers and peer volunteers through the realisation that they were 'not alone' in their experiences and emotions. Additional carer benefits included opportunities to talk freely about difficult experiences and learning how others cope. Volunteers found their role rewarding, describing satisfaction from putting their own experiences to good use. These findings highlight the isolation and exclusion experienced by current and former carers of people with dementia and draw attention to the benefits of peer support for both groups. Evidence suggests that education or peer support also did not impact on staff members' level of burnout. There was, however, a change in staff members' attitudes to working with people with dementia (Visser *et al.*, 2008). However, more research into living better with dementia is definitely needed.

We know that carers can experience significant levels of emotional stress from the demands of caring for a family member with dementia, yet their uptake of formal services tends to be lower than in other conditions related to ageing (Singh *et al.*, 2014). But an interesting tension may have now developed between personalisation of a 'care service' between carer and person living with dementia and 'friendsourcing' of pooled knowledge, behaviours and experience amongst persons living with dementia. A good account of the divide between personalisation and friendsourcing is provided by Bernstein and colleagues (2010).

Kitwood (1997) has challenged the prevailing reductionist biomedical view of dementia by postulating that seeing the person, not just the disease, is important. Smebye and Kirkevold (2013) have observed that relationships that sustain personhood are close emotional bonds between family carers and persons with dementia, and professional relationships between carers and persons with dementia. Likewise, relationships that tend to diminish personhood are task-centred relationships. In recent years, concern around the need for more person-centred approaches to dementia care has mounted (Tobin, 2003); yet, until recently, the evidence base to support these approaches has been rather small and anecdotal. Hunter and colleagues (2013) claimed to have found empirical evidence that beliefs about patient personhood have the potential to influence health providers' care decisions including decisions about pain management. They proposed that their results provided that 'having stronger positive beliefs about personhood in dementia increased the likelihood that health providers would select analgesics and non-pharmacological interventions, and decreased the likelihood of selecting psychotropic medication, in response to the vignettes' (p.284).

Understanding the current personhood of a person living better with dementia requires proper knowledge of the issues that a person has faced in the past. It has been reported by Osborne, Simpson and Stokes (2010) that 72% of the studies found significant relationships between pre-morbid personality and behaviour. In terms of specific relationships, the strongest evidence was found for a positive relationship between pre-morbid neuroticism and mood, and aggression and overall behavioural acts, thus supporting the inclusion of personality as one factor contributing to behaviour (Osborne *et al.*, 2010).

There needs to be acknowledgement of the nature of the relationships of people living better with dementia and the system generally. It is true that associations and international societies have made some headway in trying to address the educational needs of those diagnosed, but there remains a paucity of written materials and publications, workshops and conferences directed specifically at people striving to live better with dementia. Professionals and families may, altogether, underestimate the social and educational needs of people living with dementia (Snyder, Jenkins and Joosten, 2007).

'Collaboration' has been a core theme of my wish to boost the idea of dementia-friendly communities. It runs like letters through a stick of rock in the EU philosophical and legal policy of 'solidarity', enabling such successful initiatives as 'Rhapsody' described in the current thesis. Even within the biomedical model there has been an appreciation that greater collaboration permeating relationships, rather than competition, can lead to improved outcomes. The regulatory framework internationally needs to reflect this too. In a promising strategy, Mangialasche and colleagues (2012) call for the implementation of intervention programmes that take into account both the life-course model and the multi-factorial nature of the dementia syndromes. A promising initiative, notwithstanding, has been the European Dementia Prevention Initiative, an international collaboration aiming to improve strategies for preventing dementia. There was growing confidence that questions of broad societal and medical impact could be better understood if enough relevant clinical information was pooled on the effects on the brain of various factors, including psychiatric medications, drugs and alcohol abuse, dietary factors, and other factors including education and cardiovascular fitness, as well as pharmacological and behavioural interventions (Thompson *et al.*, 2014). International collaboration of research groups with experience in dementia prevention studies and well-organised logistics for these major projects are pivotal to success for future large-scale dementia prevention studies (Richard *et al.*, 2012).

Relationships are crucial to the delivery of person-centred care – for example, in the innovative 'life story' work. In Chapter 15, I looked at the triggering of football 'sporting memories' in people living well with dementia. This chapter considered the cognitive neuroscience of the phenomenon of this triggering of such memories, and proposed that such sporting memories could enhance the wellbeing also of people in the vicinity of the person with dementia.

'Telling the truth'

Relationships, including regulation and care, fundamentally depend on telling the truth. Perhaps the most cited rationale for telling therapeutic lies is to minimise potential distress and therefore potential treatment with antipsychotic medications (Mitchell, 2014). People have been more open-minded, on the whole, concerning many situations in which lying may seem, on the face of it, harmless or at least a lesser evil, and the question of whether or not to lie requires serious moral deliberation in such cases (Schermer, 2007). Hasselkus (1997) found that staff working in dementia day care settings used a variety of responses to maintain a patient's safety, including benign manipulation, lying and pretending. The issue of not telling the truth, in its various forms, is controversial and has a number of practical and ethical implications (Cutcliffe and Milton, 1996). James and colleagues (2006) have drawn up some helpful draft guidelines developed from participants' qualitative comments: for example, lies should only be told if they are in the best interest of the resident (e.g. to ease distress).

This is clearly different from 'pathological lying', which describes a clinical picture in which an individual repeatedly and apparently compulsively tells false stories; this has been reported in psychiatric disorders such as malingering, confabulation, factitious disorder and personality disorders (Dike, Baranowski and Griffith, 2005). Patients who confabulate tend to retrieve personal habits, repeated events or over-learned information and mistake them for actually experienced, specific unique events, possibly as a result of poor encoding, and over-learned information is involved in confabulation in dementia of the Alzheimer type (Attali *et al.*, 2009). Meanwhile, further research is needed to elucidate a defect of frontal lobe function that might lead to problems in reading others' emotions in behavioural variant frontotemporal dementia and pathological lying (Poletti, Borelli and Bonuccelli, 2011). As discussed by Day and colleagues (2011), the morality of lying and deception more generally has been an ongoing debate for philosophers for several years (e.g. Kant). This debate is linked to the equally heated deliberations about the actual definition of a lie, and whether or not it should be differentiated from deception. Thus far, a biomedical framing of dementia has dominated work in dementia, and there has been a reluctance to include the views about people living with dementia in research (e.g. Wilkinson, 2002).

Co-morbidity

A number of conditions can cause dementia as well as co-exist with dementia. Chapter 6 focused on delirium, or the acute confusional state, which can also co-exist or be caused by general medical conditions. Chapter 9 described one specific co-morbidity of dementia – incontinence. Dementia shortens life expectancy regardless of cause of death, and individuals with dementia, it is thought, have twice the risk of death independent of co-morbid conditions (Helvik *et al.*, 2014). Neuropsychiatric symptoms are quite common in patients with dementia, being more frequent as severity increases, and those symptoms are associated with functional impairment in the patients (Tascone *et al.*, 2008). This might contribute to people failing to receive a diagnosis of young-onset dementia, if clinicians are not trained adequately in this area. Significant co-morbidities have been discovered at autopsy in individuals with dementia.

Understanding the causes of death and associated co-morbidities in individuals with various subtypes of dementia is important in the assessment of end-of-life care in these individuals (Magaki *et al.*, 2014). Dementia and depression are among the most common conditions of the elderly, having a major impact on quality of life for patients and relatives, increased mortality and substantial health and social care costs. The relationship between depression and dementia is complex; depression has been reported to be both a risk factor and a prodrome for dementia of the Alzheimer type and other dementias, and is also a common complication of dementia at all stages (Bennett and Thomas, 2014).

There is a growing recognition that all those involved in dementia care need a greater level of expertise in managing general health problems. Several cardiovascular disorders have been suggested as risk factors for dementia, such as hypertension, hypercholesterolaemia, atrial fibrillation and heart failure; it is generally felt that correct management of these conditions can slow down cognitive decline and reduce the risk for dementia. A clear focus in future should be the interplay of medications for such conditions (e.g. Cermakova *et al.*, 2014). Co-morbid conditions can overlap with each other during the management of treatment, further mandating a case for clinical nursing specialists in 'proactive case management' (Baxter and Leary, 2011). Patients and carers can experience difficulties with the therapies prescribed for each co-morbid condition, reducing adherence to the treatment plan and consequently diminishing its efficacy (Damiani *et al.*, 2014). Innovative commissioning, through the 'prime contractor' model of encouraging plural stakeholders including the third sector, could have a constructive role here in meeting wellbeing outcomes for the National Health Service, which will be critical in the delivery of 'whole-person care'. (For an overview of the prime contractor model, see Department of Health, 2013.) There is also a coherent economic case for such proactive case management in the drive to avoid certain acute hospital admissions for people with dementia (Griffiths *et al.*, 2013).

Smith and colleagues (2014) recently reported that published randomly controlled trials poorly report medical co-morbidities and medications for people with dementia, and suggested that future trials should include the report of these factors to allow interpretation of whether the results are generalisable to frailer, older populations. Since dementia is most frequently associated with older people, people with dementia most commonly present with additional co-existing medical conditions. Such co-morbidities may include diabetes, chronic obstructive pulmonary disorder, musculoskeletal disorders and chronic cardiac failure (Helvik *et al.*, 2014). Helvik and colleagues noted that not fully appreciating the medical status and co-morbidities of cohorts means that the researchers are unable to make realistic headway. They further pointed out that interventions such as medication or physical activity may be more or less effective for some specific participant groups dependent on their co-morbidities. Therefore, it is not surprising that there will be a greater drive to report medical co-morbidities for research and service provision in future. The danger of working in 'silos' is staggering, to the extent that we are in danger of not understanding, for example, the health and social care needs of those citizens with diabetes complicated by cognitive impairment or dementia, and those with dementia complicated by diabetes (Sinclair *et al.*, 2014).

People living with dementia may be less likely to attend regular appointments or to notice or report relevant symptoms, and they may be more reliant on carers to manage and facilitate appointments (Keenan, Goldacre and Goldacre, 2014). Bunn and colleagues (2014) have found that the prevalence of co-morbid conditions in people with dementia is high. Whilst current evidence suggests that people with dementia may have poorer access to services, the reasons for this are not clear. Overall, Bunn and colleagues feel that there is a need for more research looking at the ways in which having dementia impacts on clinical care for other conditions and how the process of care and different services are adapting to the needs of people with dementia and co-morbidity. It turns out that even less is known about healthcare providers' experiences of managing people living with dementia and co-morbid health conditions, and how the presence of dementia influences the care they receive for their co-morbidity. These are areas that are currently being explored in an NIHR study on dementia and co-morbidity (Bunn *et al.*, 2013). Chapter 7 was the longest chapter in this book and took as its theme care and support networks. It included an overview of how patient-centred care is different from person-centred care, and how person-centred care differs from relationship-centred care.

Risk and uncertainty

My thesis has embraced the idea of positive risk engagement. It is inconceivable that positive risk engagement is irrelevant to successful dementia-friendly communities. This much-needed discussion is about to get 'lift off': see, for example, the excellent blogpost by Steve Morgan and Toby Williamson, 'How can "positive risk-taking" help to build dementia friendly communities?', on the Joseph Rowntree Foundation blog (2014).

Risk engagement has, in fact, been touched upon by Atul Gawande (2014) in a recent interview. The example Gawande gave is the risk of someone living well with dementia possibly spluttering on food that has not been pureed – but this risk engagement is all part of the 'eating well with dementia' experience (Chapter 8). Taking an individual approach to risk engagement is arguably the only option consistent with an approach that prioritises personhood, taking into account the decision making of a person living well with dementia in relation to other factors, including 'social, cultural, financial and family situation' (Tilse, Wilson and Setterlund, 2009, p.140). I write more generally on the policy drive for risk engagement or 'positive risk taking' in Chapter 13.

Another strand of the risk policy is whether leading a riskier lifestyle might encourage you to develop dementia. I presented the implications of this line of inquiry for private insurance markets in a session at Alzheimer Europe in 2014 (Rahman, 2014). Risk factors for dementia of the Alzheimer type have been extensively reported in the literature so far. Those examined in previous studies include advanced age, genetics, family history of dementia, female sex, low level of education, head trauma, smoking, apolipoprotein (APOE) ε4 allele, alcohol intake, diet rich in fat, systolic hypertension, cerebrovascular events, depression, dyslipidaemia, vascular risk factors, homocysteine, neurotoxic agents, oxidative stress, inflammation and infections (e.g. Cankurtaran *et al.*, 2008).

We are yet to assess properly the precise impact of non-modifiable risk factors. A recent meta-analysis study identifying the association of the ε4 allele with sporadic late-onset dementia of the Alzheimer type suggested that the ε4 allele increases the risk of sporadic late-onset dementia of the Alzheimer type, and determination of the ε4 allele in populations may be a useful tool for monitoring dementia patients and planning healthcare policies. Due to this potential relationship between APOE isoforms and dementia of the Alzheimer type, many companies have developed ε4 allele genotyping kits for prognostic diagnosis of dementia of the Alzheimer type, and evaluations of these kits with various ethnic groups have been conducted (see Kim *et al.*, 2014).

Not all the risk factors for dementia of the Alzheimer type hold true for other less prevalent dementias, but Fratiglioni, Winblad and von Strauss (2007) have helpfully set out a list of various preventative approaches to dementia of the Alzheimer type. These are, broadly, classified as 'primary', 'secondary' and 'tertiary' strategies, for instance in terms of delaying development of dementias, or reducing the impact of implications of long-term disease and disability in individuals.

Population-based studies, such as the Kungsholmen Project (Fratiglioni *et al.*, 2007), have made a great contribution to our knowledge of dementia and particularly dementia of the Alzheimer type, and these authors thought that it might be possible to delineate two preventative strategies for dementia:

» a good control of blood pressure, both in adult and late life

» an active and socially integrated life in old age.

There is a growing consensus that it is important for old people to participate in mentally as well as socially and physically stimulating activities. An active life may postpone the onset of dementia, and this might include the development of healthy social networks. Currently, the evidence does appear consistent with the widely propagated public health message that 'what is healthy for the body is healthy for the brain'. Norton and colleagues (2014) notably continue to argue that, with no proven interventions for altering the effects of genetic susceptibility to dementia of the Alzheimer type, it is important to identify and improve modifiable lifestyle risk factors for cognitive decline and dementia risk. Several recent trials have considered whether other forms of physical activity may also enhance cognition in old age (Lövdén, Xu and Wang, 2013). Involvement in mental, social and productive (e.g. gardening, volunteering) activities have also been associated with reduced incidence of dementia. Somewhat embarrassingly, however, Annette Leibing (2014, p.221) reviewed: 'In 2013, the list of risk factors and biomarkers for Alzheimer's disease are almost identical to those found in parallel publications from around 1993.'

I have already warned – with others – against 'Alzheimerisation' of policy, and this scenario is yet another very good example. It is argued that biomarkers of dementia of the Alzheimer type provide complementary information for disease staging and differential diagnosis. Determining the particular sequence and evolution of biomarker abnormality, their advocates argue, potentially provides a mechanism to stage and stratify patients throughout the full disease time course, and, in particular, during the presymptomatic phase (Young *et al.*, 2014). This might conceivably reduce heterogeneity in trial groups, match individuals to putative treatments and monitor treatment outcomes. A focus of dementia research has shifted from identification of potential risk factors to using this information for developing interventions to prevent or delay the onset of dementia as well as identifying special high-risk populations who could be targeted in intervention trials (Imtiaz *et al.*, 2014). These biomarkers are the latest in the long line of products from the pharmaceutical companies, which have thrown everything but the kitchen sink at capturing the dementia market. These products have included various interventions (Tariot *et al.*, 2004).

In Chapter 4, I looked at the issue of how different jurisdictions around the world have formulated their national dementia strategies. However, there is clearly an urgent need, challenge and responsibility to respond to multiple stakeholders (Ferreira and Adkins, 2011). Presently, among the array of impediments to prevention studies, the most critical factors are the lack of:

> (a) validated algorithms, biomarkers, and assessment tools to facilitate the identification of asymptomatic people with elevated risk for dementia of the Alzheimer type;
>
> (b) research resources or infrastructure for large scale longitudinal studies; and
>
> (c) a national/international database on asymptomatic volunteers with elevated risk who might be recruited as potential research volunteers.
>
> (Khachaturian *et al.*, 2010, p.90)

A risk in policy is whether we are able to determine with greater clarity those people who might go on to develop dementia of the Alzheimer type. And there is a potentially large market for this, especially if the English policy is successful at capturing volunteers for research trials into dementia. Fervour for this type of research does not seem to be accompanied yet by an equal fervour for engagement in living well with dementia research, apart from a few outstanding initiatives such as 'DEEP 2' (Joseph Rowntree Foundation, 2013). But progress in neuroimaging-based research has been important, particularly if there is an outside chance that we will one day be able to follow the response to therapy of people living with dementia to certain pharmaceutical interventions. There is, for example, the possibility of the 'timely intervention' of potential anti-amyloid therapeutics, suggesting that such therapy should be evaluated in mildly symptomatic or asymptomatic individuals with increased brain β-amyloid burden to assess the potential for the prevention of dementia (Pike *et al.*, 2007).

In January 2013, shortly after approval by the US Food and Drug Administration (FDA), the European Commission issued a single marketing authorisation for 'Amyvid' ([18F] florbetapir), making it possible to estimate β-amyloid neuritic plaque density in the brain when the subject is still alive (Cortes-Blanco *et al.*,

2014). It is well accepted that none to sparse neuritic plaque density measured in the region of maximal involvement in frontal, temporal or parietal cortex is inconsistent with a definitive diagnosis of dementia of the Alzheimer type in adults older than 50 years of age (Mirra *et al.*, 1991). Considering that entorhinal cortex atrophy tends to correlate well with cognitive decline only among subjects with β-amyloid, (18F) florbetapir PET makes it possible to detect dementia of the Alzheimer type pathology in the early stage, whereas MRI morphometry for subjects with β-amyloid may provide a good biomarker to assess the severity of dementia of the Alzheimer type in the later stage (Tateno *et al.*, 2014). Further evidence also suggests that both positive and negative (18F) florbetapir scans may enhance diagnostic certainty and impact clinical decision making (Zannas *et al.*, 2014). Controlled longitudinal studies are needed to confirm these data. Most people wish for a prompt diagnosis of dementia, but it is vital for each individual concerned that this diagnosis is correct as far as possible.

There is uncertainty about some of the biological features of dementia of the Alzheimer type, and unfortunately this impacts on the development of the right therapeutic interventions. For example, there may be a link between insulin resistance or sensitivity and dementias, particularly dementia of the Alzheimer type, and, if so, this might produce novel therapeutic targets (Cholerton, Baker and Craft, 2013). Also, antidepressants may have a role in helping to stop dementia of the Alzheimer type in its tracks. For example, it was recently reported that citalopram could arrest the growth of pre-existing plaques of dementia of the Alzheimer type, and reduce the appearance of new plaques by 78% (Sheline *et al.*, 2014). Furthermore, in healthy human volunteers in that study, β-amyloid production in cerebrospinal fluid was slowed by 37% in the citalopram group compared with placebo. Also, the ability to safely decrease β-amyloid concentrations is potentially important as a preventive strategy for Alzheimer's disease. The use of ACE inhibitors (ACE-Is) in older adults with dementia of the Alzheimer type has been found to be associated with a slower rate of cognitive decline independent of hypertension (Soto *et al.*, 2013). Future research is needed to explore the role of ACE-Is in long-term progression of dementia of the Alzheimer type.

So far I have described the need to embrace risk for living better with dementia. I then considered the potentially preventable risks of life which could lead to dementia. I went on to consider the risks in making the diagnosis and in developing new drug products. And risk will have a part to play in service transformation very soon. It is likely that a large-scale transformation in the way the service helps people living with dementia is likely to happen. The implications for planning are far-reaching. The agent of change must give up notions of 'control' over the process of change and should avoid language that emphasises 'overcoming resistance' (Best *et al.*, 2012).

In Chapter 10, I argued how the needs for people living better with dementia would be best served by a fully integrated health and social care service. That chapter provided the rationale behind this policy instrument in England. And a true 'whole-person care' outlook will go far beyond the health and social care sectors in time: Chapter 11 considered the profound influence of housing as a social determinant of health for a person trying to live better with dementia.

Overall conclusion

Anything can happen to anyone at any time. Despite all the best initiatives in the world, it will be unachievable to extinguish all negative perceptions about dementia. Nobody can deny the imperative for communities and society to be inclusive and accessible for people with dementia, but it is no mean feat to rationalise with more individualistic approaches ranging from personal budgets, human rights and equality law responsibilities. It really is not a question of what a person can no longer do. It is an issue of what a person can currently do, and this might include, for example, the unleashing of previously unwitnessed artistic and creative talents.

All jurisdictions converge on the right for a timely diagnosis and a right to timely post-diagnostic support, but political grandstanding over cures will be small change to those people currently wanting to live better with dementia. People who have received a diagnosis of dementia are not all consumers, and some do not even interact with health and social care services as patients. They are all persons, however, and wish for inalienable dignity and respect. Everyone knows that the diagnosis affects not just the person with dementia but their whole network of friends and family. There now must be a political will to do something about this, and this is not just a societal issue for the G7.

Silos must be abolished. For example, in considering eating better with dementia, the emphasis can no longer be on the design of 'finger snacks', but responsible thought has to be put into how certain mealtime environments work (or do not work). It is utterly pointless talking about joining initiatives to encourage 'dementia friendliness' as long as words such as 'victim' continue to litter the mainstream press. And 'leading' scientists and practitioners can unwittingly perpetuate stigma through somewhat pejorative language such as 'wanderer'; the wilful blindness to this must stop too. Living better with dementia is not just an aspiration; in many places it is legally enforceable.

I think people aspiring to live better with dementia themselves can 'turbo boost' the phenomenon of dementia-friendly communities, if they are given the opportunity to do so. There is much work to be done to ensure that they themselves benefit, as is clearly intended by the policy. There is no doubt, however, that we have come a long way from where we were. The weakest link is what is realistically achievable in the rest of the community, such as access to justice, so that people with dementia have enforceable rights under human rights or equality law, or standards of affordable housing. Enforceable legal rights enshrine autonomy and dignity. Dementia is primarily not a brand to generate competitive advantage, though we do need to keep a very careful eye on opportunity costs of allocation of scarce resources into areas of low returns. The NHS currently has a statutory duty to promote innovation, and I feel that this is especially urgent in service provision, in reducing the number of inappropriate antipsychotic prescriptions in care homes and in delivering proactive case management through clinical nursing specialists. Aspiring to live better with dementia is a unique test of our solidarity and what we actually value in life. 'We're all in this together' (George Osborne MP, Conservative Party Conference, October 2012, reported in *The Guardian* newspaper).

Dr Shibley Rahman
London
December 2014

References

Ablitt, A., Jones, G.V. and Muers, J. (2009) Living with dementia: a systematic review of the influence of relationship factors. Aging and Mental Health, 13, 4, 497–511.

Adams, S. (2006) GPs 'failing to diagnose dementia'. *The Telegraph.* Available at www.telegraph.co.uk/news/health/news/7928340/GPs-failing-to-diagnose-dementia.html (accessed 20 April 2015).

Adams, T. (2010) The applicability of a recovery approach to nursing people with dementia. International Journal of Nursing Studies, 47, 5, 626–34.

Attali, E., De Anna, F., Dubois, B. and Dalla Barba, G. (2009) Confabulation in Alzheimer's disease: poor encoding and retrieval of over-learned information. Brain, 132, 1, 204–12.

Baxter, J. and Leary, A. (2011) Productivity gains by specialist nurses. Nursing Times, 107, 30–1, 15–17.

Bennett, S. and Thomas, A.J. (2014) Depression and dementia: cause, consequence or coincidence? Maturitas, 79, 2, 184–90.

Bernstein, M.S., Tan, D., Smith, G., Czerwinski, M. and Horvitz, E. (2010) Personalization via friendsourcing. Transactions on Computer Human Interaction, 17, 2, 6.

Bertram, L., McQueen, M.B., Mullin, K., Blacker, D. and Tanzi, R.E. (2007) Systematic meta analyses of Alzheimer disease genetic association studies: the AlzGene database. Nature Genetics, 39, 1, 17–23.

Best, A., Greenhalgh, T., Lewis, S., Saul, J.E., Carroll, S. and Bitz, J. (2012) Large-system transformation in health care: a realist review. The Milbank Quarterly, 90, 3, 421–56.

Brodaty, H. and Donkin, M. (2009) Family caregivers of people with dementia. Dialogues in Clinical Neuroscience, 11, 217–28.

Bunn, F., Burn, A.M., Goodman, C., Rait, G. *et al.* (2014) Comorbidity and dementia: a scoping review of the literature. BMC Medicine, 12, 1, 192.

Bunn, F., Goodman, C., Brayne, C., Norton, S. *et al.* (2013) Comorbidity and dementia: improving healthcare for people with dementia (CoDem). Available at www.nets.nihr.ac.uk/projects/hsdr/11101707 (accessed 6 December 2014).

Cankurtaran, M., Yavuz, B.B., Cankurtaran, E.S., Halil, M., Ulger, Z. and Ariogul, S. (2008) Risk factors and type of dementia: vascular or Alzheimer? Archives of Gerontology and Geriatrics, 47, 1, 25–34.

Cermakova, P., Fereshtehnejad, S.M., Johnell, K., Winblad, B., Eriksdotter, M. and Religa, D. (2014) Cardiovascular medication burden in dementia disorders: a nationwide study of 19,743 dementia patients in the Swedish Dementia Registry. Alzheimer's Research and Therapy, 6, 3, 34.

Chassot, C.S. and Mendes, F. (2014) The experience of mental distress and recovery among people involved with the service user/survivor movement. Health (London), Oct 14, pii: 1363459314554313 [Epub ahead of print].

Cholerton, B., Baker, L.D. and Craft, S. (2013) Insulin, cognition, and dementia. European Journal of Pharmacology, 719, 1–3, 170–9.

Clark, R. (2004) Significance of Perceived Racism: Toward Understanding Ethnic Group Disparities in Health, the Later Years. In N.B. Anderson, R.A. Bulatao and B. Cohen (eds) Critical Perspectives on Racial and Ethnic Differences in Health in Late Life. Washington, DC: National Academies Press.

Cortes-Blanco, A., Prieto-Yerro, C., Martinez-Lazaro, R., Zamora, J. *et al.* (2014) Florbetapir (18F) for brain amyloid positron emission tomography: highlights on the European marketing approval. Alzheimer's and Dementia, 10, 5 Suppl., S395–9.

Cutcliffe, J. and Milton, J. (1996) In defence of telling lies to cognitively impaired elderly patients. International Journal of Geriatric Psychiatry, 11, 1117–18.

Damiani, G., Silvestrini, G., Trozzi, L., Maci, D., Iodice, L. and Ricciardi, W. (2014) Quality of dementia clinical guidelines and relevance to the care of older people with comorbidity: evidence from the literature. Clinical Interventions in Aging, 20, 9, 1399–407.

Davies, N., Maio, L., Rait, G. and Iliffe, S. (2014) Quality end-of-life care for dementia: what have family carers told us so far? A narrative synthesis. Palliative Medicine, 28, 7, 919–30.

Day, A.M., James, I.A., Meyer, T.D. and Lee, D.R. (2011) Do people with dementia find lies and deception in dementia care acceptable? Aging and Mental Health, 15, 7, 822–9.

Dementia Alliance International (2014) Online Support Groups for People with Dementia. Presented at the ADI Conference, 1–4 May 2014. Available at www.alz.co.uk/sites/default/files/conf2014/OC043.pdf (accessed 6 December 2014).

Department of Health (2013) The NHS Standard Contract: a guide for clinical commissioners. Available at www.england.nhs.uk/wp-content/uploads/2013/02/contract-guide-clinical.pdf (accessed 25 February 2015).

Dike, C.C., Baranowski, M. and Griffith, E.E.H. (2005) Pathological lying revisited. Journal of the American Academy of Psychiatry and the Law, 33, 342–9.

Dolan, J. (2013) Smoothing the Wrinkles: Hollywood, Successful Aging and the New Visibility of Older Female Stars. In C. Carter, L. Steiner and L. McClaughlin (eds) The Routledge Companion to Media and Gender. London and New York, NY: Routledge.

Drennan, G., Law, K. and Alred, D. (2012) Recovery in the Forensic Organisation. In G. Drennan and D. Alred (eds) Secure Recovery. Abingdon: Routledge.

Ducharme, F., Lachance, L., Lévesque, L., Zarit, S.H. and Kergoat, M.J. (2014) Maintaining the potential of a psycho-educational program: efficacy of a booster session after an intervention offered family caregivers at disclosure of a relative's dementia diagnosis. Aging and Mental Health, 19, 3, 207–16.

Ferreira, M. and Adkins, J. (2011) The globalisation of dementia: issues and responses in 'global ageing'. Available at www.ifa-fiv.org/global-ageing-issues-action-volume-7-1 (accessed 20 April 2015).

Fratiglioni, L., Winblad, B. and von Strauss, E. (2007) Prevention of Alzheimer's disease and dementia: major findings from the Kungsholmen Project. Physiology and Behavior, 92, 1–2, 98–104.

Gawande, A. (2014) We Have Medicalized Aging, and That Experiment Is Failing Us. Mother Jones, 7 October 2014. Available at www.motherjones.com/media/2014/10/atul-gawande-being-mortal-interview-assisted-living (accessed 6 December 2014).

Goffman, E. (1963) Stigma: Notes on the Management of Spoiled Identity. Englewood Cliffs, NJ: Prentice-Hall.

Goldman, J.S., Hahn, S.E., Catania, J.W., LaRusse-Eckert, S. *et al.* American College of Medical Genetics and the National Society of Genetic Counselors (2011) Genetic counseling and testing for Alzheimer disease: joint practice guidelines of the American College of Medical Genetics and the National Society of Genetic Counselors. Genetics in Medicine, 13, 6, 597–605.

Golics, C.J., Basra, M.K., Salek, M.S. and Finlay, A.Y. (2013) The impact of patients' chronic disease on family quality of life: an experience from 26 specialties. International Journal of General Medicine, 6, 787–98.

Greenwood, N., Habibi, R., Mackenzie, A., Drennan, V. and Easton, N. (2013) Peer support for carers: a qualitative investigation of the experiences of carers and peer volunteers. American Journal of Alzheimer's Disease and Other Dementias, 28, 6, 617–26.

Griffiths, P., Bridges, J., Sheldon, H., Bartlett, R. and Hunt, K. (2013) Scoping the role of the dementia nurse specialist in acute care. Centre for Innovation and Leadership in the Health Sciences/University of Southampton. Available at http://eprints.soton.ac.uk/349714/13/dementia%20specialist%20nurses.pdf (accessed 12 February 2015).

Guardian website (2012) George Osborne tells Tory conference: 'We're all in this together.' Available at www.theguardian.com/politics/video/2012/oct/08/george-osborne-tory-conference-video (accessed 6 December 2014).

Hasselkus, B.R. (1997) Everyday ethics in dementia care: narratives of crossing the line. Gerontologist, 37, 640–9.

Heath, I. (2013) Overdiagnosis: when good intentions meet vested interests – an essay by Iona Heath. British Medical Journal, 347, f6361.

Helvik, A.S., Engedal, K., Benth, J.S. and Selbæk, G. (2014) A 52 month follow-up of functional decline in nursing home residents – degree of dementia contributes. BMC Geriatrics, 14, 45.

Hsieh, S., Irish, M., Daveson, N., Hodges, J.R. and Piguet, O. (2013) When one loses empathy: its effect on carers of patients with dementia. Journal of Geriatric Psychiatry and Neurology, 6, 3, 174–84.

Hunter, P.V., Hadjistavropoulos, T., Smythe, W.E., Malloy, D.C., Kaasalainen, S. and Williams, J. (2013) The Personhood in Dementia Questionnaire (PDQ): establishing an association between beliefs about personhood and health providers' approaches to person-centred care. Aging Studies, 27, 3, 276–87.

Huppert, F.A. and So, T.T. (2013) Flourishing across Europe: application of a new conceptual framework for defining wellbeing. Social Indicators Research, 110, 3, 837–61.

Iliffe, S. and Manthorpe, J. (2007) Dementia: still muddling along? British Journal of General Practice, 57, 541, 606–7.

Imtiaz, B., Tolppanen, A.M., Kivipelto, M. and Soininen, H. (2014) Future directions in Alzheimer's disease from risk factors to prevention. Biochemical Pharmacology, 88, 4, 661–70.

James, I.A., Wood-Mitchell, A.J., Waterworth, A.M., Mackenzie, L.E. and Cunningham, J. (2006) Lying to people with dementia: developing ethical guidelines for care settings. International Journal of Geriatric Psychiatry, 21, 8, 800–1.

Joling, K.J., Bosmans, J.E., van Marwijk, H.W., van der Horst, H.E. *et al.* (2013) The cost-effectiveness of a family meetings intervention to prevent depression and anxiety in family caregivers of patients with dementia: a randomized trial. Trials, 14, 305.

Joseph Rowntree Foundation (2013) Dementia without Walls: Early activity and progress. Available at www.jrf.org.uk/sites/files/jrf/DWW-June2013.pdf (accessed 15 May 2015).

Keenan, T.D., Goldacre, R. and Goldacre, M.J. (2014) Associations between age-related macular degeneration, Alzheimer disease, and dementia: record linkage study of hospital admissions. JAMA Ophthalmology, 132, 63–8.

Keyes, C.L.M. (2002) The mental health continuum: from languishing to flourishing in life. Journal of Health and Social Behavior, 43, 207–22.

Keyes, S.E., Clarke, C.L., Wilkinson, H., Alexjuk, E.J. *et al.* (2014) 'We're all thrown in the same boat...' A qualitative analysis of peer support in dementia care. Dementia (London), Apr 17 [Epub ahead of print].

Khachaturian, Z.S., Barnes, D., Einstein, R., Johnson, S. *et al.* (2010) Developing a national strategy to prevent dementia: Leon Thal Symposium 2009. Alzheimer's and Dementia, 6, 2, 89–97.

Killaspy, H. (2014) Contemporary mental health rehabilitation. East Asian Archives of Psychiatry, 24, 3, 89–94.

Kim, D.H., Yeo, S.H., Park, J.M., Choi, J.Y. *et al.* (2014) Genetic markers for diagnosis and pathogenesis of Alzheimer's disease. Gene, 545, 2, 185–93.

Kitwood, T. (1997) Dementia Reconsidered: The Person Comes First. Philadelphia, PA: Open University Press.

Lancet Global Mental Health Group (2007) Scale-up services for mental disorders: a call for action. Lancet, 370, 9594, 1241–52.

Leibing, A. (2014) The earlier the better: Alzheimer's prevention, early detection, and the quest for pharmacological interventions. Culture, Medicine and Psychiatry, 38, 2, 217–36.

Lövdén, M., Xu, W. and Wang, H.X. (2013) Lifestyle change and the prevention of cognitive decline and dementia: what is the evidence? Current Opinion in Psychiatry, 26, 3, 239–43.

Magaki, S., Yong, W.H., Khanlou, N., Tung, S. and Vinters, H.V. (2014) Co-morbidity in dementia: update of an ongoing autopsy study. Journal of the American Geriatrics Society, 62, 9, 1722–8.

Mahieu, L., Anckaert, L. and Gastmans, C. (2014) Intimacy and sexuality in institutionalized dementia care: clinical-ethical considerations. Health Care Analysis, Oct 1 [Epub ahead of print].

Mangialasche, F., Kivipelto, M., Solomon, A. and Fratiglioni, L. (2012) Dementia prevention: current epidemiological evidence and future perspective. Alzheimer's Research and Therapy, 4, 1, 6.

Marino, C.K. (2015) To belong, contribute, and hope: first stage development of a measure of social recovery. Journal of Mental Health, 24, 2, 68–72.

McKenna, B., Furness, T., Dhital, D. and Ireland, S. (2014) Recovery-oriented care in older-adult acute inpatient mental health settings in Australia: an exploratory study. Journal of the American Geriatrics Society, 62, 10, 1938–42.

Meeks, S., Van Haitsma, K., Kostiwa, I. and Murrell, S.A. (2012) Positivity and wellbeing among community residing elders and nursing home residents: what is the optimal affect balance? Journals of Gerontology Series B: Psychological Sciences and Social Sciences, 67, 4, 460–7.

Mirra, S.S., Heyman, A., McKeel, D., Sumi, S.M. *et al.* (1991) The Consortium to Establish a Registry for Alzheimer's Disease (CERAD). Part II. Standardization of the neuropathologic assessment of Alzheimer's disease. Neurology, 41, 4, 479–86.

Mitchell, G. (2014) Therapeutic lying to assist people with dementia in maintaining medication adherence. Nursing Ethics, 21, 7, 844–84.

Morgan, S. and Williamson, T. (2014) How can 'positive risk-taking' help to build dementia friendly communities? Joseph Rowntree Foundation blog (blogpost dated 11 November 2014). Available at www.jrf.org.uk/publications/how-can-positive-risk-taking-help-build-dementia-friendly-communities (accessed 6 December 2014).

Norton, S., Matthews, F.E., Barnes, D.E., Yaffe, K. and Brayne, C. (2014) Potential for primary prevention of Alzheimer's disease: an analysis of population-based data. Lancet Neurology, 13, 8, 788–94.

Osborne, H., Simpson, J. and Stokes, G. (2010) The relationship between pre-morbid personality and challenging behaviour in people with dementia: a systematic review. Aging and Mental Health, 14, 5, 503–15.

Park, N.S. and Peterson, C. (2009) Achieving and sustaining a good life. Perspectives on Psychological Science, 4, 422–8.

Perry, R.J., Rosen, H.R., Kramer, J.H., Beer, J.S., Levenson, R.L. and Miller, B.L. (2001) Hemispheric dominance for emotions, empathy and social behaviour: evidence from right and left handers with frontotemporal dementia. Neurocase, 7, 2, 145–60.

Pike, K.E., Savage, G., Villemagne, V.L., Ng, S.C.A. *et al.* (2007) Beta-amyloid imaging and memory in non-demented individuals: evidence for preclinical Alzheimer's disease. Brain, 130, 2837–44.

Poletti, M., Borelli, P. and Bonuccelli, U. (2011) The neuropsychological correlates of pathological lying: evidence from behavioural variant frontotemporal dementia. Journal of Neurology, 258, 11, 2009–13.

Quaid, K.A. (2011) Genetic counseling for frontotemporal dementias. Journal of Molecular Neuroscience, 45, 3, 706–9.

Rahman, S. (2014) Poster P14.4. Would future NHS dementia care easily lend itself to private markets? Policy stream on socio-economic costs of dementia and financing of care. Alzheimer Europe Conference, Glasgow, 2014.

Reinhardt, J.P., Chichin, E., Posner, L. and Kassabian, S. (2014) Vital conversations with family in the nursing home: preparation for end-stage dementia care. Journal of Social Work in End-of-Life and Palliative Care, 10, 2, 112–26.

Richard, E., Andrieu, S., Solomon, A., Mangialasche, F. *et al.* (2012) Methodological challenges in designing dementia prevention trials: the European Dementia Prevention Initiative (EDPI). Journal of the Neurological Sciences, 322, 1–2, 64–70.

Roses, A.D. and Saunders, A.M. (1997) Clinical overdiagnosis of vascular dementia versus necropsy confirmed series. Journal of Neurology, Neurosurgery and Psychiatry, 62, 6, 677–8.

Ryff, C.D. (1989) Happiness is everything, or is it? Explorations on the meaning of psychological well-being. Journal of Personality and Social Psychology, 57, 1069–81.

Ryff, C.D. (2014) Psychological wellbeing revisited: advances in the science and practice of eudaimonia. Psychotherapy and Psychosomatics, 83, 1, 10–28.

Ryff, C.D. and Singer, B. (1998) The contours of positive human health. Psychological Inquiry, 9, 1–28.

Salem, L.C., Andersen, B.B., Nielsen, T.R., Stokholm, J. *et al.* (2012) Overdiagnosis of dementia in young patients: a nationwide register-based study. Dementia and Geriatric Cognitive Disorders, 34, 5–6, 292–9.

Sampson, E.L., Jones, L., Thuné-Boyle, I.C., Kukkastenvehmas, R. *et al.* (2011) Palliative assessment and advance care planning in severe dementia: an exploratory randomized controlled trial of a complex intervention. Palliative Medicine, 25, 3, 197–209.

Schermer, M. (2007) Nothing but the truth? On truth and deception in dementia care. Bioethics, 21, 1, 13–22.

Schrank, B., Brownell, T., Tylee, A. and Slade, M. (2014) Positive psychology: an approach to supporting recovery in mental illness. East Asian Archives of Psychiatry, 24, 3, 95–103.

Sheline, Y.I., West, T., Yarasheski, K., Swarm, R. *et al.* (2014) An antidepressant decreases CSF Aβ production in healthy individuals and in transgenic AD mice. Science Translational Medicine, 6, 236, 236re4.

Shen, L., Thompson, P.M., Potkin, S.G., Bertram, L. *et al.* (2014) Alzheimer's Disease Neuroimaging Initiative Genetic analysis of quantitative phenotypes in AD and MCI: imaging, cognition and biomarkers. Brain Imaging and Behavior, 8, 2, 183–207.

Shmotkin, D. (2005) Happiness in the face of adversity: reformulating the dynamic and modular bases of subjective wellbeing. Review of General Psychology, 9, 291–325.

Sinclair, A.J., Hillson, R. and Bayer, A.J./National Expert Working Group (2014) Diabetes and dementia in older people: a Best Clinical Practice Statement by a multidisciplinary National Expert Working Group. Diabetic Medicine, 31, 9, 1024–31.

Singh, P., Hussain, R., Khan, A., Irwin, L. and Foskey, R. (2014) Dementia care: intersecting informal family care and formal care systems. Journal of Aging Research, 2014, 486521.

Slooter, A.J., Cruts, M., Kalmijn, S., Hofman, A. *et al.* (1998) Risk estimates of dementia by apolipoprotein E genotypes from a population-based incidence study: the Rotterdam Study. Archives of Neurology, 55, 964–8.

Smebye, K.L. and Kirkevold, M. (2013) The influence of relationships on personhood in dementia care: a qualitative, hermeneutic study. BMC Nursing, 12, 1, 29.

Smith, T., Maidment, I., Hebding, J., Madzima, T. *et al.* (2014) Systematic review investigating the reporting of co-morbidities and medication in randomized controlled trials of people with dementia. Age and Ageing, 43, 6, 868–72.

Snyder, L., Jenkins, C. and Joosten, L. (2007) Effectiveness of support groups for people with mild to moderate Alzheimer's disease: an evaluative survey. American Journal of Alzheimer's Disease and Other Dementias, 22, 1, 14–19.

Soto, M.E., van Kan, G.A., Nourhashemi, F., Gillette-Guyonnet, S. *et al.* (2013) Angiotensin-converting enzyme inhibitors and Alzheimer's disease progression in older adults: results from the Réseau sur la Maladie d'Alzheimer Français cohort. Journal of the American Geriatrics Society, 61, 9, 1482–8.

Sullivan, K.A., Beattie, E., Khawaja, N.G., Wilz, G. and Cunningham, L. (2014) The Thoughts Questionnaire (TQ) for family caregivers of people with dementia. Dementia (London), Oct 2, pii: 1471301214553038 [Epub ahead of print].

Swaffer, K. (2014) Dementia: stigma, language, and dementia-friendly. Dementia, 13, 709–16.

Szasz, T.S. (2001) The therapeutic state: the tyranny of pharmacracy. Available at www.independent.org/pdf/tir/tir_05_4_szasz.pdf (accessed 20 April 2015).

Tariot, P.N., Farlow, M.R., Grossberg, G.T., Graham, S.M., McDonald, S. and Gergel, I. (2004) Memantine treatment in patients with moderate to severe Alzheimer disease already receiving donepezil: a randomized controlled trial. JAMA, 291, 317–24

Tascone, L.S., Marques, R.C.G., Pereira, E.C. and Bottino, C. (2008) Characteristics of patients assisted at an ambulatory of dementia from a university hospital. Arqivos de Neuro-psiquiatra, 66, 631–5.

Tateno, A., Sakayori, T., Kawashima, Y., Higuchi, M. *et al.* (2014) Comparison of imaging biomarkers for Alzheimer's disease: amyloid imaging with 18F-florbetapir positron emission tomography and magnetic resonance imaging voxel-based analysis for entorhinal cortex atrophy. International Journal of Geriatric Psychiatry, Jul 7, doi: 10.1002/gps.4173 [Epub ahead of print].

Thompson, P.M., Stein, J.L., Medland, S.E., Hibar, D.P. *et al.* (2014) The ENIGMA Consortium: large scale collaborative analyses of neuroimaging and genetic data. Brain Imaging and Behavior, 8, 2, 153–82.

Tilse, C., Wilson, J. and Setterlund, J. (2009) Personhood, Financial Decision Making and Dementia: An Australian Perspective. In D. O'Connor and B. Purves (eds) Decision-Making, Personhood and Dementia: Exploring the Interface. London: Jessica Kingsley Publishers.

Tobin, S.S. (2003) The historical context of 'humanistic' culture change in long-term care. Journal of Social Work in Long-Term Care, 2, 53–64.
Visser, S.M., McCabe, M.P., Hudgson, C., Buchanan, G., Davison, T.E. and George, K. (2008) Managing behavioural symptoms of dementia: effectiveness of staff education and peer support. Aging and Mental Health, 12, 1, 47–55.
Warchol-Biedermann, K., Mojs, E., Gregersen, R., Maibom, K., Millán-Calenti, J.C. and Maseda, A. (2014) What causes grief in dementia caregivers? Archives of Gerontology and Geriatrics, 59, 2, 462–7.
Wilken, J.P. and Hollander, D. (2008) Rehabilitering og recovery. En integreret tilgang [Rehabilitation and Recovery. An Integrated Approach]. København: Akademisk Forlag.
Wilkinson, H. (2002) The Perspectives of People with Dementia: Research Methods and Motivations. London: Jessica Kingsley Publishers.
World Health Organization (2014) Mental health: a state of well-being. Available at www.who.int/features/factfiles/mental_health/en (accessed 6 December 2014).
Young, A.L., Oxtoby, N.P., Daga, P., Cash, D.M. *et al.* Alzheimer's Disease Neuroimaging Initiative (2014) A data-driven model of biomarker changes in sporadic Alzheimer's disease. Brain, 137, 9, 2564–77.
Zannas, A.S., Doraiswamy, P.M., Shpanskaya, K.S., Murphy, K.R. *et al.* (2014) Impact of ^{18}F-florbetapir PET imaging of β-amyloid neuritic plaque density on clinical decision-making. Neurocase, 20, 4, 466–73.

SUBJECT INDEX

Page numbers in *italics* refer to figures and boxes.

Admiral Nurses 144–5, *147*, 194
advance care planning (ACP) 361
Age and Ageing (journal) 248
age discrimination 54
Age UK 166
alcohol, and risk of dementia 39
All-Party Parliamentary Group (APPG) on Dementia 27, *28*, 42, 67, *67–8*, 90, 92, 329–30
AlzGene database 362
Alzheimer, Alois 103
Alzheimer Europe conferences 275, 298, 299, 370
Alzheimer type dementia
 caregiving 139, 322, 362
  characteristics 56, 118, 186, 206, 245, 259, 280–1, 328, 373
  creativity 291–2, 293, 298
  dementia and 122
  diagnosis, coping with 105–8
  eating issues 167, 169, 171, 171–5
  ethical issues 29
  memory issues 304, 306, 310, 314
  prevalence 43, 102, 103
  primary care visits 136
  risk factors 19, 35–41, *36*, 270, 362–3, 368, 370–1, 373
Alzheimer's Association 29
Alzheimer's Australia 137, 152
Alzheimer's Disease International (ADI) 82–3, *83–4*, 151, 173, 175, 364
Alzheimer's Society 42
ambient-assisted living 214
American Delirium Society 114
amnesia 307, 310–11, 312
amyloid 31, *32*, 36, 41, 372–3
Amyvid 372–3
Angelou, Maya 128, 289
antidepressants 373
antioxidants 40, 171, 172
antipsychotics 91, 120, 321–34, 360, 367
 behavioural and psychological symptoms of dementia 326–7
 'call to action' 332–4, *333*
 the case for behavioural interventions 330–1
 inappropriate use of 30–1, *31*, 375
 and innovation 334–5
 stepped care model 331, *332*
 use in care homes 327–30
aphasia 295
apraxia 181, 291
architecture *see* design considerations
art 291–4
arts therapies 294, 298–9
Asian communities 71–2, 144
 see also BAME communities
AT trial 36
atrophy 43, 169, 279, 296, 298
attachment theory 130
Augustine of Hippo, Saint 81
autism 262, 291
autobiographical memories (ABM) 294, 295–6, 312–14, *314*
autonomy 87, 149, 199, 216, 235, 243, 248–9, 252, 260–4, 276, 360, 375

BAME (black, Asian and minority ethnic) communities 65–72, *67–8*, 227, 370
Beckett, Samuel 113
behavioural interventions, the case for 330–1
Beresford, Peter 268
Better Care Fund 210
big data 44–5, 100, 109, 362–3
black communities *see* BAME communities
Blackfriars Consensus Statement 34–5
BMI (body mass index) 39, 166, 173
Brain (journal) 57
brain, the
 and creativity 294–5
 and decision-making 278–9, *279*
 diseases of 43
 and eating behaviour 167–8, 169
 effect of damage to 291–3, 295–6, 297, 311
 function 43, 292, 361–2
 and memory 307, *307*, 308–17
 reserve 18, 118
 size 316
 and suffering 57
British Geriatrics Society 116

British Medical Journal 26, 27, 206
British Psychological Society 331, *332*
Burnham, Andy 193
Burns, Alistair 123

CALD (culturally and linguistically diverse communities) 70–1
  see also cultural issues
Camberwell Assessment of Needs for the Elderly (CANE) 188
Cameron, David (Prime Minister), Dementia Challenge 26–34, *28*, *33–4*
cancer 86, 107, 151, 194, 201
cardiovascular disorders 35, 38, 86, 368
  see also vascular dementia
Cardiovascular Health Cognition Study (CHCS) 172
Care Act 2014 261
Care and Repair England 235
Care Commission, Scotland 165–6
care homes
  'challenging behaviour' in 327
  and community visitors 149–50
  CQC standards 232, *232*
  design issues 235, *235–6*, 236–7
  incontinence issues 180–1, 182, 188
  mealtime environments 173–4
  moving into a care home 151–2
  nutrition standards 166
  rights issues 261–2
  social interaction 232–3
  use of antipsychotics 324–6, 327–30
Care Quality Commission (CQC) 166, 210–11, 232, *232*
caregiving 128–55
  acute hospital care 152–5
  care homes and community visitors 149–50
  clinical nursing specialists 144–5
  coordination of 88–90, *89*
  cultural diversity in 70–1
  for delirium 120–1
  dyadic relationship 132–3
  factors contributing additional pressures on *138*
  family carers 87, 142–4, 151, 153, 180–1, 248–9, 361–3
  impact of YOD 107–8
  incontinence issues 180–1
  intermediate care 150–1
  monitoring progress 90
  moving into a care home 151–2
  National Dementia Declaration Action Plan *146–8*
  network approach 136–40
  person-centred 87–8, 101, 129–32, 152, 154–5, 324, 359, 365, 366
  relationship-centred 129–32
  social networks 141–2
  support for carers 145–6, 364–5
  Triangle of Care 133–6, *134*
  views on tracking devices 248–9
  young carers 102
  see also whole-person care
Carers Trust, Royal College of Nursing (RCN) 133–4
'challenging behaviour' 107, 132–3, 149, 244, 324–5, 326–7
Charter of Fundamental Rights of the European Union 276–7
Charter of Rights for People with Dementia and their Carers in Scotland *272–3*, 273–4
Chekhov, Anton 341
chewing problems 174
citizenship 19, 45, 57–9, 207–8
clinical nursing specialists 136, 144–5, 215, 322, 368, 375
clothing 184–5
co-morbidities 114, 122, 187–8, 205, 216, 367–9
  see also individual co-morbidites
Cochrane Reviews 226
collaboration 363–6, 366
collaborative leadership 203–5
College of Occupational Therapists 253
Commissioning for Quality and Innovation (CQUIN) framework 117–18
Community Care (Direct Payments) Act 1996 267
community visitors 149–50
conclusion 356–75
  co-morbidity 367–9
  families 361–3
  medicalisation 357–8
  recovery 358–60
  relationships and collaboration 363–6
  risk and uncertainty 370–4
  'telling the truth' 367
Confusion Assessment Method (CAM) 116
consent issues 202–3, 243, 248–9, 249–51, 262
consolidation theory 312, 313
consumerism 59, 88, 129–30, 266
Corbett, Bill 307
counselling, genetic 100, 105, 363
creativity 289–300
  art 291–4
  definition 290
  music 294–9
Creutzfeldt-Jakob disease, variant (vCJD) 43
crises 185–6
cultural issues 63–75, 85–6, 143–4, *148*
cure versus care 99, 357

DAT (dementia of Alzheimer type) *see* Alzheimer type dementia
data sharing 202–3
day care 186, 367

Day, George 206
de Kooning, Willem 291
decision-making 249, 251, 277–81, 324
delirium 113–23
  and cognitive decline 118
  CQUIN framework 117–18
  improving care and financial incentives 120–1
  living well after 121–3
  NICE and 119–20
  possible predisposing factors *115*
  prophylaxis 120
Dementia Action Alliance (DAA) 30, 145–6, *146–7*, *147–8*, 332–3, *333*, 362
Dementia Alliance International (DAI) 58–9, 92, 137, 211, 364
Dementia and Neurodegenerative Diseases research network (DeNDRoN) 149
Dementia Care Mapping 342
Dementia Champions 350–2
dementia charities, 'competition' between 357
Dementia Engagement and Empowerment Project (DEEP) 58, 72, 372
dementia-friendly communities 17, 18–19, 34, 74–5, 130, *148*, 193, 236, 360, 366, 375
Dementia Friends campaign 42–4, 85, *148*, 306
Dementia Innovation Envoys 321–2
demographic issues 87, 131, 137
depression 27, 106, 108, 139, 142, 151, 179, 181, 206–7, 231, 368
Deprivation of Liberty Safeguards (DoLS) policy 261–2
design considerations 149–50, 155, 234–8, *234*, 235, *235–6*, 245–6
detrusor hyperactivity / overactivity (DOA) 182–3
diabetes 35, 38, 72, 107, 151, 205, 213, 217, 329, 369
diagnosis
  coping with 105–8
  delays in 68–9, 70, 103–4, 356
  diagnostic labels 53–4
  impact of 104–5
  improving 85–6, 373
  misdiagnosis 103, 104, 114, 368
  over-diagnosis 356–7, 358
  post-diagnostic care and support 29–31, *31*, *32*, 217, 364
  statistics 27
  timely 26–8, *28*, 86
diary-keeping 58
Dickens, Charles 25, 290
diet *32*, 40, 171
  see also eating
dignity 106, 154, 216, 247, 253, 260–1, 276–7
disAbility model of care 259, *260*
DisabledGo 259
discrimination 18, 34, 53–4, 57, 58, 59, 259, 269–71
diversity issues 18–19, 63–75
doctor–patient relationship 144, 199, 200–1, 324
Donne, John 55
dopamine 280
Down's syndrome 74, 75
dyadic relationships 132–3, 135, 139, 142
Dying Elderly at Home (DEATH) project 181
dysphagia *see* swallowing problems

e-prescriptions 333–4
early-onset dementia 37, 44, 66, 69
  see also young-onset dementia
eating 164–75, 374
  contributory factors to the development of Alzheimer's disease 171–5
  eating behaviours and volumetric neuroimaging 167–9
  the 'human sweet tooth' 169, *170*
  malnutrition 166–7
  metabolism 170
  nutrition and diet 171
  nutrition standards and care homes 166
EClipSE (Epidemiological Clinicopathological Studies in Europe) 37
8 Pillar Model of Community Support 88, *89*
electrostimulation therapy 184
emotions
  emotional arousal 309–10, *310*, 311–12, 316
  emotional gist 314–15
  music and 295, 297
empathy 342, 362
Employment Equality Acts 1998–2011, Ireland 271
employment problems 18–19, 106
empowerment 58, 72, 211, 213, 229
end-of-life care 181, 249, 322, 361, 368
  see also palliative care
ENRICH project 149
Enriched Opportunities Programme 231
environmental docility hypothesis 226, 245–6
environmental health practitioners 226
Equal Status Acts 2000–11, Ireland 271
Equality Act 2010 259, 271
ethical issues 29, 200, 206, 227, 243, 251, 252–3, 367
ethnic minorities *see* BAME communities
EU 'Rhapsody Project' 108, 366
European Commission 372
European Convention for the Protection of Human Rights and Fundamental Freedoms 251–2, 262–4
European Court of Human Rights 262

European Delirium Association (EDA) 114, 116, 119
European Dementia Prevention Initiative 366
EVIDEM-C study 187
EVOLVE evaluation tool 237
exercise 38
extra care housing 231, 236, 237

face recognition 315–16
falls, risk of 180, 205–6, 331
family carers 87, 142–4, 151, 153, 180–1, 248–9, 361–3
family conflict 200
family history, and risk of dementia 37, 362
financial issues 120–1, 145, 193, 210, 264–9, *266–7*, 324, 328, 330–1, 357–8, 358, 362, 368
football memories *see* sporting memories
framing the narrative 54–6
Francis Inquiry 150
Freud, Sigmund 297
frontotemporal dementia (FTD) / behavioural variant frontotemporal dementia (bvFTD) 100–1, 102, 167–8, 169, 170, 182, 278, 279, 292–3, 294, 298, 314, 362, 363, 367

G7 Dementia Summit 99, 108, 341, 342
G8 Dementia Summit 32, 81, 321–2
Gandhi, Mahatma 63
garments 184–5
Genetic Information Non-discrimination Act (GINA) 2008, US 271
genetics 45, 99–101, 172, 269–71, 362–3
Gerada, Clare 268
gerontology, social 32
global strategies 81–94
GPS tracking 242–53
  Dewing's process of obtaining consent 249–51
  ethical issues 243
  human rights 251–3
  spatial navigation 245–6
  stigma 253
  tagging and tracking 246–9, *246*
  'wandering': terminology issues 244–5
Greengross, Baroness Sally 20, 67
Grip on Challenging Behaviour programme 327
Guardian (newspaper) 100, 375

Hale, Lady 261
hallucinations 293
Harvard Business Review 322, 347, 348, 349
Health Education England (HEE) 207
health field concept 228, *228*
Health Foundation 150–1, 264
health insurance 89, 370
health rainbow 228, *229*
hearing loss 206
holistic approach 64, 93, *93*, 196–7
hospitals
  acute care 152–5
  discharge from 150
  reducing avoidable admissions 150, 154–5, 368
housing 225–38
  architectural considerations 234–8, *234*, *235–6*
  care homes 232–3, *232*
  extra care 231, 236, 237
  policy 230
  public health and social determinants 227–30, *228*, *229*
  as a social determinant of health 226–7
Human Genome Project 269, 357
human rights 251–3, 258–83
  autonomy, dignity and the Deprivation of Liberty Safeguards policy 260–4
  dignity 276–7
  disability and dementia 274–6
  genetic discrimination 269–71
  personal budgets and self-directed support 264–9, *266–7*
  rights-based approaches 271–4, *272–3*
  risk factors 277–81, *279*, 281–2
Human Rights Act 1998 263
Huntington's disease 102, 270, 363
hydrocephalus 182, 186–7
hyperphagia 168–9
hypertension 35, 38, 72, 151, 368

incontinence 152, 179–89, 206
  aids 187
  co-morbidity 187–8
  cognition and 181
  communication 185
  crises 185–6
  day care 186
  in different dementias 186–7
  evaluation 183
  garments 184–5
  management 184
  and moving into a care home 188
  predictors 182–3
  prompted voiding 187
Independent Commission for Whole Person Care (ICWPC) 203, 205
inequalities, of health 41–2
  see also housing
information cascades 165
innovation 321–3, 334–5, 343–4, 375
  see also antipsychotics
Institute for Public Policy Research 195
insulin 31, *32*, 170, 373
insurance 89, 370
intellectual difficulties, persons with 74–5
International Continence Society 180, 187–8
Iowa Gambling Task 279

Jameson Allen, Tony 304–5
John Snow, Inc. 195–6, *196*
Joseph Rowntree Foundation 58, 150, 370, 372
Judge Institute, Cambridge 205

Kant, Immanuel 367
King, Billie Jean 350
King's Fund 216
Klüver-Bucy syndrome 168
Kornfeld-Matte, Rosa 276
Kungsholmen Project 371

Lancet Neurology (journal) 35
Lang Leav 242
leadership 341–53
  collaborative 203–5
  Dementia Champions 350–2
  leading 'change' 345–50, *350*
  NHS policy 343–5
Leav, Lang 242
Leon Thal Symposium 34
Lewy body disease (DLB) / diffuse Lewy body disease (DLBD) 44, 102, 122, 180, 186, 293
LGBT (lesbian, gay, bisexual and transgender) communities 72–3, *148*
lying, therapeutic and pathological 367

McKeown, Thomas 228
Macmillan Nurses 144
malnutrition 165, 166–7
Malnutrition Task Force 166–7
Malnutrition Universal Screening Tool 165
media, attitude towards dementia 54–6
Medical Research Council Cognitive Function and Ageing Study (MRC CFAS) 56
medicalisation 357–8
medication
  and incontinence 182–3
  new 81
  personalised 100–1, 357
  see also antipsychotics
Mediterranean Diet (MeDi) 40, 171
memory clinics 27, 35, *147*
memory issues 43, 58, 294–5, 295–6, 299
  types of memory 305–6, *305*, *306*
  see also sporting memories
Mental Capacity Act 2005 232–3, 262, 274, 281
Mental Health Act 2007 262
Mental Health Foundation 262
metals, risk from 40–1
metaphors 54–6
misdiagnosis 103, 104, 114, 368
motor neurone disease 170
movement 183
music 183, 294–9
music therapy 298–9
musicophilia 297–8

Nabokov, Vladimir 297
National Council for Palliative Care *147*, 149
National Dementia Declaration *146–7*
National Dementia Strategy for England 26, 85, 117, *146–8*, 265–6, 325, 330
National Health Service (NHS), England
  CQUIN framework 117–18
  End of Life Care Programme *147*, 149
  financial issues 27, 193, 210, 267
  Horizon Scanning Centre 101
  Institute for Innovation and Improvement 30, 332–3, *333*
  Leadership Academy 343
  management 26, 94, 266, 322, 343–5, 368
  Outcomes Framework 215
  personal budgets 264–9
  Standard Contract 118
National Housing Federation 235
National Institute for Health and Care Excellence (NICE) 81, 116, 119–20, 166, 217, 325, 326
National Institute on Aging 29
National Mental Health Development Unit 133
national policies 82–94
  critical issues 84–91, *89*
  development 82–4, *83–4*, 91–2
  guidance points *83–4*
  implementation *84*, 92–4, *93*
National Service Frameworks 101, 150, 188, 325
Need-Driven Dementia-Compromised Behaviour model 132
Need for Nutrition Education/Innovation Programme (NNEdPro) 165
neural networks 31, *32*, 306–7, 308–16, *314*, 324
Neuropsychiatric Inventory 168
New Statesman (magazine) 346
Nuffield Foundation 264, 277
nursing homes *see* care homes
nutrition 166, 171
  malnutrition 165, 166–7
  see also eating issues
Nutrition Education and Leadership for Improved Clinical Outcomes (NELICO) 165

obesity 39
odour processing 307, 316–17
omega-3 fatty acids 40, 172
Osborne, George 375

pain management 206, 365
palliative care 99, *147*, 155
  see also end-of-life care
parity of esteem 206–7
Parkinson's disease 136, 186, 280, 293, 328
patient-centredness 197–201
Peake, Mervyn 293
peer support groups *147*, 364–5

person-centred care 87–8, 101, 129–32, 152, 154–5, 324, 359, 365, 366
personal budgets 264–9, *266–7*
personhood 55, 57–8, 87–8, 101, 129–30, 195, 364, 365, 370
Pharma 19, 81, 348, 357
physical activity 38
physical health issues 205–6
polypharmacy 116, 120
pre-morbid behaviour and personality 365–6
prejudice 53, 72
prevalence 82, 86, 92, 102–3, 324, 362
PREVENT trial 35–6
preventative strategies 34–41, 371–2
prime contractor model 368
Prime Minister's Dementia Challenge 26–34, *28*, *33–4*
prion disease 102
proportionality 251, 263
psychological stress 38–9
  see also stress
psychological symptoms 41, 194, 326–7
public health 227–30, *228*, *229*
Public Health England 42

Ravel, Maurice 295
recovery, policies on 358–60
relationship-centred care 129–32
restraints 247–8, 327
'Rhapsody' project 108, 366
Ribot's law / Ribot's gradient 311
risk issues 34–41, *36*, 56, 74, 85–6, *138*, 238, 244, 244–5, 277–81, *279*, 281–2, 362–3, 368, 370–4
risperidone 120, 325
Roberts, Chris 356
Rogers, Carl 195
Ronaldo, Cristiano 304
Rotterdam study 40
Royal College of Nursing (RCN) 152–5
Royal College of Psychiatrists 27, 207, 209
Royal Pharmaceutical Society 332–3

Sartorius, Norman 52
Saul, John Ralston 225
schizophrenia 52, 328, 329
Scully, Maureen 347
self-care / self-management 197, 200, 211–14, *213–14*, 215, 217, 264–9, *266–7*
semantic dementia (SD) 167–8, 170, 292, 296, 297–8, 307, 362
Senses Framework 131, 299
serotonin 169
Shakespeare, William 51, 290
'Side by Side' programme 106
silos, policy 42, 189, 194, 205, 347, 369, 374
singing 299
Single Assessment Process 179–80
smell, sense of 307, 316–17
smoking, and risk of dementia 39
Snow, Judith 258
social capital 136, 142, 350, *350*
Social Care Institute for Excellence (SCIE) 174, 260
social change, campaigning for 57–9
social determinants of health 41–2, 193, 226–7, 227–30, *228*, *229*, 230
social experience concept 140
social gerontology 32
social networks 37, 141–2, 204, 334, 371
social recovery 358–60
spatial navigation 245–6
spirituality 64, 197
sporting memories 304–17
  football memories 307–8, *308*
  neural networks 306–7
  neural substrates for visual football memories 308–16, *310*
  smell aiding football memories 316–17
  types of memory 305–6, *305*, *306*
Sporting Memories Network 304–5, 307–8
stepped care model 331, *332*
stigma 51–6, *53*, 65, 86, 106, 197, 253, 360
stress 132, 183, 194, 235, 324
  carer 70, 108, 129, 142, 327, 365
  psychological 38–9
stroke 38, 82, 86, 100, 122, 292, 297, 331
suffering 56–7
support
  8 Pillar Model of Community Support 88, *89*
  for carers 145–6, 364–5
  peer support groups 147, 364–5
  post-diagnosis 29–31, *31*, 32, 217, 364
  self-directed 264–9, *266–7*
swallowing problems 167, 174

tagging *see* GPS tracking
tau 31, 39, 101, 170
technologies
  assistive 214
  innovative 91, 323
10/66 Dementia Research Group 69
TENS stimulation 184
therapeutic approaches 31, *32*
Three-City cohort study 40
tracking *see* GPS tracking
transtheoretical model (TTM) 346
triadic relationships 133–6, *134*, 144–5
Triangle of Care 133–6, *134*
trilateration 246, *246*
truth, telling the 367
Twain, Mark 98

United Nations (UN), Convention on the Rights of Persons with Disabilities 18, 87, 258, 274–5
United States Constitution 252
Universal Declaration on the Human Genome and Human Rights 269
US Food and Drug Administration (FDA) 326, 328, 372

Vanderbilt Law Review 271
vascular dementia 38, 39, 43, 66, 102, 172, 182
visual realism 292
vitamins 40, 172, 173
volumetric neuroimaging 168
voxel-based morphometry (VBM) 168

'wandering' 70, 140
  terminology problems 16, 363, 374
  see also GPS tracking
Wanless, Derek 215–16
Ware Invitational Summit 91
weight issues 39, 166, 169, 173, 175, 206, 329
Wellbeing and Health for People with Dementia (WHELD) initiative 204–5
whole-person care 193–218, 368
  assistive technology and ambient-assisted living 214
  background 194–6
  care coordinators 207–9, *208*, *209*
  collaborative leadership 203–5
  data sharing 202–3
  holistic viewpoint 196–7
  multi-disciplinary teams and 202
  parity of esteem for mental health 206–7
  person- vs patient-centredness 197–201, *198*
  physical health conditions 205–6
  policy considerations *201*
  primary care 210
  self-management and self-care 211–14, *213–14*
  social care 210–11
  'year of care' initiative 214–17
Williams syndrome 297
Williamson, Toby 262
Woolf, Virginia 164
World Alzheimer Report 151
World Dementia Council 18, 92
World Health Organization (WHO) 43, 227, 229, 230, 356
World Psychiatric Association 52, 360

'year of care' initiative 214–17
young-onset dementia 368
young-onset dementia (YOD) 19, 43, 98–109
  coping with a diagnosis 105–8
  cure versus care 99
  current policy 101–3
  delay in diagnosis 103–4
  genetics, 'big data' and personalised medicine 99–101
  overall impact on individual and partner 104–5

zinc 40–1

AUTHOR INDEX

Page numbers in *italics* refer to figures and boxes.

Aalten, P. 194
AARP 233
Aarsland, D. 325, 326
Ablitt, A. 70, 364
Abma, I. 121
Aboriginal and Torres Strait Islander Healing Foundation Development Team 64
Adams, K.B. 143
Adams, S. 107, 362
Adams, T. 131, 359
Addis, D.R. 313
Adelman, R.D. 135, *138*, 144
Adelman, S. 69
Adkins, J. 372
Aguero-Torres, H. 151
Ahlskog, J.E. 38
Ahmed, S. 116, 118, 119
Ahtiluoto, S. 72
Alagiakrishnan, K. 174
Alarcón, R.D. 86
Alaszewski, H. 281
Albert, M.S. 29, 206
Algase, D.L. 244, 246
Alisky, J.M. 323
All-Party Parliamentary Group (APPG) on Dementia 27, *28*, 42, 65, *67–8*, 92, 329–30
Allan, L. 180
Alred, D. 359
Alvarez, P. 307, 312
Alvaro, L.C. 276
Alzheimer Scotland 88, *89*, 266
Alzheimer's Association 45, 137
Alzheimer's Australia 55, 92, 93, 152
Alzheimer's Disease International 83, 92, 104, 145, 151, 173, 175
Alzheimer's Society 42, 236
Amabile, T.M. 290
Amaducci, L. 295
American Psychiatric Association 114, 291
Amieva, H. 141
Anckaert, L. 364
Andersberg, P. 247
Anderson, A.K. 309
Anderson, D. 326
Anderson, N. 290
Andrews, S. 71
Andrieu, S. 35
Aneshensel, C. 73
Arai, A. 107
Archbold, P.G. 142
Archer, D. 203
Argyle, E. 231
Armari, E. 101
Arnheim, G. 55
Arseven, A. 115
Arthur, D.G. 244
Arto Rajala, A. 323
Ask, H. 140
Atchison, T.A. 205
Attali, E. 367
Attoe, R. 243
Audit Commission 265
Australian Department of Health 86
Australian Health Ministers' Conference 88
Australian Institute of Health and Welfare 155
Authors undisclosed (*Vanderbilt Law Review*) 271
Aveling, E.L. 351
Aveyard, B. 233
Awata, S. 137
Aylward, E.H. 74
Ayres, S. 214
Azermai, M. 88, 325

Backhouse, T. 324, 327–8
Bail, M. 253
Bailey, M. 231
Baker, L.D. 372
Baker, M. 106
Baldwin, C. 243
Balint, E. 198
Ballard, C. 325, 326
Ballenger, J. 56
Balteş, F.R. 297
Bambra, C. 41, 225
Banerjee, S. 25, 30–1, 42, 69, 82, 185, 225, 321, 325, 352
Baran, M. 105
Baranowski, M. 367
Barberger-Gateau, P. 40, 171
Bardsley, M. 210
Barley, V.M. 107
Barnard, C. 58
Barnes, C. 212
Barnes, T.R. 328, 333
Barron, E.A. 114
Bartlett, F.C. 56
Bartlett, R. 57, 58, 130
Barton, A. 206
Basaglia-Pappas, S. 296
Basso, A. 295
Bastawrous, M. 137
Bates, M.S. 107
Batsch, N.L. 52, *53*, 59
Battilana, J. 349
Baxter, J. 368

Bazinet, R.P. 172
BBC News 259
Beail, N. 74
Beard, R.L. 59, 294
Beattie, A.M. 103, 108
Beattie, B.L. 249
Beck, A.P. 345
Becker, D. 251
Beckman, S.L. 204
Beer, C. 352
Beerens, H.C. 151
Behuniak, S.M. 58
Benbow, S.M. 54, 66
Bender, M. 130
Benford, R.D. 56, 332
Beninger, R.J. 280
Bennett, S. 206–7, 368
Bennett, V. 244
Beresford, P. 59, 265, 269
Berkhout, A.M. 175
Bernstein, M.S. 59, 365
Berntsen, D. 312
Berrios, G.E. 103, 182
Bertram, L. 362
Best, A. 374
Bettens, K. 172
Bevan, H. 347, 352
Beydoun, H.A. 39
Beydoun, M.A. 39
Bhanji, R.A. 174
Bhattacharyya, S. 66, 101
Bickerstaffe, S. 195, 203, 209
Biessels, G.J. 35
Bigby, C. 276
Bikhchandani, S. 165
Billings, J.A. 247
Billings, P.R. 269
Binney, R.J. 307
Bisla, J. 324
Bjørneby, S. 237
Black, S.E. 37
Blackburn, D.J. 38
Blackstock, K.L. 85
Blessed, G. 103
Blood, A.J. 295
Bo, K. 184
Boettger, S. 120
Boeve, B.F. 102, 104
Boller, F. 295
Bond, J. 32
Bonuccelli, U. 367
Borelli, P. 367
Borroni, B. 101
Boudrault, C. 172
Bourn, C. 226
Boustani, M. 70
Bower, P. 198, 199, 210
Bowling, A. 32, 141
Bowman, C.E. 276
Boyd, A. 333
Braak, E. 280
Braak, H. 280
BRACE 348
Braddock, D. 74
Bradford Dementia Group 231
Bradley, M.M. 311
Brand, M. 280
Brandon, D. 133
Braun, M. 143
Brayne, C. 82
Brearley, C. 281
Breibart, W. 120, 121
Bremberg, S. 248
Brennan, M. 73
Breteler, M.M. 39
Bridges, J. 153, 351
British Geriatrics Society 116
British Psychological Society 327, 331, *332*
Britton, B. 98–9, 187
Brocklehurst, J. 182
Brodal, A. 316
Brodaty, H. 26, 102, 140, 143, 200, 326, 362
Bronfenbrenner, U. 233
Brooker, D. 231, 342
Brooks, J. 268
Brotman, S. 73
Brotons, M. 298
Brown, R. 294–5
Bruce, V. 315
Brunet, M. 28
Brunnström, H. 43
Bryden, C. 17
Buchman, A.S. 39
Buck, H.G. 197
Buckwalter, K.C. 132, 325
Budrys, V. 294
Buisson, E. 149
Bujak, J.S. 205
Bunn, F. 369
Bupa 145, 151
Burant, C.J. 212
Burgener, S.C. 54
Burgess, P.W. 314
Burnham, W.H. 309
Burns, A. 26, 64, 103
Burns, L.R. 205
Burton, A.M. 315
Burton, E. 237, 238
Burton, J. 144
Busemeyer, J.R. 280
Bush, A. 74
Bush, S.H. 119
Bushe, G.R. 345, 347
Butler, M. 194
Butt, J. 64
Byrne, P. 198–9

Cabeza, R. 296, 311
Cacioppo, J.T. 141
Caddell, L.S. 55, 104, 212
Cahill, S. 253
Cai, W. 184
Caldwell, C.E. 290
Callahan, C.M. 143
Cameron, A. 203
Cameron, K. 322, 323
Camic, P.M. 299
Campbell, A. 180
Campbell, D. 100
Campbell, J.C. 131, 282
Campbell, S. 185
Campo, M. 233
Candy, B. 174
Cankurtaran, M. 370
Cannon, W.B. 309
Cant, B. 72
Cantley, C. 150
Cantor, M. 73
Capitani, E. 295
Carbonneau, H. 322
Care Commission 165–6
Care Quality Commission (CQC) 166, 210–11, 232, *232*, 324
Carers Trust, Royal College of Nursing (RCN) 129, 133, *134*, 144
Carey, G. 230
Caron, C. 322
Carpentier, N. 140
Carr, D. 249
Carr, S. 265
Carreon, D. 149
Carroll, G.R. 165
Carruthers, I. *33–4*
Carter, A.I. 140
Casciaro, T. 349
Cass, B. 102
Cassel, E.J. 200

Casten, R.J. 64
Centre for Welfare Reform 88
Cermak, L.S. 314
Cermakova, P. 368
Chakravarty, A. 293
Challis, C. 316
Chan, K.Y. 85
Chan, S.W. 144
Chang, M. 38
Chapin, K. 298
Chappell, N.L. 138, 234
Charles, C. 200
Charon, R. 135
Charpentier, P.A. 119
Charter of Fundamental Rights of the European Union 276–7
Chassot, C.S. 359
Chaudhury, H. 233
Chaufan, C. 98
Chen, R. 226
Chen, T. 89
Cheng, A. 70
Chenoweth, B. 73
Cherry, D.L. 352
Chesbrough, H. 334
Chetty, S.K. 323
Chinthapalli, K. 267
Cholerton, B. 372
Chonchurhair, N.A. 114
Choo, W.Y. 139
Christensen, C.M. 322, 343
Christmas, M. 75
Chryssanthopoulou, C. 66
Chung, J.C. 87
Chung, L.C. 144
Clancy, D. 231
Clare, L. 55, 104, 130, 211, 212, 276
Clark, C.N. 297
Clark, H. 267
Clark, R. 361
Clark, V.P. 315
Clarke, A. 151, 197
Clarkson, P. 180
Clayman, M.L. 135
CLBC 274
Clegg, A. 116
Clemerson, G. 102, 105–6
Clore, G.L. 309
Coetzer, G.H. 345
Cohen, C.A. 139
Cohen, D. 18
Cohen, E. 237
Cohen-Eliya, M. 251
Cohen-Mansfield, J. 55, 324, 330
Cohen, M.E. 243
Cohen, N.J. 307
Cohen, S. 132, 139
Coile, R.C. 204
Cole, L. 180, 185
College of Occupational Therapists 253
Collins, C. 194
Collins, P.A. 226
Combes, H. 72
Commonwealth Fund 88
Commonwealth of Australia 93
Conklin, J. 351
Conner, M. 350
Connolly, S. 87
Conservative Party 22
Conway, M.A. 312, 313, 314
Cook, C. 174
Cooke, H.A. 232, 234
Cooley, S.J. 247
Cools, H.J. 175
Coons, H.L. 202
Cooper, C. 70, 71, 72
Coppola, G. 172
Coriell, M. 132
Cornegé-Blokland, E. 325, 326
Corrigan, P.W. 54
Corsonello, A. 328
Cortes-Blanco, A. 372
Cottrell, V. 51, 58
Covinsky, K.E. 181
Craft, S. 170, 372
Craig, C. 289
Crammond, B. 230
Cranswick, K. 137
Crawley, H. 164, 169, 175
Creese, B. 325, 326
Crespy, D.A. 205
Cronin-Stubbs, D. 206
Croom, B. 142
Crossley, M.L. 324
Crossley, N. 324
Croucher, K. 231
Crutch, S.J. 291, 291–2
Cummings, J.L. 82, 140, 167, 292
Cunningham, C. 122
Cunningham, E.L. 31, *32*
Cunningham, H. 75
Curb, J.D. 69
Currie, G. 351
Cushman, L.A. 245
Cutcliffe, J. 367

Dagerman, K. 325
Dahlgren, G 228, *229*
Dalton, A. 75
Dalton, J.M. 136
Damiani, G. 368
Dasgupta, M. 114
Dauphinot, V. *138*
Davies, N. 361
Davies, P. 114
Davies, S. 131
Davies, S.L. 149
Daviglus, M.L. 35
Davis, D.H. 120, 122
Davis, G.F. 165
Davis, R. 199
Davis, S. 149
Day, A. 64
Day, A.M. 367
Day, K. 149
de Ajuriaguerra, J. 291
De Bellis, A. 248
De Boer, M.E. 276
De Civita, M. 135
de Haes, H. 200
De Lepeleire, J. 27, 214
De Martino, B. 309
de Medeiros, K. 233
De Meyer, A. 205
De Rosa, E. 309
de Vugt, M.E. 130, 142, 143, 327
Defanti, C.A. 249
Degner, L.F. 352
Delancey, J.O.L. 184
Delany, N. 108
Delazer, M. 280
Delgado, M.R. 311
Deloitte 210, 334
Dementia Action Alliance (DAA) 30, *146–7*, *147–8*, 332–3, *333*
Dementia Alliance International (DAI) 58–9, 364
Dementia Services Development Centre 234
Dementia UK 66

Department of Health 29–30, *31*, 34, 65, 66, 68, 69, 72, 74, 101, 117, 149, 150, 179, 188, 199, 200, 202, 203, 207, 209, 210, 214, 215, 216, 237, 264, 265, 266, 281, 281–2, 325, 345, 368
DeRienzis, D. 103
Desmond, D.W. 38
Desrosiers, J. 322
Devi, G. 37
Devine, M. 185
Devore, E.E. 40
Dewing, J. 144, 244, 250–1
Diabetes UK 217
DiClemente, C.C. 346
Diderichsen, F. 226
Dike, C.C. 367
Dillane, J. 182
DiNatale, Johnson, B. 185
Dingjan, P. 243
Dixon-Fyle, S. 195
DNA Web Team 276
Dobkin, P.L. 135
Dodd, K. 75
Dodds, P. 245
Dolan, J. 357
Donelan, K. 138
Donkin, M. 102, 362
Donnelly, M. 249
Doran, T. 121
Dosman, D. 137
Dougherty, T.-M.P. 334
Downs, M. 27, 180
Doyle, P.J. 233
Drance, E. 132
Draper, B. 351–2
Drennan, G. 359
Drennan, V.M. 180, 185, 186
Drentea, P. 139
Dröes, R.-M. 276
Duarte, N.T. 334
DuBeau, C.E. 184, 188
Dubet, F. 140
DuBois, B. 243
Ducharme, F. 361
Duchen, L.W. 167
Duffy, C.J. 245
Duffy, S. 258
Dunlap, S. 204
Dupuis, S.L. 132
Dutton, R. 231
Ebersbach, G. 293
EClipSE 37
Edquist, C. 323
Edvardsson, D. 87, 130, 152, 197
Edward, H.G. 174
Edwards, A.B. 137
Eeles, E. 113–14, 119
Eidelman, S. 72
Ekelund, P. 179
Ekman, P. 297
El-Murad, J. 290
Ellis, K. 267
Ellis, R.P. 89
Eltis, K. 246, 251
Embrett, M.G. 230
Emilsson, U.M. 89
Engel, S.A. 199, 200
Ennis, E.M. 197
Equality and Human Rights Commission 252, 259
Ericsson, I. 233
Eriksson, S. 205–6
Estabrook, C.A. 352
EU 'Rhapsody Project' 108
Eustace, A. 142
Evandrou, M. 65
Evans, S. 237

Fainstein, C. 187
Fairburn, C.G. 168
Fairman, S. 347, 352
Farah, M.J. 315
Féart, C. 171
Feightner, J. 37
Feinberg, L.F. 251
Ferraro, F.R. 85
Ferreira, M. 372
Ferri, C.P. 86
Fetherstonhaugh, D. 87
Fick, D.M. 123
Field, E.M. 141
Finkel, S. 326
Firth, L. 136
Fisk, J.D. 249
Fitch, W.T. 289
Flatley, M. 153
Fletcher, P.D. 297
Foebel, A.D. 326
Folkman, S. 70
Follett, M.P. 346
Fong, T.G. 118
Forder, J. 264
Forstelund, L. 331
Fortinsky, R.H. 212
Fossey, J. 106, 149, 331
Foster, D.P. 107
Fox, N.C. 81
Fozard, J.L. 247
Francisco, A. 64
Fratiglioni, L. 371
Frawley, P. 276
Freeth, S. 102
French, J. 58
Freyne, A. 107
Fried, L.P. 181
Friedson, E. 199
Friesen, W.V. 297
Füller, J. 18
Furst, M. 108

G8 Summit Declaration 321–2
Gabbay, J. 188
Gabrieli, J.D. 309
Gafni, A. 200
Gamsu, D.S. 107
Ganz, M. 332, 346, 348
Gao, S. 37
Garand, L. 52
Gardener, S. 171
Gardiner, P. 131
Gastmans, C. 277, 364
Gaugler, J.E. 137
Gauthier, I. 315
Gauthier, S. 29
Gawande, A. 370
Genomic Data Sharing 100
George, D.R. 56
George, L.K. 199
Giannakouris, K. 137
Giblin, F.J. 270
Gibson, C. 121
Gibson, F. 282
Gibson, G.D. 70
Giebel, C.M. 82
Gill, D. 113
Gilleard, C. 88
Gillette-Guyonnet, S. 35
Gilmour, H. 282
Girard, T.D. 120
Gitlin, L.N. 237
Gladwell, M. 204
Glasby, J. 267
Glassman, R.N. 18
Gleckman, H. 99
Gleicher, D. 230

Gleichgerrcht, E. 278, *279*
Glendinning, C. 267, 268, 269
Glover, J.C. 244
Glymour, M.M. 226
Godden, S. 150
Goffman, E. 52, 54, 56, 130, 197, 360
Goh, A.M. 269, 270
Golander, H. 55
Goldacre, M.J. 369
Goldacre, R. 369
Goldberg, D. 74
Goldman, J.S. 363
Goldsilver, P.M. 322
Golics, C.J. 361
Goodchild, C. 268
Goodman, C. 149, 350–1
Goodson, J.R. 334
Goodwin, N. 202, 207, 208
Gordon, N. 291
Gore, R.L. 122
Gorno-Tempini, M.L. 168
Gort, A.M. *138*
Graham, K.S. 313
Grant, G. 131
Grant, R.L. 206
Grassi, E. 295
Green, D. 281
Green, R.C. 56
Green, S. 53, 54
Greenberg, D.L. 312
Greene, J.D. 315
Greene, M.G. 135
Greenhalgh, T. 322, 344
Greenwood, N. 137, 364
Gregory, C. 342
Grenier, A. 140
Greve, H.R. 165
Gridley, K. 268
Griffith, E.E.H. 367
Griffith, R. 262
Griffiths, P. 368
Grimley Evans, J. 248
Gruneir, A. 329
Gruneir, M.R. 322
Guan, J.-Z. 172
Guardian website 375
Guétin, S. 298
Gupta, A.K. 335
Gustafson, D.R. 39

Ha, J. 280
Haase, H. 41
Habell, M. 259
Hachinski, V. 72
Hägglund, D. 180, 184
Hahn, C. 352
Hailstone, J.C. 297
Hall, G.R. 132, 325
Hall, N.M. 312
Hall, R.J. 113
Hallberg, I.R. 90
Hampton, A.N. 280
Hancock, G.A. 188
Hannah, M.T. 165
Hansen, M.T. 204
Hanson, E.J. 151
Haque, S. 313
Haralambous, B. 71
Harari, D. 188
Harding, R. 139, 140
Harris, L.F. 64
Harris, M. 202
Harris, P.G. 104
Hart, V. 265
Harvey, R.J. 108
Hasegawa, J. 180
Hasselkus, B.R. 367
Hauser, R.M. 249
Hawkins, R.L. 142
Hawkley, J.C. 141
Haxby, J.V. 315
Haycox, A. 99
Hayes, M.V. 226
Health Foundation 129, 150, 153, 154, 210, 264, 265
Heath, I. 358
Heaven, A. 120
Hébert, R. 38
Hecaen, H. 291
Heggestad, A.K. 277
Hein, C. *115*, 120
Heller, L. 18, 81, 214
Heller, T. 18, 81, 214
Hellström, I. 233
Helvik, A.S. 205, 368, 369
Henderson, V.W. 245
Hendrie, H.C. 85
Hennessy, S. 328
Henry, W.D. 116
Herman, P.M. 195
Hermans, D.G. 247, 248
Heru, A.M. 143
Hewer, R.L. 138
Heywood, F. 237
Hick, R. 74
Higgins, D. 227
Higgs, P. 88
Hilgeman, M.M. 142
Hillier, L.M. 114
Hinchliffe, A.C. 129
Hirasawa, Y. 181
Hirsch, M.A. 136
Hirsh, D. 187
Hirshleifer, D. 165
Hirstein, W. 290, 291
HM Government 68, 87
Hobfauer, R.K. 206
Hocking, E. 164, 169, 175
Hodges, J.R. 314, 315
Hoe, J. 351
Hofman, A. 39
Holford, P. 172
Holland, A.C. *279*, 297, 313
Holland, A.J. 74
Holland, W. 26
Hollander, D. 358
Hollander, M.J. 138
Holman, C. 350–1
Holman, H. 212
Holmes, J.D. 114
Hölttä, E.H. *115*
Hoof, J. 231
Hope, K.W. 144
Hope, R.A. 168
Hope, T. 168, 250, 252
Hopkins, R.O. 312
Horimoto, Y. 180
Horizon Scanning Centre 101
House, A.O. 114
House of Lords 247, 262
Housing Learning and Improvement Network *234*, 235, 236, 237
Houwelingen, H.C. 175
Hovens, I.B. 122
Hsieh, S. 296, 362
Hsu, M. 280
Htay, U.H. 247
Huang, H.L. 142
Huang, T.L. 172
Hubbard, R. 73
Hudson, D.L. 243
Hughes, B. 103
Hughes, J.C. 243, 244, 246, 253
Hughes, T.F. 171
Hulko, W. 57
Humphrey, K. 315
Hunter, P.V. 365
Hunter, R. 153
Huppert, F.A. 359

Hurley, A.C. 245
Hussein, S. 54
Hutchins, R.M. *246*
Hutchinson, N. 74
Huybrechts, K.F. 329
Hynan, L.S. 40

Ibarra, H. 204
Iemmi, V. 92
Igbedioh, C. 188
Iguchi, A. 180
Ikeda, M. 167, 168
Ikegami, N. 131
Ilies, R. 343
Iliffe, S. 26, 54, 72, 180, 185, 193, 197, 322, 344, 363
Iltanen-Tähkävuori, S. 185
Imtiaz, B. 37, 372
Independent Commission for Whole Person Care (ICWPC) 203, 205
Innes, A. 32, 82, 92, 128, 154, 253
Innovations in Dementia 72
Inoue, K. 169
Inouye, S.K. 115, *115*, 119
Insel, N. 309
Insel, P. 325
Ionicioiu, I. 28
Iqbal, A. 143
Iris, M. 68–9, 70
Irish, M. 314
Isaac, C. 102, 105–6
Isaacs, R. 291–2
Isern, J. 345

Jack, R. 133
Jacobs, S. 267
Jacobs, W.J. 245
Jacome, D.E. 297
Jaglal, S. 139
James, I.A. 367
James, M. 315
James, W. 309
Janata, P. 296
Janicki, M.P. 74, 75
Jansen, K.J. 346
Jansen, S.J.T. 201
Janßen, C. 230
Jarmolowicz, A. 101
Jasinarachchi, K. 150
Jenewein, J. 120
Jenkins, C. 366
Jenkins, C.R. 33
Jirovec, M.M. 182
Johannessen, A. 106, 106–7
Johansson, L. 38
Johl, N. 70
Johnson, E.J. 18
Johnston, R.A. 315
Joling, K.J. 361, 362
Jolley, D. 37
Jones, A. 107
Jones, G.M.M. 306
Jones, G.V. 70, 364
Jones, L. 174
Jones, R.N. 226
Jones, R.W. 211
Jong-Wook, L. 227
Joosten, L. 366
Jorm, A.F. 37
Josefowitz, N. 58
Joseph Rowntree Foundation 150, 370, 372
Josephs, K.A. 102, 104
Josephson, B.R. 295
Judge, T.A. 343

Kahana, Z. 251
Kaiser, S. 108
Kalaria, R.N. 39, 92, 121
Kalsy-Lillico, S. 74
Kammer, S. 298, 299
Kapur, N. 293
Kar, N. 66, 326
Karnieli-Miller, O. 72
Katz, M.L. 204
Kaufman, G. 290
Kaufmann, E.G. 199, 200
Kawamura, K. 247
Kay, D.W. 107
Kazer, M.W. 197
Keady, J. 104, 108, 135, 151, 233
Kearney, M. 196
Kearns, W.D. 247
Keast, R. 230
Keenan, T.D. 369
Keene, J. 168
Kehne, J.H. 39
Kellaher, L. 174
Kelleher, D. 107
Keller, H.H. 174
Keller, L.J. 173
Kellett, U. 87
Kelley, B.J. 102, 104
Kelley, W.M. 315
Kelly, J.F. 202
Kemshall, H. 281
Kendrick, M.J. 274
Kensinger, E.A. *279*, 297, 313
Kercher, K. 212
Kerr, D. 75
Kertesz, A. 291
Keyes, C.L.M. 359
Keyes, S.E. 364
Khachaturian, Z.S. 34, 372
Khalfa, S. 297
Kibayashi, K. 245
Kickbusch, I. 230
Kiecolt-Glaser, J.K. 143
Killaspy, H. 360
Killick, J. 289
Kim, D.H. 370
Kim, J.W. 39
King, M. 73
King, N. 290
King's Fund 216
Kingston, P. 101
Kinney, J.M. 129
Kirk, A. 291
Kirk, L.J. 74
Kirkevold, M. 365
Kitwood, T. 57, 58, 130, 151, 211, 324, 364, 365
Kivipelto, M. 39
Kjellstrom, S. 233
Kloeters, S. 279
Kmietowicz, Z. 27
Knapp, M. 66, 92
Knauss, J. 59
Knight, A. 227, 228
Knight, B.G. 70
Knocker, S. 73
Koch, T. 26, 54, 72, 197, 322
Koehn, S.D. 132
Koester, R. 244
Koger, S.M. 298
Köhler, L. 137, 141
Kolanowski, A.M. 132
Kopelman, P.G. 39
Korczyn, A.D. 103
Kort, H.S.M. 231
Kotter, J.P. 348, 349
Kovach, C.R. 132
Kowalski, C. 230
Kozak, J.-F. 132
Kozin, M. 294
KPMG 208

Kramer, M.W. 205
Kratzer, J. 334
Krieger, J. 227
Krishnamoorthy, A. 326
Krishnamoorthy, E.K. 82
Kristensen, S.R. 117
Kroenke, K. 206
Kroll, N.E. 307
Krull, A.C. 69
Kulik, J. 294–5
Kümpers, S. 89
Kurian, M. 174
Kuruppu, D.K. 102
Kuzuya, M. 180

La Fontaine 72
La Placa, V. 227, 228
LaBar, K.S. 296, 311
Labudda, K. 280
Laeng, B. 292
Lai, C.K.Y. 244
Lai, F. 75
Laing, W. 149
Lakey, B. 139
Lalonde, M. 228, *228*
Lambert, A. 72, 315
Lancet Global Mental Health Group 359
Landau, R. 248, 249, 251
Lane, H.P. 55
Lane, L. 195
Lapane, K.L. 329
Laraway, A. 74
Larsson, M. 316
Lauque, S. 173
Laurila, J.V. *115*
Lautenschlager, N.T. 37
Lautrette, A. 249
Law, K. 359
Lawley, D. 113, *115*, 116, 333
Lawrence, V. 70
Lawton, M.P. 226, 245–6
Lazarus, R.S. 70
Leary, A. 368
LeDoux, J.E. 316
LeDuc, L. 139
Leech, D. 344
Legh-Smith, J. 138
Leibing, A. 371
Leonard, B.E. 39
Leonard, M. 115, 116
Leppert, J. 180
Letter to the Prime Minister 42
Leung, F.W. 185, 187
Leurent, B. 116, 118, 119
Levenson, R. 297
Levine, B. 296, 314
Lewin, S.A. 130
Lewis, G.H. 228, 229
Liberzon, I. 315
Lieb, W. 40
Lievesley, N. 64, 66
Ligthart, S.A. 35
Limb, M. 267, 268
Lin, F.R. 206
Lin, L.C. 175
Lin, N. 350
Lincoln, P. 35
Lindsay, J. 38
Lingler, J.H. 136
Link, B.G. 52
Linsk, N.L. 200
Liperoti, R. 326, 328
Litch, B.K. 204
Littlechild, R. 267
Liu, G. 138
Liu, H.Y. 143
Liu, S. 226
Livingston, G. 66, 70
Lloyd, B.T. 140
Locadia, M. 201
Lockeridge, S. 107
Logsdon, R.G. 244
Loiselle, L. 132
Long, B. 198–9
Lopez, O.L. 142
Lorig, K.R. 212
Louw, S.J. 244, 246, 253
Lövdén, M. 371
Loveday, B. 342
Low, L.F. 68
Lucas, C. 237
Lucas, J.A. 328
Lucas, M. 180
Lupton, D. 27
Luscombe, C.E. 89
Luscombe, G. 102, 103–4
Lussier, M. 181
Lutz, C.J. 139
Lyketsos, C.G. 140
Lyman, K.A. 32
Lynn, M.R. 33
Lyons, K. 143

Ma, D.W.L. 172
McCabe, L.F. 86
McCabe, M.P. 136
McCarthy, R.A. 315
McCormack, B. 87, 130, 197
McCosh, L. 180
McCoy, D. 150
McCrae, N. 352
McCullagh, C.D. 37
McDaniel, A.H. *170*
McDonald, A. 272, 274
McDonald, R. 117, 120, 121
Mace, N. 180
McEwen, M. 197
McGettrick, G. 275
McGuinness, B. 82
Mack, W. 245
McKee, K. 133
McKee, M. 268–9
McKenna, B. 359
McKeown, J. 151
McKhann, G.M. 29
McKinnon, M.C. 296
McKinsey Centre for Business Technology 100
McLachlan, S. 55
McLaren, S. 231
MacLean, P.D. 316
MacLullich, A.M. 113, 121
Macmillan 144
McNess, G. 105
Macovei, M. 261
McShane, R. 244, 252
Magaki, S. 368
Magnus, R. 292
Maguire, E.A. 313
Mahieu, L. 364
Mahoney, D.F. 70
Mahoney, E.K. 245
Mainsbridge, A. 269
Maisog, J.M. 315
Malmberg, B. 186
Malnutrition Task Force 166–7
Mandell, A.M. 56
Manderson, B. 208
Mandler, G. 314, 316
Manes, F. 278
Mangialasche, F. 85, 366
Manly, J.J. 85
Mann, A.M. 116
Mann, D.M. 103
Manns, J.R. 312
Manthorpe, J. 32, 54, 73, 82, 92, 105, 106, 173, 193, 211, 232, 247, 281, 344, 363

Marcantonio, E.R. 116, 121
Marcusson, J. 140
Marino, C.K. 359
Markowitsch, H.J. 280, 316, 317
Markus, H.S. 100
Marmot, M. 227, 228, 229
Marquardt, G. 234, 235
Marr, D. 292, 313
Marshak, R.J. 347
Marshall, M. 149
Marslen-Wilson, W.D. 315
Martens, M.A. 297
Martin, C. 154
Martin, F. 197, 211, 213
Martin, M. 143
Martire, L.M. 142
Masaki, K.H. 69
Masi, C.M. 34
Mason, M. 236
Mather, L. 211
Matrix Evidence 331
Matsuzawa, T. 289
Matthews, B.R. 102
Matthews, F.E. 56, 82
Maurer, K. 142
Måvall, L. 186
Maxwell, J. 196, *196*
Mayou, R. 113
Mayrhofer, A. 350–1
Mead, N. 198, 199, 210
Meagher, D. 115, 116
Means, R. 237
Medeiros de A Nunes, V. 149
Meeks, S. 359
Meeten, F. 299
Meeter, M. 312
Melkas, S. 122
Meltzer, D.O. 100
Mendes, F. 359
Mendez, M. 104
Mennell, S. 167
Mental Welfare Commission for Scotland 261
Meri Yaadai Dementia Team 71
Merks-Van Brunschot, I. 207, 208
Meyer, J. 153
Meyer, L.B. 297
Meyerson, D.E. 347–8
Mgekn, I. 172
Michelfelder, I. 334
Milano, W. 169
Miles, S. 248
Miley, K.K. 243
Miller, B.L. 293
Mills, J.K. 118
Milne, A. 27, 66, 71
Milne, H. 247
Milner, B. 308, 312
Milton, J. 367
Minhas, J.S. 118
Mirra, S.S. 372
Miskelly, F. 247, 248
Mitchell, G. 367
Mitchell, L. 237, 238
Mithen, S.J. 297
Mitka, M. 326
Mittelman, M. 52, *53*, 59
Mohamed, S. 137
Moise, P. 134
Molinari, V. 244
Möller, A. 106, 106–7
Monastero, R. 41
Moniz Cook, E. 211, 214
Montgomery, P. 245, 249
Moon, H. 143
Moore, K.H. 184
Moore, W.R. 73
Moorman, S.M. 249
Morandi, A. 116, 119, 120, 122–3
Morgan, D.G. 120
Morgan, E. 113, 119
Morgan, S. 370
Moriarty, J. 68, 73
Moroney, J.T. 38
Morris, B.W. 203
Morris, C.H. 168
Morris, J.C. 29
Morriss-Kay, G.M. 290
Moscovitch, M. 307
Moss, S. 74
Mount, B. 196, 298
Mountain, G.A. 211
Moyer, D. 59
Moyle, W. 82, 90
Muers, J. 70, 364
Mukadam, N. 70, 85
Mukaetova-Ladinska, E.B. 121
Mulley, A. 200
Mulley, G. 206
Mummery, C.J. 168
Munro, S. 298
Murcott, A. 167
Murman, D.L. 327
Murray, J.A. 18
Musher, D. 187
Myferi Williams, C. 299
Nadel, L. 245, 307
Nåden, D. 247
Nadler, A. 54
Nakanishi, M. 90, 93
Nakashima, T. 90, 93
Namazi, K.H. 185
Narayan, S. 143
National Audit Office 27, 66, 117
National Council for Palliative Care 149
National Housing Federation 234, 235, *235–6*
National Institute for Health and Care Excellence (NICE) 81, 114, 116, 119–20, 166, 217, 325, 326
National Institute for Health Research 101
National Institute for Mental Health 324
National Institute for Mental Health in England (NIMHE) 345
Nauta, W.J.H. 316
Nay, R. 87
Naylor, M.D. 91
Neary, D. 314
Neary, S.R. 70
Neilsen, E. 345
Nelson, C.A. 315
Nelson, R.R. 334
Neundorfer, M.M. 139
Newbronner, L. 145, 268
Newens, A.J. 107
Ngandu, T. 37, 39
NHS Confederation 29, 266, 268
NHS End of Life Care Programme 149
NHS England 117, 117–18
NHS Institute for Innovation and Improvement 30, 331, 332–3, *333*
NHS Leadership Academy 343
Nickerson, R.S. 290
Nielsen, S.L. 309
Nielsen, T.R. 65
Nieuwenhuis, I.L. 313, *314*
Nilstun, T. 248
Nobili, A. 154
Nogawa, H. 298
Nolan, M.R. 108, 130, 131, 135, 233
Nordenfelt, L. 277

Norton, S. 35, 82, 371
Nortvedt, P. 277
Nourhashemi, F. 154
Nuffield Council on Bioethics 250, 251, 277
Nuffield Trust 208, 210, 264

Obert, S. 345
Oboh, L. 334
Ochsner, K.N. 296
O'Connell, C.M. 70
O'Connor, D.O. 57, 58
O'Doherty, J.P. 280
O'Donnell, B.F. 188
O'Driscoll, A. 18
O'Dwyer, C. 87, 88
O'Hanlon, S. 114, 122, 333
Ohman, A. 309
O'Keefe, J. 245
O'Keeffe, S.T. 113, 114
Olafsdóttir, M. 140
Oldman, C. 237
Oliver, M. 87
Olsson, H. 180
O'Malley, G. 121
O'Malley, L. 231
Omar, R. 296, 297
O'Neill, D.J. 253
O'Neill, K. 322, 323
Ormel, J. 206
Orrell, M.W. 141, 185, 188
Ortony, A. 309
Osborne, H. 365–6
Ouslander, J. 183, 187
Oveisgharan, S. 72

Pai, M.C. 245
Pak-Hin Kong, A. 323
Paller, K.A. 315–16
Palmer, J.L. 151
Panegyres, P.K. 101, 108
Panksepp, J. 294
Panza, F. 39
Pari, G. 280
Park, N.S. 359
Parker, K. 248
Parkinson, R. 183
Parmar, J. 140
Parsons, T. 199
Partanen, J. 323
Partridge, J.S. 115
Passini, R. 245
Passmore, A.P. 31, *32*
Patel, P. 74
Paton, J. 73
Patterson, C. 37
Patterson, T. 70
Peacock, S. 211
Pearlin, L.I. 137
Pearson, L. 70
Pedone, C. 328
Peel, E. 139, 140
Peisah, C. 200
Peralin, L.I. 70
Perera, G. 115
Perretta, J.G. 280
Perry, R.J. 362
Persson, G. 114
Pertez, I. 297
Peters, R. 38
Petersen, G. 249
Petersen, K.A. 247
Petersen, R.C. 81
Peterson, C. 359
Petrea, I. 82, 83, *83–4*, 91, 92, 94
Phelan, J.C. 52
Phelps, E.A. 309, 311, 312
Phil, R. 107
Philip, J. 55
Phillips, M.L. 310, *310*
Phillipson, L. 54
Piccolo, R.F. 343
Piefke, M. 312
Pieisah, C. 324
Piercy, M. 291
Pike, K.E. 372
Pimlott, N.J.G. 140
Pinkston, E.M. 200
Piquet, O. 169
Platzer, H. 73
Pleydell-Pearce, C.W. 314
Ploeg, J. 352
Poggesi, A. 187
Poletti, M. 367
Policy Research Unit in Commissioning and the Healthcare System 264
Poline, J.B. 203
Pollock, A. 150
Polos, L. 165
Pons-Vigués, M. 230
Porat, I. 251
Pot, A.M. 82, 83, *83–4*, 91, 92, 94
Powell, P.H. 184
Power, A. 274
Prasad, A.S. 41
Premi, E. 101
Price, B.H. 278
Price, E. 73
Price, J.D. 248
Prince, M.J. 66, 69, 81, 82, 86
Pringle, D. 139
Pritchard, J. 281
Prochaska, J.O. 346
Public Enquiry Unit 215–16
Public Health England 34, 38
Pulsford, D. 324
Pung, C. 345
Pusey, H. 153, 214
PwC 203
Pynoos, J. 237

Quadrio, C. 200
Quaid, K.A. 363
Quin, R. 211
Quinn, C. 130, 144
Quinn, R. 172
Qureshi, H. 133

Rabins, P. 180
Radley, A. 107
Rafferty, J. 154
Rahman, S. 17, 18, 20, 34, 55, 63, 88, 100, 155, 185, 195, 214, 236, 261, 277, 278, 279, *279*, 370
Rai, J. 183
Raj, S.P. 335
Ramachandran, V.S. 290, 291
Randall, G.E. 230
Rankin-Hill, L. 107
Rankin, K.P. 292
Ransmayr, G.N. 186
Rao, H. 165
Rapaport, J. 276
Rapoff, M.A. 135
Rascovsky, K. 167
Ratnavalli, E. 100
Raven, B. 58
Ray, S. 165
Ray, W.A. 328
Ready, D.A. 347
Redman, R.W. 33
Reed, D.R. *170*
Reese, S.D. 56
Reid, C. 232, 234

Reid, R.C. 234
Reinhardt, J.P. 361
Reinken, J. 180
Rempel-Clower, N.L. 311
Repper, J. 151
Resnick, N.M. 182, 183
Reutens, D.C. 297
Reynolds, D. 54
Ribot, T. 310–11, 312
Richard, E. 366
Richards, D. 214
Richards, M. 72
Richardson, T.J. *138*, 143
Richter, T. 326, 331
Riegel, B. 135
Ringman, J.M. 172
Rink, L. 41
Rioux, M.H. 19
Ritchie, C.W. 36
Ritchie, K. 36
Riva, G. 259
Robert, P. 26
Roberts, C. 136
Robertson, J. 106
Robinson, C.A. 232, 234
Robinson, J. 68
Robinson, L. 247, 253, 322
Robotham, S.L. 118
Rockwood, K. 38, 114
Rogers, J. 266
Rohrer, J.D. 297
Roland, M. 121
Rolland, Y. 244
Romeo, R. 92
Roozendaal, M. 207
Rose, P. 73
Rosen, H.J. 168
Rosenbloom, M.H. 278
Rosenheck, R.A. 328
Rosenvinge, H. 108
Roses, A.D. 358
Ross, H. 151
Rossington, J. 73
Rossor, M.N. 102, 104, 291, 291–2
Roth, M. 103
Rovner, B.W. 64
Rowe, M.A. 244
Rowlands, J.M. 211
Royal College of General Practitioners 214, 215
Royal College of Nursing (RCN) 152
Royal College of Physicians 214
Royal College of Psychiatrists 207, 209
Royal Commission on Long Term Care 231
Royal Pharmaceutical Society 332–3
Rozario, P.A. 103
Rubin, D.C. 294, 312
Rundgren, A. 179
Runnymede Centre for Policy on Ageing 64
Rusanen, M. 39
Ryan, C.E. 143
Ryan, T. 131
Ryff, C.D. 359

Sachdev, P.S. 64
Sacks, O. 297
Saczynski, J.S. *115*
Sahlas, D.J. 293
Sakakibara, R. 182, 183, 186
Sakamoto, R. 122
Salem, L.C. 358
Salimpoor, V.N. 297
Salovey, P. 295
Sampson, E.L. 102, 104, 116, 117, 118, 119, 174, 322, 361
Samsi, K. 232
Sandman, P.O. 130, 152, 197
Sapolsky, R.M. 39
Sarason, I.G. 309
Saunders, A.M. 358
Saunders, P.A. 233
Sauter, S. 230
Saxena, S. 113, *115*, 116
Scarmeas, N. 40, 171
Schalk, R. 207
Schein, E.H. 164, 345
Schermer, M. 367
Schleimer, S.C. 335
Schmahmann, J.D. 278
Schmidt, K.L. 136
Schmieg, P. 234, 235
Schmitz, T.W. 309
Schneider, L. 325
Schnelle, J.F. 182, 185, 187
Schofield, P. 269
Schrank, B. 360
Schrauf, R.W. 68–9, 70
Schultz, M. 197
Schulz, R. 51, 58, 136, 139, 142
Schumacher, K.L. 142
Schur, H.V. 107
Schwabenland, C. 19
Schwarzinger, M. 134
Scott, C.J. 206
Scottish Dementia Champions Managed Knowledge Network 351
Scottish Development Centre for Mental Health 289–90
Scottish Government 91, 272, *272–3*, 273–4, 289–90
Scoville, W.B. 308
Sculman, A.D. 335
Seabrooke, B. 71
Seelaar, H. 101
Seeley, W.W. 289
Senge, P. 165
Serino, S. 259
Setterlund, J. 370
Shaji, K.S. 129
Shallice, T. 314
Shany-Ur, T. 57
Sharif, N. 68
Sharot, T. 311
Shastry, B.S. 270
Sheehan, B. 237, 238
Sheline, Y.I. 372
Shen, L. 363
Shi, Y. 227
Shimizu, K. 247
Shinoda-Tagawa, T. 244
Shippy, A. 73
Shmotkin, D. 360
Shojo, H. 245
Shyu, Y.I. 143
Siddiqi, N. 114
Signoret, J.L. 295
Silkinson, J. 252
Silva, S.A. 130
Silverstone, F.A. 206
Simon, F. 245–6
Simpson, J. 107, 365–6
Sinclair, A.J. 216–17, 369
Singer, B. 359
Singer, J.A. 295
Singh, P. 365
Sinz, H. 280
Skevington, S.M. 211
Skills for Care/Skills for Health 217
Skladzien, E. 324
Skoog, I. 39, 114, 140
Slasberg, C. 269
Sleegers, K. 172

Slettbø, A. 277
Slooter, A.J. 362
Smebye, K.L. 365
Smith, S.J. 297
Smith, T. 369
Smyth, K.A. 139
Smythe, A. 344
Snow, D.A. 56, 332
Snyder, A.W. 291, 293
Snyder, L. 366
So, T.T. 359
Soares, J.J. 309
Social Care Institute for Excellence (SCIE) 174, 260, 276
Sofi, F. 38
Sontag, S. 55
Soto, M.E. 372
Soyinka, A. 333
Spencer, B. 73
Sperling, R.A. 36
Sperlinger, D. 108
Spilsbury, K. 212
Sporting Memories Network 307
Spreng, R.N. 101
Squire, L.R. 307, 312
Srivastva, S. 345
Stanley, N. 233
Starbuck, W.H. 351
Stechl, E. 199–200
Steel, A. 82, 90
Stein, K. 245
Stein-Shvachman, I. 103
Stephens, M.A.P. 129
Stern, Y. 18, 37, 118
Stevens, A. 188
Stewart, B.J. 142
Stewart, J. 226
Stewart, R. 115
Stirling, C. 140
Stokes, C. 72
Stokes, G. 365–6
Stokes, L.A. 72
Stooksbury, D. 244
Stott, N. 199
Stout, J.C. 280
Strachan, P.H. 135
Strategy& 202, 208
Straus, S.M. 328
Stuckey, J.C. 139
Stump, C. 149
Sturmberg, J. 154
Sugarman, J. 249
Sullivan, K.A. 361
Sullivan, L. 274
Sung, H.C. 183
Sutton, M. 117
Svoboda, E. 296
Swaffer, K. 104–5, 136–7, 259, *260*, 360
Szasz, T.S. 358
Szewczyk, B. 41

Tabet, N. 172
Tahir, T.A. 113, 119
Takahata, K. 291, 292
Takashima, A. 313, *314*
Takehara-Nishiuchi, K. 309
Taket, A. 72
Tan, D. 181, 183
Tanaka, H. 298
Tanaka, Y. 298
Tanenbaum, S.J. 129
Tangney, C.C. 171
Tariot, P.N. 372
Tascone, L.S. 368
Tateno, A. 372
Taylor, N.S.D. 265
Taylor, S.E. 107
Teece, D.J. 323
10/66 Dementia Research Group 86
Teri, L. 182
Teuber, H.L. 315
The, A.-M. 276
The Princess Royal Trust for Carers 134
Thomas, A.J. 206–7, 368
Thomas, B. 227
Thompson, C.A. 212
Thompson, G.N. 352
Thompson, P.M. 366
Thompson, R. 324, 351
Thompson, R.G. 296
Thompson Coon, J. 327
Thomson, H. 226
Tilse, C. 370
Tilvis, R.S. 188
Timmins, N. 352
Timpson, T. 322
Tindall, L. 105, 106
Tingle, J. 262
Tischler, V. 33
Tobin, S.S. 365
Todd, R.M. 307
Tolbert, P.S. 165
Tolhurst, E. 101
Tomlinson, B.E. 103
Tomlinson, F. 19
Toot, S. 181, 185
Tooth, L. 129
Topo, P. 185, 298
Torres, A. 18
Tranvåg, O. 247
Traynor, V. 144
Tremblay, A. 121
Trigg, R. 211
Truswell, D. 65, 66
Trzepacz, P.T. 115
Tsang, S.W. 169
Tu, M.C. 245
Tulving, E. 305, 314
Turk, V. 75
Turner, D. 66

Udell, L. 74–5
UK Health Prevention Forum 34, 38
Um, M.Y. 134
Underwood, G. 315
Unison 195
United Nations (UN) 226, 258, 269, 274
University of Sheffield 294
US Courts 252
US Supreme Court 252
Uzzi, B. 204

Valcour, V.G. 69
Valentina, E. 197
Van Broeckhoven, C. 172
van de Ven-Vakhteeva, J. 329
Van Der Gaag, M. 142
van der Ham, K. 207
van der Lee, J. 139
van der Linde, R.M. 41
Van Dick, R. 346
Van Dijk, R. 346
van Duijn, C.M. 37
van El, C.G. 45
Van Gorp, B. 56
van Hoof, J. 206, 237
van Otterloo, A. 167
Vanhaverbeke, W. 334
Vardy, E. 122
Vedin, I. 172
Velilla, N.M. 116
Vellas, B. 35

Venturato, L. 82, 90
Vercruysse, T. 56
Verhey, F.R. 130, 142
Verity, C.M. 43
Vernooij-Dassen, M. 214
Vickrey, B.G. 352
Vileland, T. 33
Villars, H. 154
Visser, S.M. 365
Volicer, L. 245
Vollenberg, M. 207
von Strauss, E. 371

Waarde, H. 231
Wade, D.T. 138
Wagner, U. 311
Wais, P.E. 309
Walker, M.H. 141
Wallin, A. 249
Walsh, S. 102, 105–6
Walter, J.S. 184
Wang, H.X. 37, 371
Wang, Y. 39
Wanganeen, R. 64
Warchol-Biedermann, K. 362
Ward, G. 115
Ward, R. 185
Warren, J.D. 102, 104, 297
Warren, M.W. 40
Warrick, D.D. 165
Warrington, E.K. 315
Watchman, K. 74
Watson, G.S. 170
Watson, R. 173, 175
Watson-Wolfe, K. 334
Waugh, A. 352
Waugh, F. 238
Weatherhead, I. 173, 175
Webb, R.J. 184
Webber, M. 141, 142, 265
Weber, L.R. 140
Weiner, M.F. 40, 119
Weingarten, S.R. 212
Weinstein, J. 59
Weintraub, D. 280
Welch, I. 165
Wells, T.J. 182
Welsh, S. 246
Werner, P. 72, 103
Werner, S. 249, 251
Wessely, S. 52
West, D.G. 290
West, J. 334
West, M. 345, 351
Westendorp, R.G. *115*
Westphal, A. 243
Whall, A.L. 132
Whalley, L. 105
Whear, R. 174
Wheeler, J.S. 184
Whelan, T. 200
Whitaker, R. 204, 325
White, C. 268
White, E.B. 245, 249
Whitehead, M. 228, *229*
Whitehouse, P.J. 56
Whitlatch, C.J. 143, 251
Whitwell, J.L. 168
Wiersma, E. 132
Wight, M. 143
Wikberg, M. 185
Wilemon, D. 335
Wilken, J.P. 358
Wilkinson, C. 351
Wilkinson, H. 74, 75, 367
Wilkinson, R. 227
Wilks, S.E. 142
Willander, J. 316
Williams, B.W. 245
Williams, D.D.R. 106
Williams, K. 173, 175
Williams, R.S. 75
Williams, S. 151
Williamson, G.M. 142
Williamson, T. 58, 370
Willig, S. 298–9
Wills, T.A. 139
Wilson, J. 370
Wilson, P.D. 184
Wilson, R.C. 150
Wilson, S.J. 297
Wilson, S.N. 203, 204
Wimo, A. 82
Winblad, B. 130, 152, 197, 371
Wise, J. 27
Witlox, J. 115
Wittenberg, R. 69
Wolf Klein, G.P. 206
Wong, C.L. 114
Wong, F.K. 144
Woods, B. 200
Woods, R.T. 130, 306
World Health Organization (WHO) 41, 43, 53, 132, 226, 229, 356
Wortmann, M. 85
Wu, S.C. 175
Wyver, P.C. 130
Xiao, L.D. 137
Xu, W. 371

Yalla, S.V. 182
Yamaguchi, H. 141
Yamamoto, K. 247
Yang, C.T. 143
Yap, P. 181, 183
Year of Care Partnerships 215
Yonelinas, A.P. 314
Young, A. 315
Young, A.L. 371
Young, J.B. 116, 119
Young, K.W. 173
Young, R.S. 115
Yovel, G. 315–16

Zannas, A.S. 372
Zarit, J.M. 292
Zarit, S.H. 137
Zatorre, R.J. 295, 296, 297
Zecca, L. 40
Zeilig, H. 55
Zgola, J.M. 298
Zhan, L. 70
Zhong, S. 227
Zimmerman, S. 149
Zucker, L.G. 165
Zuidema, S

CPI Antony Rowe
Chippenham, UK
2018-11-06 17:04